W0050813

DOCUMENTA OPHTHALMOLOGICA

PROCEEDINGS SERIES

Editor

HAROLD E. HENKES

VOL. II

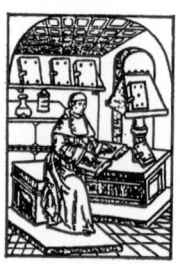

DR. W. JUNK B.V., PUBLISHERS, 1973
THE HAGUE   THE NETHERLANDS

Xth I.S.C.E.R.G. SYMPOSIUM

Editor

JEROME T. PEARLMAN

Los Angeles, 1972 August 20–23.

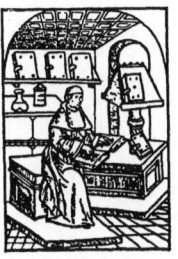

DR. W. JUNK B.V., PUBLISHERS, 1973
THE HAGUE   THE NETHERLANDS

ISBN-13: 978-90-6193-142-3   e-ISBN-13: 978-94-010-2697-0
DOI: 10.1007/978-94-010-2697-0

CONTENTS

vi

INTRODUCTORY REMARKS BY HONORED GUEST:
HERMANN M. BURIAN, M.D.

A year or so ago my friend JERRY PEARLMAN asked me whether I would be willing to say a few words to set the stage for this Symposium. Not being able to decline any request of Jerry's, I accepted with pleasure. But you will realize my somewhat anxious surprise when a circular letter appeared a couple of months ago, stating that I had accepted to be the honored guest—a distinction of which I knew nothing. Of course, I am very grateful to Jerry, with whom I spent a few happy years in Iowa, that he wanted to single me out in this fashion, but I am also keenly aware that I deserve this honor infinitely less than many another person present here.

Actually, this is a very opportune occasion to take a look backward as well as forward. This is the 10th symposium organized under the auspices of the ISCERG. And while not yet of age, our ISCERG has reached the lovely age of puberty, being 14 years old. As I look around, I think with sadness of the absence of one of our Founder Fathers, ADOLPHE FRANCESCHETTI, who is no longer with us, but I am happy that all others have been spared through many vicissitudes.

While our ISCERG was created 14 years ago, clinical ERG is older. Believe it or not, it is almost 30 years old—27 years to be exact. For it is in 1945 that appeared the monograph of KARPE, the Father of clinical ERG, which was at the beginning of it all. And we must go even farther back, to 1941 when RIGGS designed his contact lens electrode which made routine human, and therefore clinical ERG possible and which in one modification or another is still one of our basic tools.

Allow me at this point to indulge in a little personal reminiscing. I was recuperating from a severe illness in 1948 when, by what accident I do not know, the first issue of Vol. I of the J. of EEG & Clinical Neurophysiology fell into my hands, containing an article by MONNIER on human ERG. My recovery was speeded, for I was inspired. I had found the method which would answer the question which had occupied me for 10 years, whether the seat of the lesion in functional amblyopia was retinal, as some thought or in the CNS. I lived in Boston at the time and DR. DENNY-BROWN kindly let me have a corner in the laboratory of his Department of Neurology at the Boston City Hospital. Being quite naive in these matters, I had my difficulties in setting up the equipment, and the like. I might mention here in passing that at that time I went to Europe and ran into my old friend, Prof. HANS GOLDMANN, for the first time after the war. I told him about my problems with ERG and he said to me, "Why don't you go and learn from HAROLD HENKES in Rotterdam how to do ERGs?" Unfortunately, at that time this was not possible for me.

However, the initial problems were overcome, especially after I moved to Iowa and was able to establish a fine electro-physiologic laboratory. And then a number of things immediately became clear. The state of the art at that time was such that ERG could not give the answer to the amblyopia problem because of the inability to produce focal ERGs, due to the factor of stray light and for

1

other technical reasons. But I was hooked! I became increasingly fascinated with ERG, and it became evident to me that to make full use of the ERG technique for clinical studies more sophisticated procedures were required than had previously been employed.

It became obvious that the electrical retinal response was first of all determined by two major factors: the stimulation provided and the state of adaptation of the eye. While I was and remained an ophthalmologist, and neither wanted nor could in any way compete with neurophysiologists, I had to investigate for my own satisfaction the importance of these and other parameters. Their significance was such that I felt quite dissatisfied with much of the literature on clinical ERG and with such statements that "the ERG of the patient was normal", when no indications were given under what conditions the ERG was obtained.

What I am saying here may sound very trite after 20 years, but at the time it was far from trite. Today, the functional testing in clinical ERG, as developed over the years, has become routine.

Of course, I cannot go into any of the details of the history of clinical ERG, but want to point out that it has two aspects, a practical one and a theoretical academic one. From the practical standpoint ERG has confirmatory rather than primary diagnostic value. It is in the nature of this method that it has been of greatest usefulness in vascular anomalies and toxic states of the retina, in degenerative diseases particularly of the retinal periphery and carrier states, and in infants. On the other hand, from an academic standpoint, ERG studies in certain abnormal conditions, for example in achromatopsia and other forms of color deficiencies were most significant in contributing to an understanding of the ERG itself.

Such, at least, was the situation until a few years ago. Meanwhile refined techniques have greatly added to the possibilities offered by ERG. I refer especially to the various methods which now make it possible, partly thanks to computer techniques, to produce more or less focal ERGs. There is also the promising field of the clinical study of the oscillatory potentials.

Furthermore, entirely new techniques have come up which singly, or in combination with ERG, would seem to add greatly to the usefulness of the electrophysiologic methods. These techniques are the EOG and the VER. Many among us are making use of these methods, as evidenced also by some of the papers on the program of this symposium. I wonder whether the time has not come to change the name of our Society from ISCERG to International Society for Clinical Electro-Physiology of the Visual System. I know that such a suggestion, made some years ago, was rejected as premature. Possibly the time has come now to consider seriously such a change.

In spite of all the difficulties, I have never given up on the amblyopia problem. The more refined electrophysiologic methods allow one now, I believe, to answer the question with which I started. Methods avoiding stray light, including the use of patterned stimuli as applied in the laboratory of Dr. LAWWILL in Louisville, Kentucky, in which I have had the privilege of working during the last few months, have given definite evidence that the electrical response of the retina of the amblyopic eye does not differ from that of the fixating eye.

2

But we know that the VER elicited through stimulation of the amblyopic eye differs materially from that elicited through stimulation of the fixating eye. These data would seem to vindicate the old view that the seat of the basic lesion in functional amblyopia is central rather than in the retina.

Now for a look forward! What is the future of clinical ERG? The devoted work of those engaged in clinical ERG has covered to a great extent the possibilities which this methodology offers from a purely ophthalmologic standpoint. Unless some entirely new methods appear on the scene, it is unlikely that new paths will be broken in this field. However, I see a vast and important application of ERG in the field of medicine in general. As we all know, the retina partakes of innumerable neurologic diseases, of diseases of the hematopoetic and circulatory systems, of abnormalities of the endocrine systems, etc., etc., without there being necessarily ophthalmoscopically visible changes. Yet, pathophysiologic changes expressed in more or less subtle alterations of the electric responses of the retina occur in many of these conditions, which may be pathognomonic and, indeed, diagnostically helpful. I believe that close cooperation with neurologists and internists, gathering electrophysiologic data in a great variety of diseases may be very rewarding. It was, therefore, with great pleasure that I noted that Dr. PEARLMAN had chosen as one of the topics of this Symposium 'ERG in Systemic Diseases.' I wish to emphasize that I had nothing to do with the selection of this topic, but it may well hark back to the time when Dr. PEARLMAN studied with me the effect of thyroid disease and artificially induced hyperthyroidism on the ERG.

The second topic which he has selected, 'Retinal Vascular Disease', is a classical one in which the application of ERG techniques is particularly attractive. This has been clear from the very beginning of clinical ERG in the work of KARPE and HENKES.

Lastly, Dr. PEARLMAN has proposed the topic of 'Light Induced Retinal Changes.' This is a very up to date subject and one which is biologically and practically of immense interest. Life can exist only within very narrow limits of the parameters required for its maintenance. This also applies to light. In the absence of light one cannot see, but such important items as the light tonus of the central nervous system, the effect of light on the gonads, etc., are also missing. Yet, a relatively slight excess of light is destructive to the retina. From a practical standpoint it is a very important subject because of the high luminances which we apply today in ophthalmology diagnostically as well as therapeutically.

Thus, I think that the topics chosen by Dr. PEARLMAN, as well as the additional topics developed through the papers submitted by our members, have much fascination, and I am sure that I am not alone in looking forward with anticipation to an interesting and gratifying meeting.

HERMANN M. BURIAN, M.D.

Department of Ophthalmology
University of North Carolina Medical School
Chapel Hill, North Carolina

3

VISUAL ELECTROPHYSIOLOGY OF MYOTONIA CONGENITA

H. LEE STEWART, M.D. & M. L. RUBIN, M.D.

(San Francisco)   *(Gainesville)*

ABSTRACT

Myotonia congenita is a rare disorder of skeletal muscle which is included in the differential diagnosis of myotonia dystrophica and paramyotonia. These three disorders plus benign hypteronias, can be clinically confused and are thought by some investigators to represent the spectrum of a single disease. Because of the dominant mode of inheritance of these disorders, it is important to be able to differentiate myotonia dystrophica since its prognosis is considerably more limited than the other disorders. The ophthalmologist is in a better position to do this than the neurologist because of the distinctive nature of the eye findings. Visual electrophysiology provides important differential diagnostic criteria between myotonia dystrophica and myotonia congenita. Two patients and their family history are presented as examples of myotonia congenita. Visual electrophysiology including electroretinograms, dark adaptation, and electrooculograms are reported for these two patients. It constitutes the first report in the literature of these findings.

INTRODUCTION

Myotonia congenita was the first of the myotonias to be described. THOMSEN, whose name is associated with the disease, described the condition in his family in 1876. Although he was antedated by (1874) LEYDEN, he himself had the disease and described it over four generations of his own family. Myotonia, a peculiar failure of relaxation of skeletal muscle following voluntary contraction or mechanical, electrical or chemical stimulation; muscular hypertrophy; an autosomal dominant inheritance pattern; and normal longevity characterize the disease (CAUGHEY & MYRIANTHOPOULOS, 1963). Paramyotonia was described as a separate entity by EULENBERG in 1886. It is characterized by myotonia following exposure to low temperatures after which the contracted muscles remain in a paretic state (CAUGHEY & MYRIANTHOPOULOS, 1963). It is similar to myotonia congenita in that it is congenital and inherited in an autosomal dominant pattern (STEPHENS, 1953). Atypical cases of myotonia congenita were frequently described until 1909 at which time dystrophia myotonica was described as a separate entity by BATTEN & GIBB (1909) and simultaneously by STEINERT (1909). It was thought to be different from myotonia congenita because of the relatively late onset, muscular atrophy of the face, forearms, and sternomastoid muscles, gonadal atrophy and frontal balding. Shortly thereafter, a number of authors noted the presence of cataracts, a finding which has become a hallmark of the disorder (GREENFIELD, 1911). Subsequently, it has been recognized that this disorder carries a far more guarded prognosis and significantly more morbidity than the two previously described syndromes (ADIE &

5

GREENFIELD, 1923). Adequate statistics are not available, but all three disorders must be considered rare with dystrophia myotonic recognized as by far the most common of the three disorders (CAUGHEY, 1958b). Dystrophia myotonica, transmitted in a dominant fashion, probably by a polyphenous gene, with tremendous variability of expression, can be easily confused on a clinical basis with myotonia congenita. For this reason, genetic counseling may be very difficult because of the uncertainty of diagnosis. Considerable disagreement occurs in the literature in terms of distinguishing the three disorders. WALTON & NATTRASS summarized the controversy and suggested that these are separate syndromes clinically, but that occasional cases cannot clearly be placed into either classification (1954). Recently, JUNGE has exhaustively examined the ocular findings of these three disorders and suggested that the clinical distinction may be made more easily on this basis than on any other (1966). BURIAN & BURNS have also commented on the widespread ocular findings in myotonic dystrophy (1966).

CASE REPORTS

The present paper reports a family suffering from myotonia congenita, two of whose members were examined for abnormalities of visual electrophysiology. The family to be reported was traced through four generations although only members of the latest two generations were examined. (See Fig. 1). The first member of the family thought to have myotonic symptoms died at the age of 82 after a lifelong history of muscle cramps which were first noted in childhood. To the best of the present family's knowledge there was no history of cataracts, muscular atrophy, frontal balding or gonadal dysfunction. This woman was reported to have died at 82 of a cerebral vascular accident. She had five children, only one of whom was overtly affected by the disorder. At the second generation level, there were three normal daughters, one normal son, and one affected daughter who died at age 39 years, after a septic miscarriage. This daughter had three daughters and two sons. Of this third generation, all three daughters were affected but not the twin sons. There are a total of eleven individuals at the fourth generation level, five male and six female. In the fourth generation a total of three of the six female and three of the five male individuals are known to have the disease. In addition, one of the males died at age two weeks of pneumonia, and it was not known whether he was affected. Curiously, there are no males affected until the fourth generation. Consanguinity was not demonstrated in this family. It is of interest that all affected members of the family have known of their disorder since birth, or shortly thereafter. Also, no history was found of early cataracts, frontal balding, decreased longevity, muscle wasting or mental or social retardation. Those individuals in the third and fourth generations that were examined demonstrate the difficulty in separating myotonia congenita from dystrophia myotonica on a purely clinical basis. The two living afflicted members of the third generation and four of the six afflicted members of the fourth generation were examined by us. One member of the third generation and one member of the fourth generation underwent extensive electrophysiologic testing.

6

The first patient, J. B. R., is a 55 year old black female who states that she was born with a "muscle disease". The muscle disorder in this patient manifested itself by an intermittent inability to initiate coordinated motor activity. She was mentally alert and an excellent historian. She denied any symptoms suggestive of endocrine dysfunction with the exception of being unable to bear

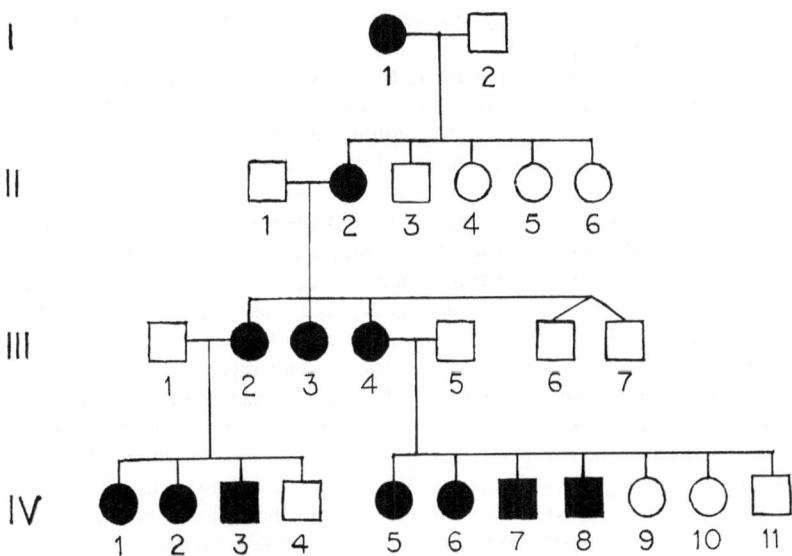

Fig. 1:
I. 1. 82, deceased, affected 2. 86, deceased
II. 1. 71, deceased. 2. 39, deceased, affected. 3. 75, L & W. 4. 80, L & W. 5. 82, L & W. 6, 76, deceased.
III. 1. 42, L & W. 2, 36, L & W, affected (Patient 2). 3. 55, L & W, affected (Patient 1). 4. 35, deceased, affected. 5. 55, L & W. 6. 33, L & W. 7. 33, L & W.
IV. 1. 13, L & W, affected (Patient 4). 2. 16, L & W, affected (Patient 5). 3. 14, L & W, affected (Patient 6). 4. 6, L & W. 5. 19, L & W, affected. 6. 34, L & W, affected. 7. 20, L & W, affected (Patient 3). 8. 32, L & W, affected. 9. 24, L & W. 10. 27, L & W. 11. 2 weeks, deceased.

children. However, she apparently had normal menstrual periods. She stated that the myotonic symptoms had not appreciably changed throughout her life. She specifically denied muscular wasting; however, she stated that in the last few years, she thought she possibly had become weaker. On examination, she was well developed with no evidence of frontal balding, hatchet facies, slurring of speech, or evidence of muscular atrophy. Physical examination revealed a generalized myotonia both active and mechanical. It was especially prominent in the orbicularis oculi. There was no ptosis. Intraocular pressure was 15.0 mm. Hg. OU by applanation tonometry. She was myopic with a −2.50 sphere OD, and −3.00 sphere OS. Her vision was correctable to 20/20 OU. Cataracts were not present, although there were a few aqueous cysts OU. Examination of the fundus revealed no ophthalmoscopic abnormalities. Pupillary reactions were normal and there was no restriction of ocular motility. There was, however, a difficulty with gross pursuit movements in both eyes. She did not demonstrate frank tropia when given sufficient time to fixate bifoveally. She was able to achieve $\frac{8}{9}$ on the WIRT stereo acuity test. The inability to pursue accurately a moving target was especially noticeable with vergence movements. No levator atrophy was demonstrated.

Patient 2, the sister of patient 1, (H. L. K.) is a 36 year old black female complaining of recent onset of weakness in her hands. She stated that she had a congenital history of myotonic symptoms in all muscles which resulted in frequent falls. She stated that the severity of her disease waxed and waned and was adversely affected by anxiety, but she denied any symptoms due to temperature or weather variations. She stated that these involuntary contractions of muscular groups were relieved by alcohol and relaxation. The patient was mentally alert and an excellent historian. She denied a family history of chronic weakness, wasting or mental deficiency, and was unaware of cataracts or endocrine disorders in the family. There was no known cardiac disease in the family. She stated that her affected children had myotonic symptoms of the eyes and eyelids from the time of birth. Physical examination revealed a well developed, well nourished, muscular black woman appearing her stated age. Examination of the cardiovascular system was normal. There was no evidence of frontal balding or hatchet facies. There was marked myotonia of the eyelids, tongue, thenar and hypothenar eminences, and the majority of the muscles in the extremities. Her grip was myotonic, as was her gait. No ptosis was noted. No weakness was noted of sternomastoid, levator or facial muscles. Sensation, reflexes and coordination were normal. There was significant hypertrophy of the proximal muscle groups. No distal wasting was noted in any of the muscle groups; however, there was some weakness of the intrinsic muscles of the hand. Ophthalmologic examination revealed a visual acuity of 20/20 OU distance and near. As previously mentioned, she had classic myotonia of the orbicularis oculi muscles and no evidence of levator weakness. There was no restriction of extraocular motility. She achieved 9 out of 9 in WIRT stereo acuity test. Color vision was normal, and visual fields were normal. Pupils were normally reactive OU to gross examination and pupillometry. Patient 2 had a difficulty similar to Patient 1 with pursuit movements; however, the difficulty was much less marked. Slit lamp examination revealed essentially clear lenses OU. Intraocular tension was 16.0 mm Hg. OU by applanation. Examination of the fundus was unremarkable. Enophthalmus was not present. Schirmer's test was normal. Psychological testing revealed a woman of better than average intelligence for her peer group. Visual electrophysiology will be discussed later. Laboratory data reveals normal gamma globulins, negative VDRL, borderline FTA, normal electrocardiogram, normal X-rays of the chest and skull, normal serum BUN and SGOT, calcium, and electrolytes. CPK was elevated on two occasions. A normal hemogram and 2 hour PC sugar were recorded.

An electromyogram revealed myotonia in all muscles tested. Muscle biopsy revealed some borderline HO thick fibers with minimal evidence of rolling of nuclei. No ringbinden were present. A lipo-protein electrophoretogram was found to be within normal limits, as were further tests of serum immunoglobulins.

The third patient, E. G. W., was a 21 year old black male, who is a nephew of Patients 1 and 2. He was first seen at our institution at age 13 years, when the diagnosis of Thomsen's disease was made on the basis of family history, muscular hypertrophy and generalized myotonic symptoms. Esotropia was also noted at that time. The description of the patient's myotonia, when he was first seen characterized it as a nonprogressive stiffness involving all skeletal-muscular groups. The stiffness was relieved by exercise. The symptoms, present since birth, were non-progressive. The patient was again seen at age 21 in the neurology clinic. Essentially, there were no new symptoms. He specifically denied any history of weakness, frontal balding, or sexual difficulties. He described the myotonia as being relatively constant and little affected by temperature or alcohol. He was a sophomore student in college doing B average work. Physical examination revealed an extremely well developed black male with marked muscular hypertrophy of all muscle groups. Examination of the genitalia was within normal limits. No abnormalities were found on examination of cardio-vascular, pulmonary, or intestinal systems. Neurologic examination revealed an intelligent, well oriented articulate young male. Percussion myotonia of the eyelids and tongue was noted and in some of the muscles of the extremities. There was no atrophy of any muscular group noted. The patient's gait and coordination were judged to be normal. Sensory examination was completely normal. No abnormalities of motor coordination or reflexes were noted. Eye examination revealed no ptosis and no weakness of the levator muscles. There was marked myotonia of the orbicularis oculi. Visual acuity was 20/80 at distance OU corrected by a −3.75 sphere OD, −3.00 sphere OS. He was able to read 20/20 at near. Extraocular motility revealed a relatively constant 15 diopter alternating esotropia. The patient suppressed bilaterally and alternated freely. Pupils were normal to gross reaction OU. Pupillometry will be discussed later. Intraocular tension was 15.0 mm Hg OU by applanation. Visual fields were found to be full OU with no central defects on careful testing. No cataractous changes were found in either eye. Fundoscopy was entirely within normal limits. No enophthalmus was noted. Schirmer's test was negative. Ocular pursuit movements were grossly normal, but were found to be abnormally slow on careful testing. Findings on visual physiology will be discussed later.

Patients 4, 5, and 6 are the children of patient 2 and will be discussed as a group. Ages of the children are 13, 14, and 16 years, and they all were in good health. All exhibited myotonic eyelid phenomenon with no ptosis or weakness of the levator. There was generalized hypertrophy of all muscle groups with percussion myotonia present. All had normal visual acuity without correction and normal extraocular motility. No cataractous changes were found on slit lamp examination. Pursuit responses were grossly normal in all. One younger brother, age 6, was apparently unaffected by the disease and had none of these findings.

9

Dark adaptation was performed on a Goldmann-Weekers Adaptometer with preadaptation to 6,000 Lux for 5 minutes. Electroretinograms were performed on dilated eyes topically anesthetized using a Burian-Allen contact lens electrode. Signals were amplified using a wide band solid state preamplifier displayed on a Tektronics 564 memory oscilloscope. They were also simultaneously examined with a Fabri-Tek 1064 digital signal averager. Photopic responses were made at 10 foot-candle illumination and dark adaptive responses after 15 minutes of

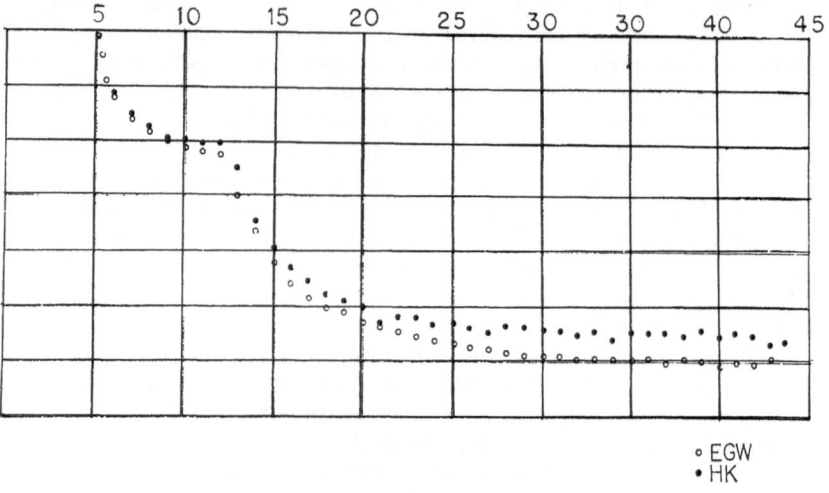

∘ EGW
• HK

DARK ADAPTATION RATE

Fig. 2. Dark adaptation rates for E. G. W. (patient 3) and H. L. K. (patient 2).
Both are well within normal limits.

dark adaptation. Electrooculograms were performed essentially in the method described by Arden (1966) using a modified Goldmann-Weekers Adaptometer. Pupillometry was performed by recording pupillary reactions on infra-red closed circuit television video tape. The video tape was then replayed frame by frame and direct measurements were made of the size of the pupil plotted against time in milliseconds. An estimate of macular function was determined with a macular glare tester which employs a visual acuity discrimination test after exposure to 9,000 Lux for 5 seconds. Normal values are well standardized at 15 seconds or less for this exam. Examination of pursuit movements were made using Beckman nystagmogram electrodes, a Dynamics Instruments DC preamplifier and a horizontal, sinusoidally oscillating target. Eye movement recordings were made on a model 220 Brush recorder. Color vision was tested with the Hardy-Rand-Rittler AO pseudoisochromatic plates under a Macbeth easel.

10

Dark adaptation curves were found to be entirely within normal limits in the four eyes of Patients 2 and 3. In order to make the standard test more sensitive (Burian & Burns, 1966), a blue filter was used over the 2° target in the Gold-mann-Weekers Adaptometer. No delay in scotopic dark adaptation was noted

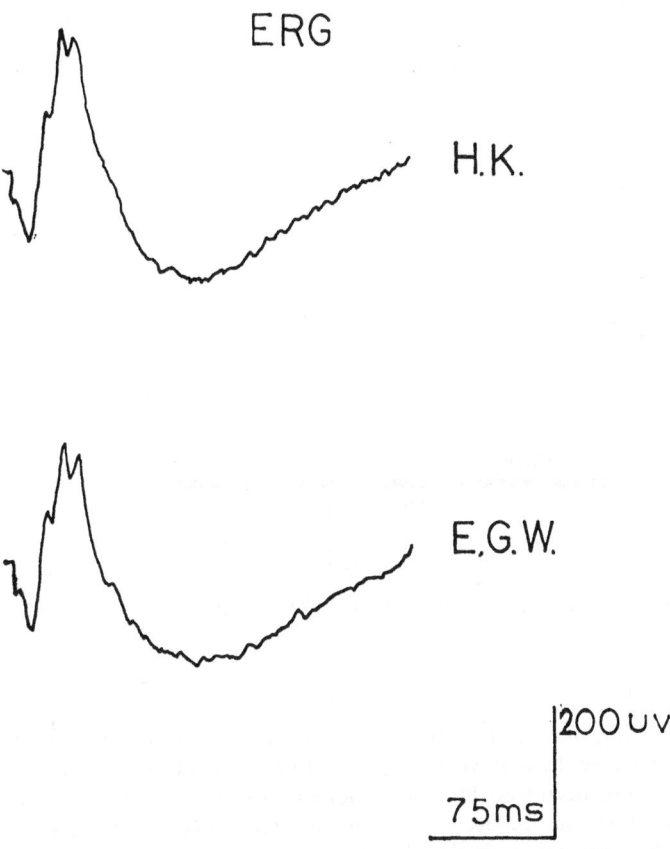

Fig. 3. Scotopic Electroretinograms for patients 2 and 3. Photopic values (not shown) are within normal limits also.

(see Fig. 2). Electroretinograms, under all conditions, were well within normal limits (see Fig. 3). Electrooculograms for both patients demonstrated a normal configuration with appropriate dark trough and elevation in the light (see Fig. 4). The tracings of the pursuit movements of the eyes (see Fig. 5) revealed that even slowly moving targets were poorly followed by both subjects. With the target moving 15° from either side of primary position, a rate of $\frac{1}{3}$ cycle/sec frequent saccadic movements were required to maintain fixation. Normally, under these conditions of testing, a frequency of twice this amount or more would elicit smooth eye movements (VON NOORDEN et al., 1964). Color vision testing was normal for both patients.

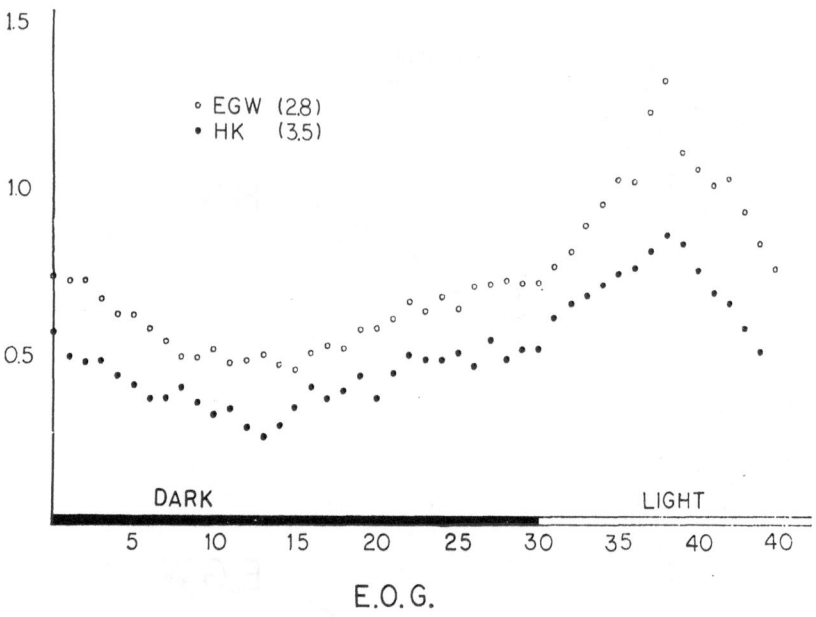

Fig. 4. Electrooculograms for patients 2 and 3. Both values are within normal limits for this lab.

DISCUSSION

Considering the fact that there is no family history of cataracts, progressive muscular atrophy and weakness, frontal baldness, ptosis, atrophy of the orbicularis oculi, decreased life expectency due to the disease, physical or mental retardation; and because of the marked family history of congenital myotonia and the widespread finding of muscular hypertrophy, this family must be considered fully typical of myotonia congenita. As has been noted in other families with this disorder, however, there are individuals who demonstrate some of the findings of dystrophia myotonia (MAAS & PATERSON, 1950). Since the chances of having affected offspring is virtually 50%, and since dystrophia myotonica carries with it a significantly more morbid prognosis than myotonia congenita, it would be helpful to the clinician in genetic counseling to be able to clearly distinguish the two disorders. Table I is a listing of symptoms or findings which help to discriminate between the two disorders. The information for the table was obtained from the paper by JUNGE (1966), or by BURIAN (1966).

12

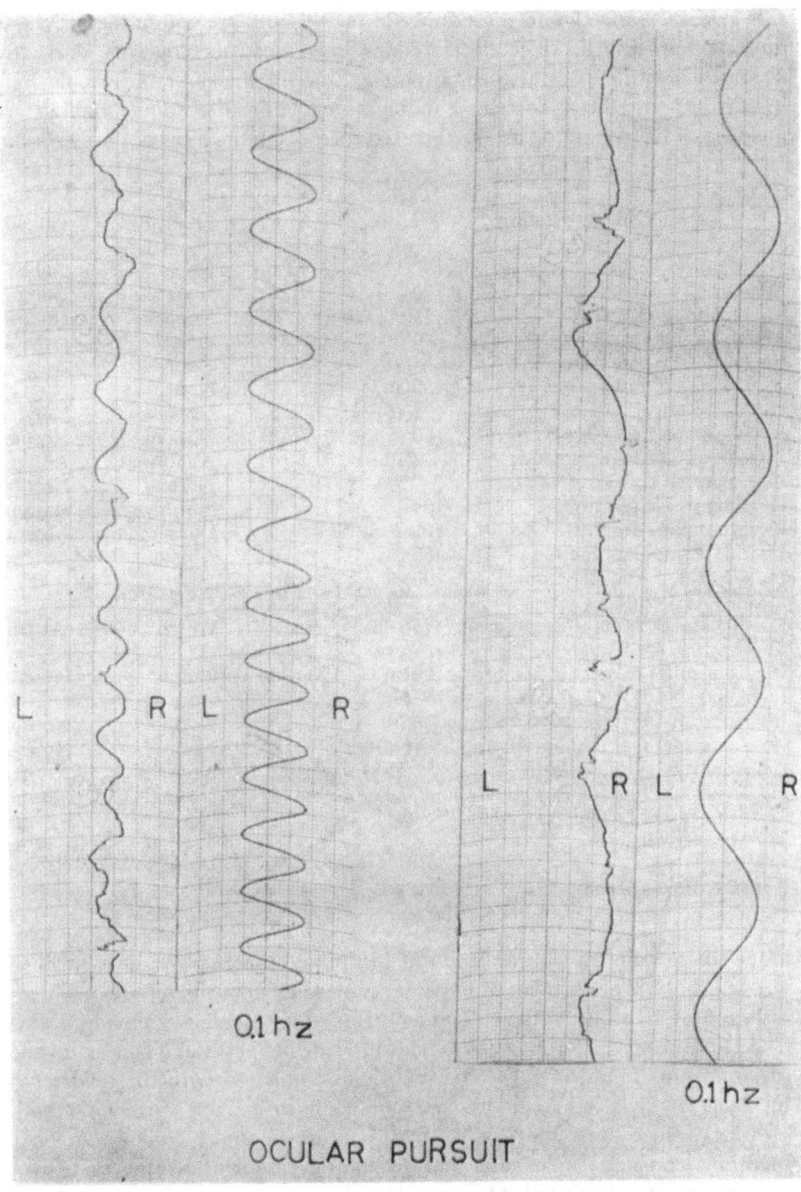

Fig. 5. Ocular pursuit movements for patient 2. They demonstrate that even at 0.1 hz smooth pursuit is interrupted by saccadic refixations. The expanded tracing shows overshooting and random instability. Both patients failed to follow the target smoothly even at slower oscillation speeds. Velocity of saccadic movements was normal.

13

It is evident that a significant number of the findings are within the province of the ophthalmologist. Since electroretinograms, electrooculograms, dark adaptation, visual fields, pursuit movements, pupillometry, and macular glare testing had not been described in myotonia congenita, these findings were included at the end of the list for these 2 patients. On the basis of the eye findings

Table I. *Incidence* (Percent)*

Characteristic or Finding	D.M.	M.C.	Patient 2	Patient 3
1. Myotonic Cataract (age 20)	100(100)	0	None	None
2. Atrophy Orbicularis Oculi	96	0	None	None
3. Ptosis	73(80–90)	0	None	None
4. Myotonia Orbicularis Oculi	0	80	Present	Present
5. Ocular Hypotension	84(76)	0	None	None
6. Enophthalmus	50(80)	0	None	None
7. Strabismus	2(16)	750	None	None
8. Pupillometry	100	40	Normal	Normal
9. Abnormal Ocular Pursuit	2(100)	?	Abnormal	Abnormal
10. Schirmer Test Positive	(55)	?	Normal	Normal
11. Progressive Myotonia	100	0	Stationary	Stationary
12. Muscular Atrophy	100	0	Questionable	Absent
13. Endocrine Dysfunction	80	0	Absent	Absent
14. Decreased Life Expectancy	90	Near Normal		
15. Physical & Mental Retardation	70–80	Near Normal	Absent	Absent
16. Congenital Myotonic Symptoms	Rare	100	Present	Present
17. Abnormal E.R.G.	83(96)	?	Normal	Normal
18. Abnormal E.O.G.	36(0)	?	Normal	Normal
19. Abnormal Dark Adaptation	84(96)	?	Normal	Normal
20. Abnormal Visual Field	82(55)	?	Normal	Normal
21. Abnormal Fundus Pigmentation	(30)	?	Normal	Normal
22. Abnormal Macular Appearance	(44)	?	Normal	Normal
23. Macular Glare	?	?	Normal	Normal

* Junge, 1966–(Burian & Burns, 1966)

alone, these patients would clearly fit in the myotonia congenita syndrome. It was felt that the abnormalities of ocular pursuit movements represented a manifestation of myotonia rather than any extraocular muscle atrophy or weakness. The relationship of the normal pursuit movements and the increased incidence of strabismus found in myotonia congenita compared with the relatively low incidence in dystrophia myotonica is difficult to explain with any certainty. However, since the symptoms of myotonia are far more common at birth in myotonia congenita it suggests that normal development of binocular function may in some way be retarded by the myotonia. In their discussion of the abnormal pupillary responses found in dystrophia myotonica, Thompson et al. favor a central lesion as the basis for the sluggish pupils (1964). It is of interest, therefore, that Patient 2 who was noted to exhibit a few of the signs of a dystrophic syndrome had clearly less brisk pupillary responses than Patient 3, although both would be considered normal (see Fig. 6).

14

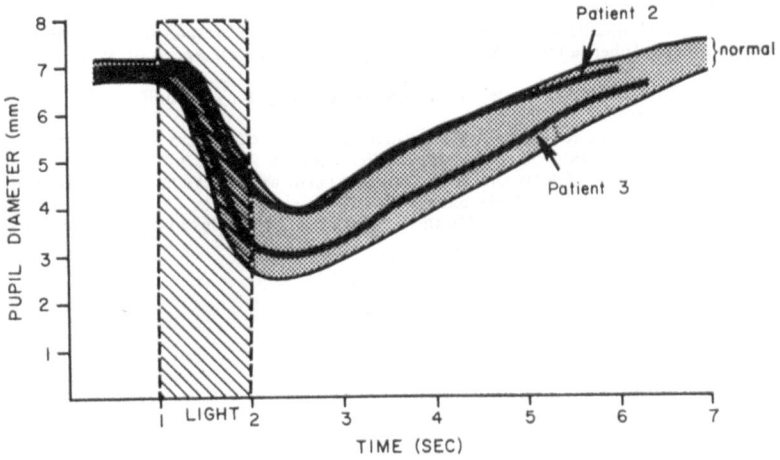

PUPILLOMETRY

Fig. 6. Pupillograms for patients 2 and 3. Both are within normal limits for this laboratory.

SUMMARY

A family afflicted with myotonia congenita is described in which two of its members were examined for visual electrophysiologic abnormalities. Electroretinograms, electrooculograms, dark adaptation, macular glare, and pupillometry were all found to be within normal limits. Ocular pursuit movements were inclined to be abnormal in both subjects. On the basis of visual electrophysiology of these two patients, it would appear that differences exist between myotonia congenita and dystrophia myotonica, and these are most evident in the ophthalmologist's realm.

REFERENCES

ADIE, W. J. & GREENFIELD, J. G. Dystrophia myotonica. *Brain* 46:*73–127* (1923).
ARDEN, J. G. B. & KELSEY, J. H.: New clinical test of retinal function based upon the standing potential of the eye. *Brit. J. Oph.* 46:*449–467* (1962).
BATTEN, F. E. & GIBB, H. P. Myotonia atrophica. *Brain*, 32:*187–205* (1909).
BURIAN, H. M. & BURNS, C. A. Ocular changes in myotonic dystrophy. *Tr. Am. Ophth. Soc.* 64:250–273 (1966).
BURIAN, H. M. & BURNS, C. A. Electroretinography and dark adaptation in patients with myotonic dystrophy. *Am. J. Oph.* 61:*1044–1054* (1966).
CAUGHEY, J. E. Relationship of dystrophia myotonica and myotonica congenita. *Neurology* 8:*469* (1958b).
CAUCHEY, J. E. & MYRIANTHOPOULOS, N. C. Dystrophia myotonica and related disorders. Thomas, Springfield (1963).
EULENBERG, A. Über eine Familiare, durch 6 Generationen verfolgbare Form congenitaler Paramyotonie. *Neurol. Centra lbl.* 5:*265–72* (1886).
GREENFIELD, J. G. Notes on a family of myotonia atrophica and early cataract with a report on an additional case. *J. Rev. Neurol. Psychiat. Einberg* 9:*169* (1911).
JUNGE, J. Ocular changes in dystrophia myotonica, para-myotonica and myotonia congenita. *Docum. Ophth.* 21:*1–115* (1966).

15

LEYDEN, E. Klinik der Rückenmarkskrankheiten. Bd. I, Berlin p. 128 (1874).

MAAS, O. & PATERSON, A. S. Myotonia congenita, Dystrophia myotonica, and Paramyotonica: reaffirmation of their identity. *Brain* 73:*318–336* (1950).

STEINERT, H. Myopathologische Beiträge. *Dtsch. Ztschr. f. Nervenh.* 37:*58–104* (1909).

STEPHENS, F. S. Inheritance of Diseases Primary in the Muscles. *Am. J. of Medicine* 15:*558–569* (1953).

THOMPSON, H. S., VAN ALLAN, M. W. & VON NOORDEN, G. K. The pupil in myotonic dystrophy. *Invest. Oph.* 3(3) *325* (1964).

THOMSEN, J. Tonische Krampfe in Willkurlich Beweglichen Muskeln in Folge von Ererbter Psychischer Disposition. *Arch. f. Psychiat. Nervenken.* 6:*702* (1876).

VON NOORDEN, G. K., THOMPSON, H. S. & VAN ALLEN, M. W. Eye movements in myotonic dystrophy. *Invest. Oph.* 3(3) *314*–324 (1964).

WALTON, J. N. & NATTRASS, F. S. On the classification, natural history, and treatment of the myopathies. Brain 77:*169–231* (1954).

ERG AND EOG IN DIABETICS PRE AND POST PHOTOCOAGULATION

THEODORE LAWWILL,* M.D. & PATRICK R. O'CONNOR,* M.D.

Extensive electroretinographic studies of diabetic retinopathy have been made by several authors. FRANCOIS & DE ROUCK (1954), KARPE, KORNERUP & WULFING (1956), using flash stimulus techniques, found decreased ERG amplitude in cases with more advanced retinal disease and no particular changes in early cases. Similarly, a depression in the EOG L/D ratio in severe cases was noted by ARDEN, BARRADA & KELSEY (1962). The analysis of the amplitudes of the wavelets superimposed on the b-wave as introduced by YONEMURA, AOKI & TSUZUKI (1962) has proven slightly more applicable to the clinical study of diabetic retinopathy as shown by SIMONSEN (1968).

This study investigates the effect of retinal destruction by photocoagulation upon the ERG and EOG. The patients studied were those with diabetic retinopathy who had one eye treated with photocoagulation.

PATIENTS

The patients selected for treatment in our clinic represented a narrow portion of the wide spectrum of severity of diabetic retinopathy. They were, in general,

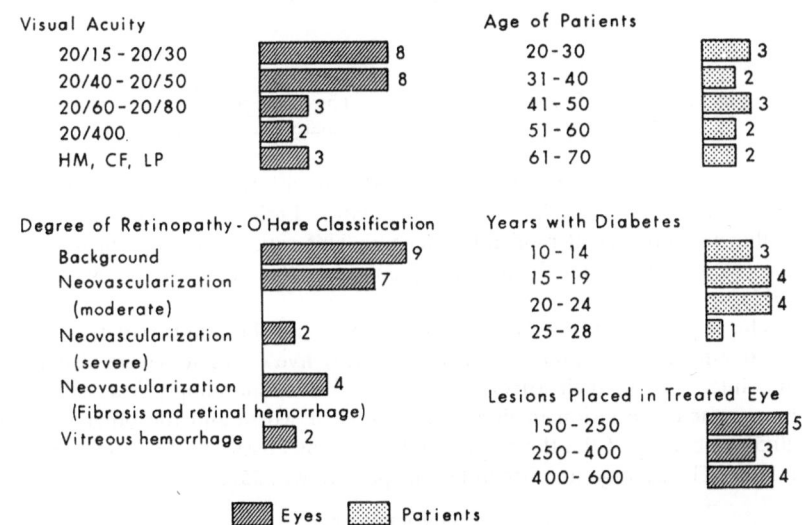

Fig. 1. Summary of the clinical conditions of the patients' eyes and the number of photocoagulation lesions placed for treatment of diabetic retinopathy.

* From the Department of Ophthalmology, University of Louisville School of Medicine. This study was supported in part by USPHS Research grant EY-00412 and Training grant EY-00023 from the National Eye Institute. Reprint requests to THEODORE LAWWILL, MD 301 East Walnut Street, Louisville, Kentucky 40202.

17

patients with early changes with background retinopathy, some vascular changes and occasional early proliferative disease. The patients were graded with the O'Hare classification evaluating multiple fundus areas (DAVIS et al., 1969). All patients were also studied by fluorescein angiography. Our standard ERG and EOG examinations were performed on both eyes before and after treatment.

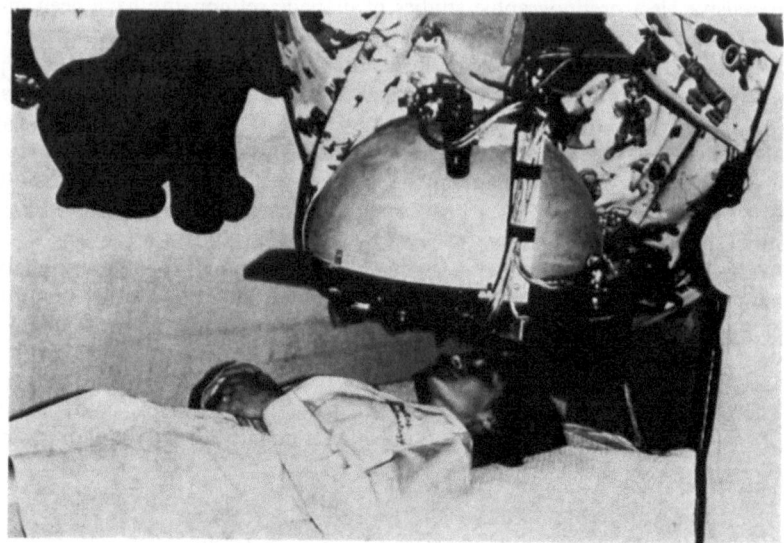

Fig. 2. Clinical ERG stimulus apparatus. The circus pictures are to make the surroundings more acceptable to the many children we examine.

One eye each of 12 patients was treated, ten with the xenon photocoagulator and 2 with the argon laser photocoagulator. Lesions were placed with one millimeter spot size at moderate intensity. This causes a lesion which destroys the receptor layer and disrupts the pigment epithelium (TOWNES & WATZKE, 1972).

The clinical condition of the patients' eyes and the number of lesions used for treatment are summarized in Fig. 1. Only five eyes had severe visual loss, and interestingly, their ERG's were not all correspondingly low. Of the 12 eyes treated, the vision in three was 20/400 or worse and the other nine had 20/50 or better. Of the three eyes showing fibrous tissue proliferation, one was treated. The average number of lesions per eye was 356.

PROCEDURE

Our standard ERG procedure has nine stimulus conditions. The patients' pupils are dilated and modified Burian-Allen contact lens electrodes placed in each eye (LAWWILL & BURIAN, 1966). The patient is preadapted to a luminance level of 100 ft-L provided by an indirectly lighted hemisphere whose inside surface is painted flat white (Fig. 2). Stimuli are presented as flashes from xenon

18

flash tubes which indirectly light the same hemisphere. Six filters are available to modify the intensity and color of the flashes.

After preadaptation the luminance in the hemisphere is lowered to 10 ft-L. On this background three different stimuli are presented, a deep red flash, a brighter red flash and a white flash. Each stimulus is presented at 30 second

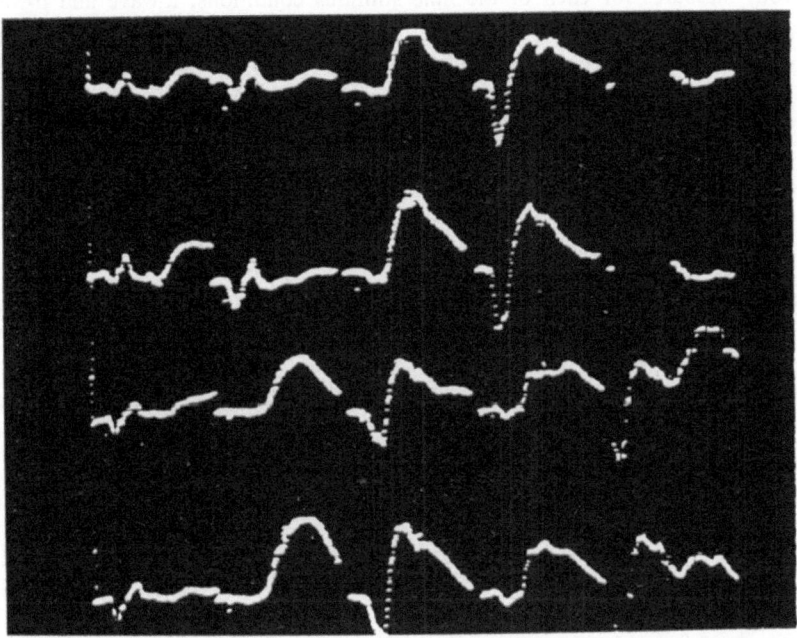

Fig. 3. Oscilloscope display of normal responses for each eye under the 9 standard conditions and flicker as stored in the digital computer.

intervals until three artifact free responses are obtained. The patient is then dark adapted for 20 minutes. Four successively brighter stimuli are presented and then the two red stimuli are presented.

The electrical response is recorded on FM analog tape and also on paper. The analog responses are digitized and stored on magnetic tape for closer analysis. Fig. 3 is a view of the nine responses for each eye as they are stored in the computer. Amplitudes and latencies are measured from the paper chart and the measurements stored in the digital computer for statistical evaluation.

Our EOG technique is similar to that described by Arden (ARDEN et al., 1962). Electrodes are placed at the inner and outer canthi and the change in electrical potential is measured as the patient moves his eyes back and forth through a constant angle. This potential is measured in the dark adapted condition and after viewing a lighted screen for 12 minutes. The result is recorded as the light over dark ratio in percent.

The first comparison available from the resulting data is for the ERG's and EOG's of the normal and diabetic patient. Shown in Figs. 4 and 5 are the means and standard deviations for normal and diabetic eyes, a- and b-waves for the 9 conditions and EOG percent rise. Analysis of variance was performed for four measures for each of the nine stimulus conditions, a-wave and b-wave

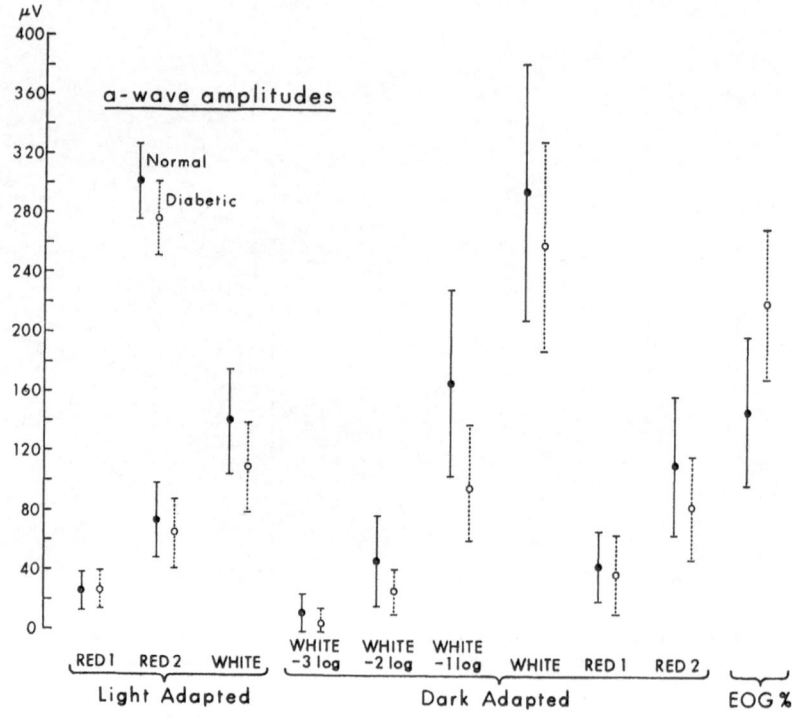

Fig. 4. The a-wave amplitudes mean and standard deviations for normal and diabetic eyes for the standard stimulus conditions. EOG percent light rise is plotted using the numbers from the μV scale.

amplitudes and a- and b-wave latencies. Of the 18 amplitude measures, 8 were statistically lower in the diabetic eyes at the 99 % level of confidence, 3 at the 95 % and 1 at the 90 % level. The other six showed differences which were not as significant. While this analysis is not completely acceptable because of repeated measures, the evidence is overwhelming that diabetics with retinopathy have lower amplitude ERG's than normal patients. This is in cases with good visual acuity and fairly early disease.

There was no correlation between visual acuity and ERG amplitudes, and the eyes with proliferative disease had ERG amplitudes both above and below

20

the mean. There was no correlation between the stage of retinopathy on a clinical grading system and ERG amplitudes or latencies.

For the effects of photocoagulation on ERG and EOG, a 2 factor repeated measures analysis of variance was used in a four cell design. The four cells contained the treated and untreated eyes pre and post treatment. The amplitudes and latencies of the a- and b-waves were analyzed separately. Shown in Figs. 6 and 7 are the means and standard deviations for the four cells for the a- and

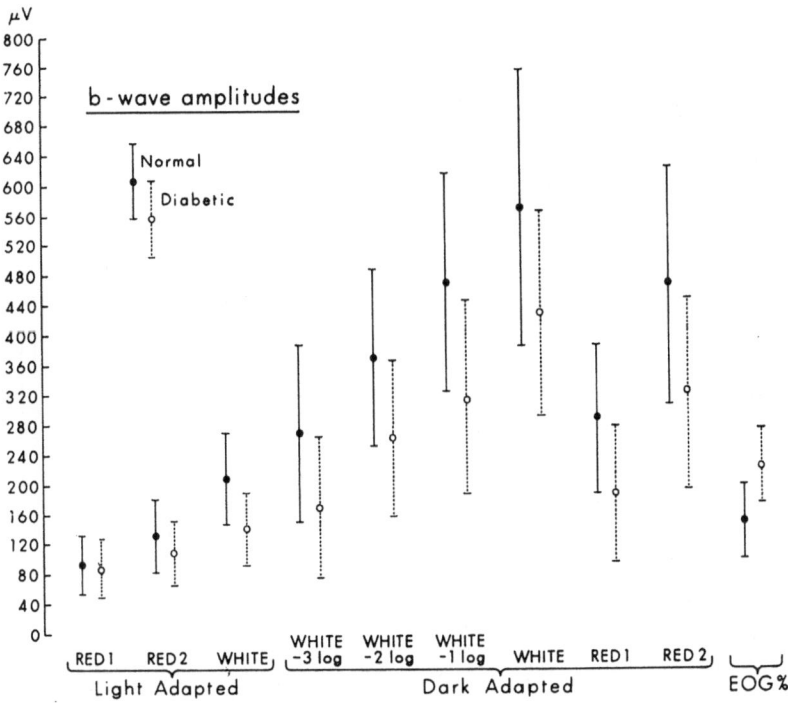

Fig. 5. The b-wave amplitudes mean and standard deviations for normal and diabetic eyes for the standard stimulus conditions. EOG percent light rise is plotted using the numbers from the μV scale.

b-waves and the EOG percent rise. In the case of amplitudes and EOG light rise in the treated eyes, all measures except one decreased after photocoagulation. Only 9 of these 19 were significant decreases at the 90% level, but the mean amplitude in the fellow untreated eyes in no case decreased. And, the interaction was significant in 10 out of 19 measures after excluding the repeated measures factor. Multivariant analysis with repeated measures correction shows that the a- and b-wave amplitudes are not significantly different in the treated eyes pre and post photocoagulation, but the interaction term is significant at the 95%

21

confidence level. This implies that the small decrease in the treated eyes is significant.

CONCLUSION

We conclude, therefore, that there is a significantly lower than normal ERG amplitude in the diabetic eye which has early retinopathy, but we note that this decrease is not sufficient to be valid for individual cases. In our small series covering a narrow spectrum of degree of retinopathy, there was no significant correlation between ERG or EOG and the degree of retinal involvement.

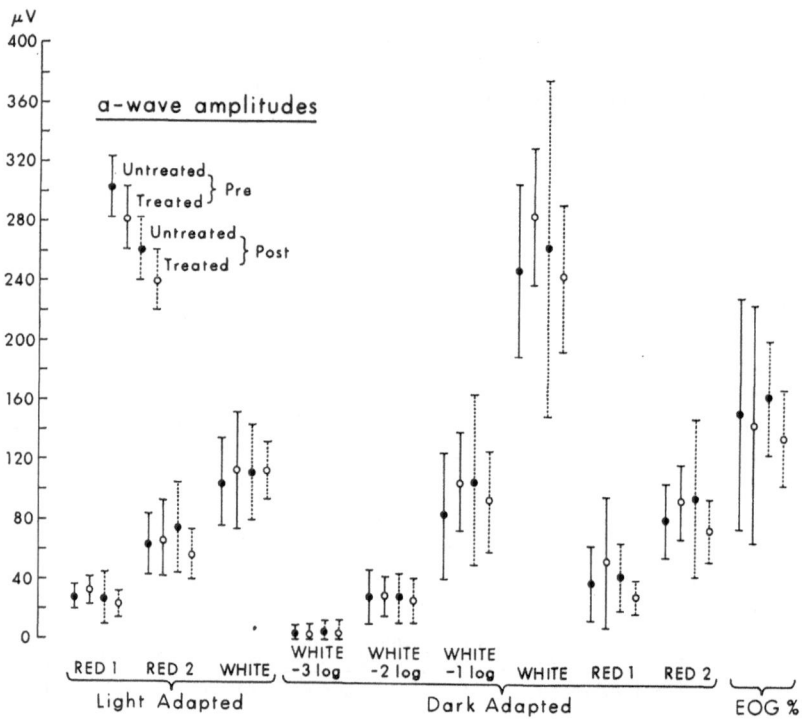

Fig. 6. The a-wave amplitudes mean and standard deviations for diabetic eyes in four groups, untreated eyes before and after treatment of the fellow eye and the treated eye before and after treatment.

The effect of photocoagulation is to reduce the amplitude of the a- and b-waves an average of 10% when the photocoagulated area averages 2.8 cm². The variability of this result does not allow prediction in any individual eye but gives an idea of the average effect. In general, the percentage decrease in ERG amplitude is less than the percentage of total retina photocoagulated.

SUMMARY

Electroretinographic and electrooculographic examination was made of eyes with diabetic retinopathy before and after treatment with photocoagulation.

There was a significant difference between the ERG amplitudes of all patients with retinopathy and normal patients, but no correlation was found with degree of retinal involvement. A statistically significant difference in a- and b-wave amplitudes of about 10% was found when approximately 20% of the retina was photocoagulated.

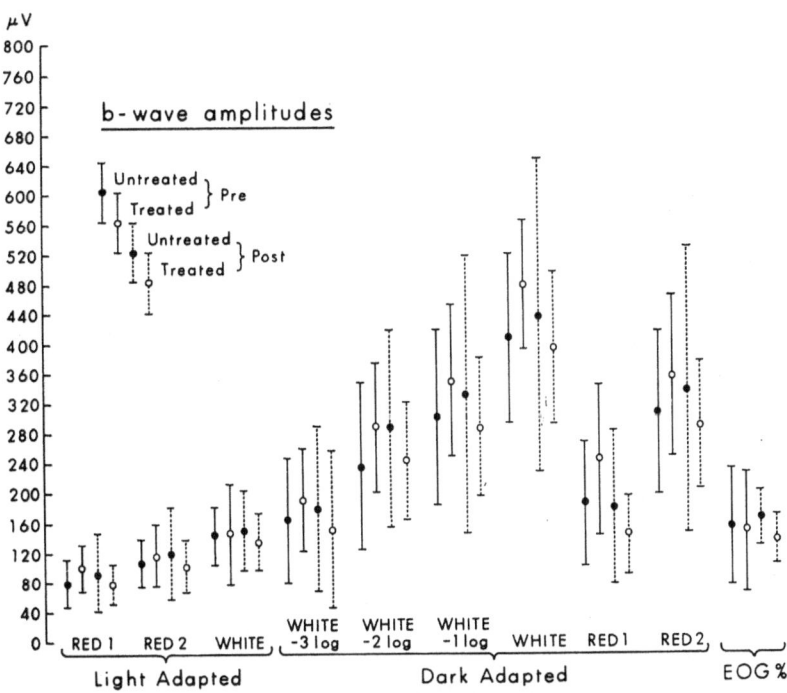

Fig. 7. The b-wave amplitudes means and standard deviation for diabetic eyes in four groups, untreated eye before and after treatment of the fellow eye and the treated eye before and after treatment.

REFERENCES

ARDEN, G. B., BARRADA, A. & KELSEY, J. H. New clinical test of retinal function based upon the standing potential of the eye. *Brit. J. Ophthal.* 46:449–467 (1962).

DAVIS, M. D., NORTON, E. W. D. & MYERS, F. L. Symposium—Treatment of diabetic retinopathy, Washington, D.C. United States Government Printing Office, 7 (1969).

FRANCOIS, J. & DE ROUCK, A. L'electroretinographie dans la retinopathie diabetique et dans la retinopathie hypertensive. *Acta ophthal. Kbh.* 32:391–404 (1954).

KARPE, G., KORNERUP, T. & WULFING, B. The clinical electroretinogram VIII: The ERG in diabetic retinopathy. *Acta ophthal. Kbh.* 36:281–291 (1956).

LAWWILL, T. & BURIAN, H. M. A modification of the Burian-Allen contact lens electrodes for human electroretinography. *Amer. J. Ophthal.* 61:1506–1509 (1966).

SIMONSEN, S. E. ERG in diabetics. ISCERG Symp. Ghent 1966, The Clinical Value of Electroretinography, 403–412, Karger, Basel/New York, (1968).

TOWNES, D. E. & WATZKE, R. C. Xenon photocoagulation of the papillomacular bundle, *Arch. Ophthal.* 87:679 (1972).

YONEMURA, D., TSUZUKI, K. & AOKI, T. Clinical importance of the oscillatory potential in the human ERG. *Acta ophthal. Kbh. Suppl.* 70:115–123 (1962).

23

ELECTROPHYSIOLOGICAL STUDIES IN PATIENTS WITH ARTERIO-VENOUS COMMUNICATIONS OF THE RETINA*

A. E. KRILL, D. B. ARCHER & A. F. DEUTMAN

(Chicago, Illinois)

ABSTRACT

The purpose of this report is to describe electrophysiological findings in five patients with arterio-venous communications of the retina.

METHOD

An electroretinogram was done in all five patients. The ERG was done with the subject supine. The active electrode was a Burian-Allen recording contact lens. Binocular recordings were obtained. An indifferent electrode was centered on the forehead above the nose. The light adaptation source used was a 61-degree field provided by a 60 watt, 130 volt tungsten filament, illuminating a plastic diffuser in front of the bulb. This source produced a 'white' light of 590 foot-lamberts luminance. The test stimulus was a Grass model PS-2 photostimulator providing an estimated maximum illumination at the position of the subject's eye of 450,000 footcandles with the lamp centered about 18 inches away from the subject's eye. The brightest light stimulus was obtained by using a maximum intensity setting on the instrument, and eight dimmer light stimuli, each differing by one-half log step, were obtained by interposing a series of four-inch square neutral density filters in front of the lamp. Control of eye position was attempted by having the subject fix on a 1.5 mm. red fixation bulb placed below the center of the lamp.

The electrodes led to a specially constructed junction box from which all impulses were conducted into two parallel systems. One of the two systems was used for single-flash evaluation. This system consisted of two RM 122 Tektronix low-level preamplifiers connected to a dual-beam type 512 Tektronix oscilloscope. The single-flash responses on the oscilloscope were photographed with a Tektronix C-13 oscilloscope camera. Single-flash photopic responses were obtained with the highest intensity light stimulus and the room lights on. Single-flash scotopic responses were obtained in total darkness after five minutes of light adaptation to the light source described above. The methodology is described in detail elsewhere (KRILL, 1966; KRILL et al., 1971).

The second system to which impulses from the junction box led was used for recording flicker responses. The impulses were led to a Nuclear Chicago data

* Supported in part by Public Health Service Grants EY-00523 and RR-55 from the National Institutes of Health, Grant G-455 from Fight For Sight, Inc. and by a NATO-fellowship.

25

retrieval computer, model 7100, and recorded on a type 700 4A Hewlett-Packard X-Y plotter. Responses were obtained with the room lights on, using the second highest or highest intensity light stimulus at each frequency. Responses to stimuli ranging from 1 to 70 flashes per second were obtained. Fifty responses were summated at each frequency.

An electrooculogram (EOG) was done in four patients (Cases 1, 2, 3, and 4). The technique for testing and normal data are described elsewhere (KRILL, 1966; KRILL et al., 1971). In evaluating the record, the average amplitude of each test period was measured and the ratio of the maximum light-adapted to minimum dark-adapted response was calculated and compared with similar ratios from a normal control group. Ratios less than 1.85 were considered definitely abnormal.

Dark-adaptation studies, as outlined elsewhere, (KRILL & MARTIN, 1971) were done in two patients (Cases 4 and 5). Rapid sequence fluorescein angiography was completed in all five patients utilizing a Zeiss fundus camera. A Baird-Atomic B4 filter was placed in the incident light pathway and a Baird-Atomic B5 filter before the film plane. The details of the procedure are reported elsewhere (ARCHER et al., 1970).

PATIENTS

Cases 1 through 4 had 20/20 acuity in both eyes. Case 5 had 20/20 acuity in the normal right eye and 20/25 acuity in the left eye with an arterio-venous communication. All patients had normal visual fields and neurological evaluation, except for case 5 who showed a left paracentral scotoma. The eyegrounds of each patient, as well as all other clinical information, are described in great detail elsewhere (ARCHER et al.) and therefore will only be briefly described in this report. In all five patients the eyegrounds without a shunt appeared normal and, therefore, will not be referred to.

Case 1 was a 35-year-old white male with an arterio-venous communication in the right macula. A large number of dilated capillaries and venules were observed at the right macula and superior paramacular area, extending to the major superior and inferior temporal veins. The majority of these vessels drained into a large retinal vein running horizontally, just below the level of the fovea (Fig. 1A). This vein appeared to drain directly into the central retinal vein. The retinal arteries subserving the vein were likewise prominent and dilated, often passing within a few microns distance from the fovea. There were no retinal hemorrhages, microaneurysms or exudates, nor any sclerosis of the arteries supplying the involved sector of retina. The right optic disc was mildly hyperemic, especially temporally, where a small dilated plexus of capillaries was evident on the disc surface.

The exact site of arterio-venous communication could only be determined with certainty during the early phase of fluorescein angiography (Fig. 1B). During the arterial phase of angiography, a direct communication between the retinal arteries and veins was distinguished (Fig. 1B-arrow). The communications between small arterioles and venules were without the interposition of a capillary network. Filling of the major retinal vein inferior to the fovea occurred one

26

second after the first appearance of dye in the retinal arterial tree, indicating an accelerated rate of flow in this location.

Case 2 was an 11-year-old white male with an arterio-venous communication in the right macula. An abnormally dilated vein coursed across the macula in a tortuous fashion to join the superotemporal retinal vein just short of its entrance into the central retinal vein (Fig. 2A). This dilated vein closely bordered the

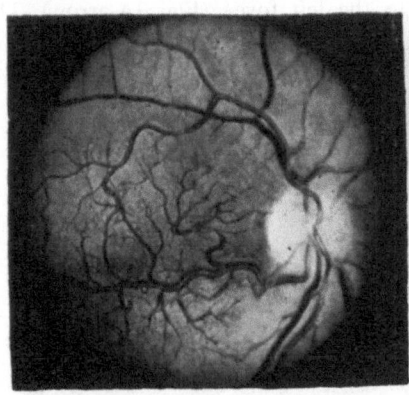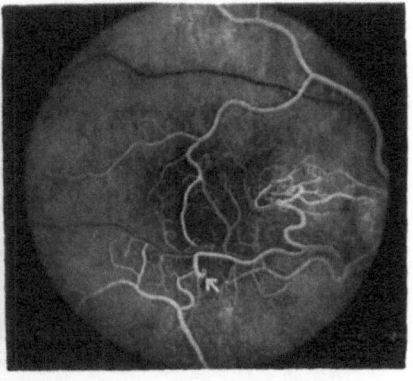

a

b

Fig. 1A and B. Black and white photograph of right posterior eye-grounds of Case 1 (1A). A complex of dilated veins and venules is apparent at the right macula. A large dilated vein courses just inferior to the fovea to drain into the central retinal vein at the optic disc. The exact site of the arterio-venous communication is not apparent.

Arterial phase angiogram (1B) of area demonstrated in 1A. Rapid filling of the dilated vein traversing the inferior macula results from a small arterio-venous communication just inferior to the fovea (arrow in 1B). A second small arterio-venous communication is present just temporal to the optic disc.

inferior fovea. A network of tributary veins and venules arranged over the macula drained into the dilated parent vessels. The retinal arteries at the posterior pole were of normal caliber. A sudden enlargement of the macular vein as it made a right angle turn from a horizontal to a vertical course, just nasal to the fovea, suggested the presence of an arterio-venous communication in this region. No hemorrhages, exudates, or microaneurysms were apparent.

The precise site of arterio-venous communication could only be delineated during the arterial phase of fluorescein angiography (Fig. 2B). A moderate sized arterio-venous communication, located just inferior to the fovea with a diameter of approximately 30–50 microns was noted. Dye was rapidly shunted from the macular branch of the inferior temporal artery via this abnormal communication into the central retinal vein. The high velocity of blood in the efferent vein was reflected by the arterial nature of dye flow, i.e., the fluorescent column of blood occupied the axial portion of the vessel, surrounded by dye-free

27

peripheral blood, whereas normally a peripheral laminar arrangement of fluorescein is seen during initial filling of the retinal veins.

Case 3 was a 19-year-old white female with an arterio-venous communication superior to the left macula (Fig. 3A). Greatly dilated and tortuous veins were noted over most of the posterior eye-grounds, but most prominently in the superior temporal eyegrounds (Fig. 3A). There appeared to be a direct arterio-venous communication between the major superior temporal artery and vein located one disc diameter superior to the left fovea (Fig. 3A-arrow). The

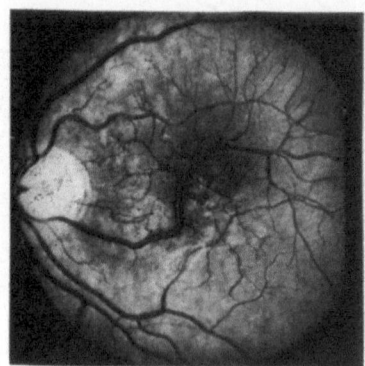 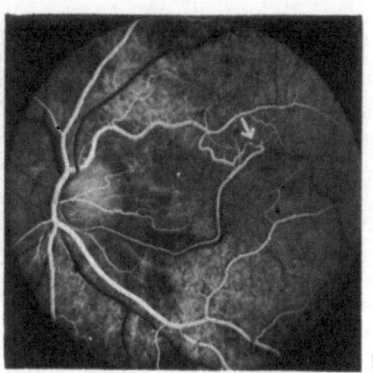

a   b

Fig. 2A and B. Right posterior fundus of Case 2 (2A). A tortuous dilated vein follows a sinuous course across the right macula to cross the optic disc at its superotemporal portion. Note how a sudden enlargement of the vein occurs as it turns from a horizontal to vertical direction. The exact site of the arterio-venous communication is not obvious.

Early retinal-venous phase angiogram (2B) of same area in 2A. The exact site of the arterio-venous communication can be easily seen (arrow in 2B). At the point of the arterio-venous communication a sudden increase in vascular caliber occurs. Fluorescein occupies the axial compartment of the dilated efferent vein.

dilated vessels became much less conspicuous as the equatorial retina was approached. The peripheral vessels appeared entirely normal. None of the involved vessels were sheathed or demonstrated early signs of arteriosclerosis. No hemorrhages, exudates, or microaneurysms were observed. The left optic disc was hyperemic but displayed sharp margins with no evidence of elevation.

Fluorescein angiography emphasized the large arterio-venous communication in the superotemporal quadrant of the left eye, particularly during the arterial phase of angiography (Fig. 3B). The superotemporal artery was significantly dilated and directly communicated with a markedly dilated vein which drained into the central retinal vein. The caliber of the vessel at the site of the communication measured some 150–200 microns (Fig. 3B-arrow). There was a

28

rapid transit of dye through the arterio-venous anomaly, and the flow characteristic of the dye column was arterial. There was a generalized dilatation of arterioles and venules throughout the posterior fundus, although no further sizeable arterio-venous communications were detected. There was full perfusion of the retinal capillary bed in the neighbourhood of the large arterio-venous shunt.

Case 4 was a 14-year-old black male with a large arterio-venous communication located in the supero-nasal aspect of the fundus (Fig. 4A). A grossly dilated and tortuous retinal artery could be traced from the optic disc, and its origin from the central retinal artery, to the supero-nasal equatorial retina (Figs. 4A

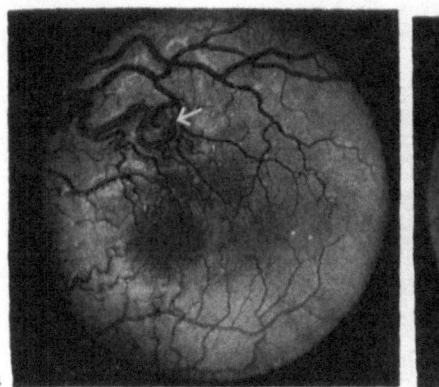 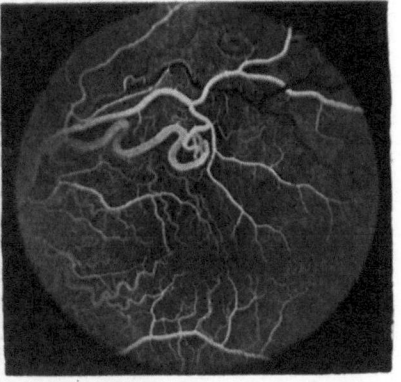

a   b

Fig. 3A and B. Black and white photograph of the left macula of Case 3 (3A). Note the dilated, tortuous superior temporal vein. An area suggestive of an arterio-venous communication is noted one disc diameter superior to the left fovea (arrow).
Early retinal venous phase angiogram (3B) of same area as in 3A. There is accelerated filling of a macular branch of the left superotemporal vein from the sizeable arterio-venous communication above the left macula.

and B). The parent artery divided into two major branches (arrow in 4A) which formed two direct communications with two large dilated veins some seven to eight disc diameters from the optic disc (arrows in Fig. 4B). At the sites of communication there was an increase in caliber of both the arteries and veins. The communicating vessel lumen diameters measured some 2–300 microns. The two dilated branch veins joined to form the major supero-nasal vein which joined the central retinal vein. The dilated artery and its two major branches were of irregular caliber and displayed pronounced beading, kinking and tortuosity along their course. There was sheathing of the supero-nasal artery and its origin adjacent to the optic disc. The communicating veins were likewise grossly dilated and showed considerable beading along their courses. These vessels were extensively sheathed along much of their length. The anomalous veins were colored bright red, indicating high oxygen saturation of the blood

29

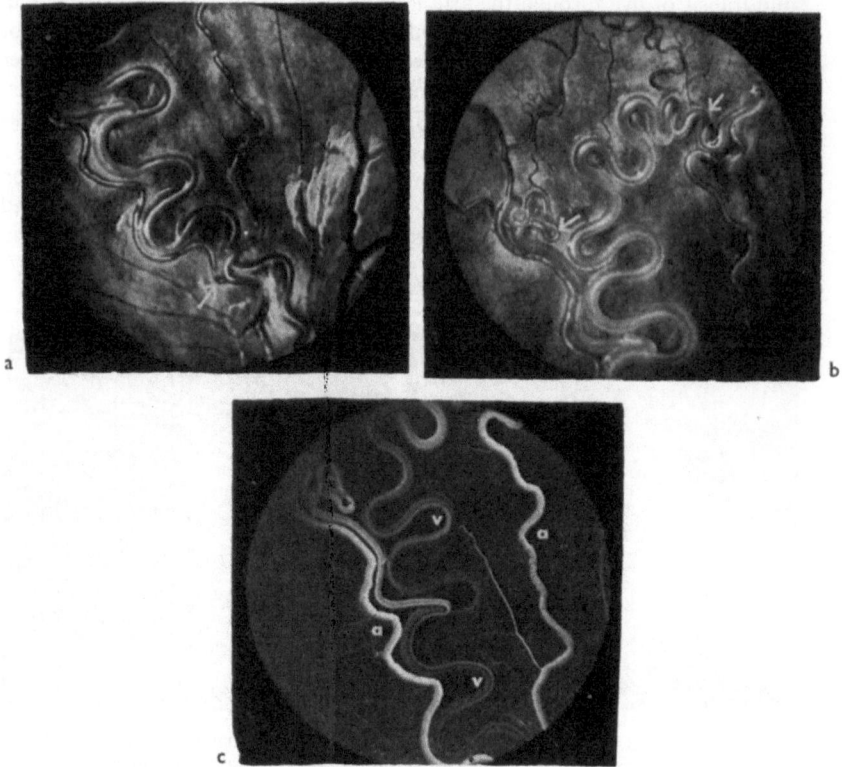

Fig. 4A, B and C. Black and white photographs of area in Case 4 superior and nasal to left optic disc (4A and B). Parent artery divides into two branches (arrow in Fig. 4A). Each branch forms a communication with large dilated veins (arrows in 4B). Note the sudden increase in the caliber of the arteries at the point of transition of artery to vein.

Mid-retinal venous phase angiogram (4C) of a segment of the arterio-venous communication shown in 4A and B. The two feeding arteries are marked *a*, and the veins *v*. There is accelerated filling of the communicating veins.

therein. The undilated tributaries of the larger vessels exhibited the normal dark hue of less saturated venous blood. The optic disc was mildly hyperemic in the region of the abnormal vessels, but had well defined borders and was not elevated. The retinal vessels in the remaining quadrants were normal.

Fluorescein angiography (Fig. 4C) strikingly demonstrated the arterio-venous communications. Dye rapidly filled the arterial side of the malformation in the early phases of angiography. The more inferior communication is illustrated in Fig. 4C.

Case 5 was a 26-year-old black female with a complex arterio-venous malformation arranged along the left inferotemporal vessels extending some 4–5 disc diameters from the optic disc (Fig. 5A). A grossly dilated infero-temporal artery and vein were distinguished at the left optic disc and for a short distance beyond. At this point these major vessels merged into a convoluted mass of vessels where it became difficult to identify arterial and venous components. Substantial hemorrhage had occurred within the retina and into the nerve fiber layer overlying much of the arterio-venous malformation, when first seen in 1962; therefore, many of the dilated tortuous vessels displayed extensive sheathing of their walls. No edema, hemorrhage, or exudates were present when the

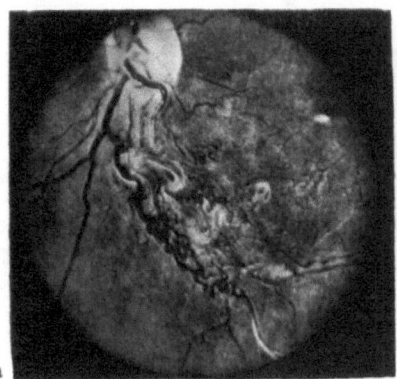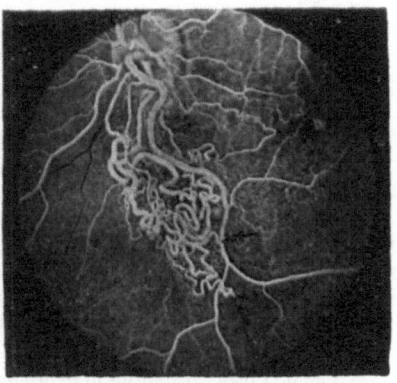

a   b

Fig. 5A and B. Black and white photograph of left inferior posterior eye-grounds of Case 5 (5A). The inferotemporal retinal vessels merge into a mass of convoluted attenuated arteries and veins in which arterial and venous components become difficult to discern. There is some sheathing of the major retinal vessels inferotemporal to the optic disc. Large numbers of venous collaterals extend from an area distal to the arterio-venous malformation across the horizontal raphé to join with fellow veins in the superotemporal quadrant.
Early retinal venous phase angiogram (5B) of same area shown in 5A. Several sites of arterio-venous communication can be discerned, and one is marked with an arrow.

patient was last seen in 1972, although there was some pigment irregularity near the fovea. Large, well-formed venous collaterals were apparent in the region of the arterio-venous communications. These channels communicated with the superotemporal veins, crossing the horizontal raphé. There was no obvious sign of vascular decompensation within the arterio-venous malformation or newly developed collaterals. The optic disc had discrete borders and was not elevated. The retinal vessels in the remaining quadrants of the fundus were normal.

Fluorescein angiography demonstrated multiple arterio-venous communications (one is identified by arrow in Fig. 5B).

31

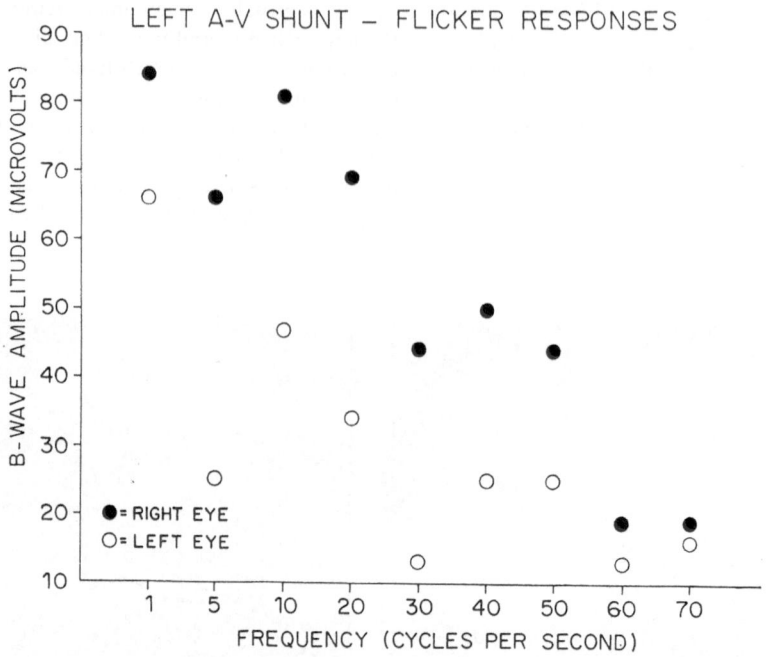

Fig. 6. Flicker responses in light-adapted eyes of Case 3. Fifty responses were summed at each frequency and values were read off X-Y plotter. Responses are notably smaller from involved left eye.

RESULTS

Electroretinogram

In four of the five patients (Cases 1, 3, 4, and 5) summated flicker responses were decidedly smaller from the eye with the arterio-venous communication. The data from three of the four patients (Cases 3, 4, and 5) are shown in Fig. 6–8. In Case 2 the responses were smaller from the normal eye (Fig. 9).

In two patients (Cases 1 and 5) all scotopic b-wave responses were smaller from the involved eye (Fig. 10 and 11). However, Case 2 had smaller scotopic b-wave responses from the normal eye (Fig. 12). The scotopic b-wave responses were equal from the two eyes in the other two patients (Cases 3 and 4). The scotopic a-waves were about the same from the two eyes in all patients. No definite conclusions could be made regarding the oscillatory potentials.

Electrooculogram

In two patients (Cases 3 and 4) abnormal ratios were obtained from the abnormal eye, whereas normal ratios were obtained from the normal eye (Fig. 13A and B).

32

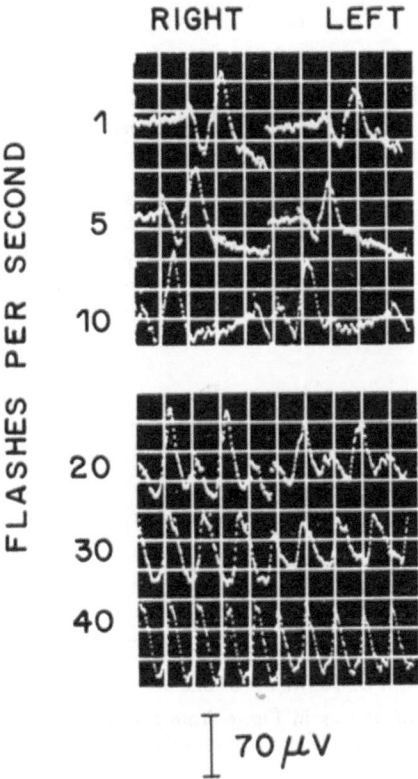

LEFT A-V SHUNT
FLICKER RESPONSES

RIGHT   LEFT

FLASHES PER SECOND

1

5

10

20

30

40

70 μV

Fig. 7. Flicker responses in light-adapted eyes of Case 4. Fifty responses were summed at each frequency and photographed from face of computer. Responses are distinctly smaller from involved left eye.

In two other patients (Cases 1 and 2) decidedly abnormal, but equal, ratios were obtained from both eyes (Fig. 14). In all patients an abnormal ratio was due mainly or solely to a smaller than normal light rise.

Dark adaptation

There was no difference in any aspect of dark adaptation in the two patients (Cases 4 and 5) studied.

33

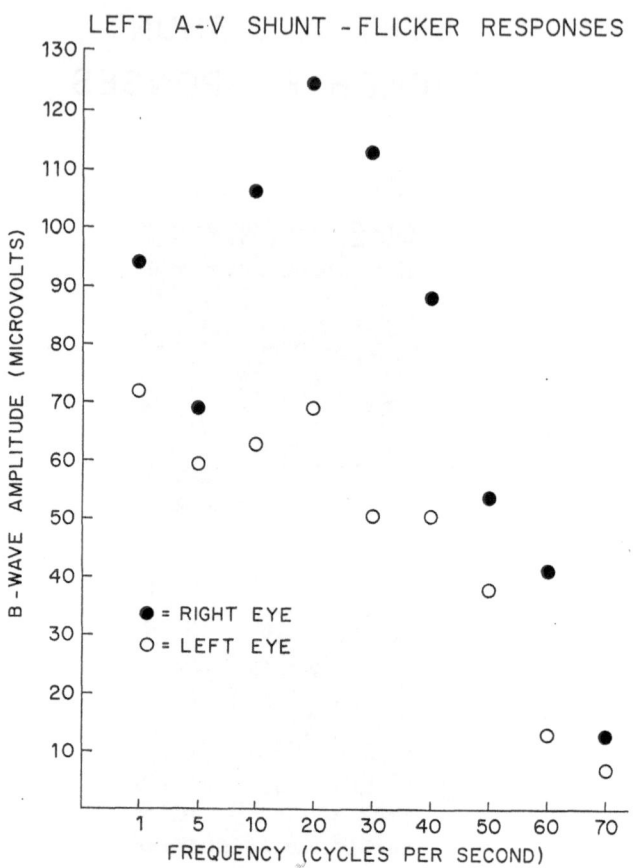

Fig. 8. Same type of plot as in Fig. 6 from eyes of Case 5. Responses are notably smaller from involved left eye.

DISCUSSION

Arterio-venous communications are easily visualized when large and single, but may be difficult to detect when small or multiple. Fluorescein angiography is of great value in demonstrating the site of communication in such cases, as has been noted elsewhere (ARCHER et al.).

The occurrence of a reduced amplitude ERG from human eyes with significant vascular alteration is well known. This reduction, which is mainly or only of the b-wave, has been cited in a whole host of clinical diseases of the retinal or more proximal vasculature, including sickle cell retinopathy, hypertension with arteriolar sclerosis, Coats' disease, central and branch retinal arteriolar obstructions, some cases of central vein obstruction, and carotid artery obstruction (KRILL, 1959; KARPE & UCHERMANN, 1955; KARPE & GERMANIS, 1962; VANNAS, 1960; HENKES, 1954, 1957; KRILL, 1962; WULFING, 1963). In animal experiments

34

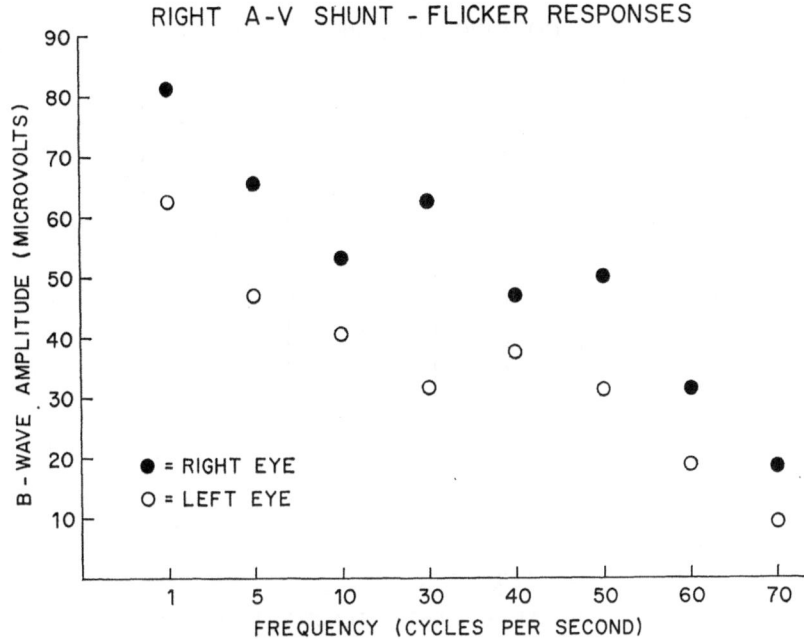

Fig. 9. Same type of plot as in Fig. 6 from eyes of Case 2. Responses are definitely smaller from left eye which has normal eyegrounds.

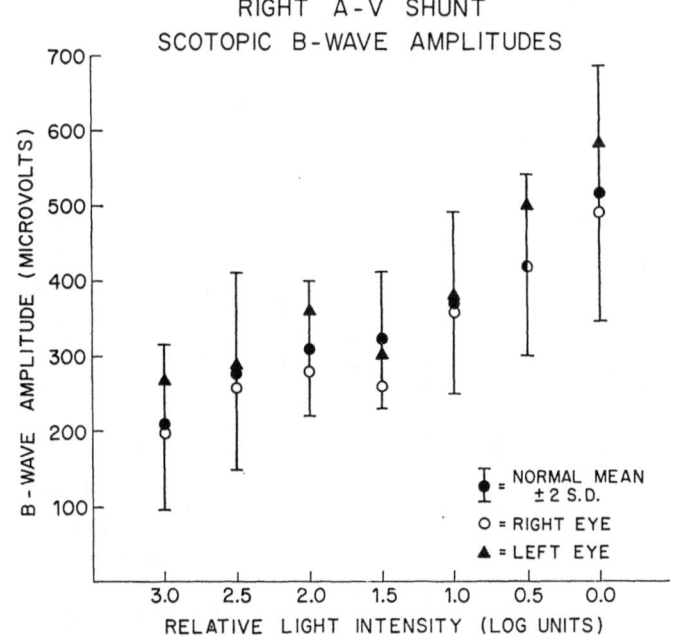

Fig. 10. A plot of b-wave amplitudes from both eyes of Case 1 compared with a normal control group (normal mean plus or minus two standard deviations). Amplitudes are smaller from involved right eye.

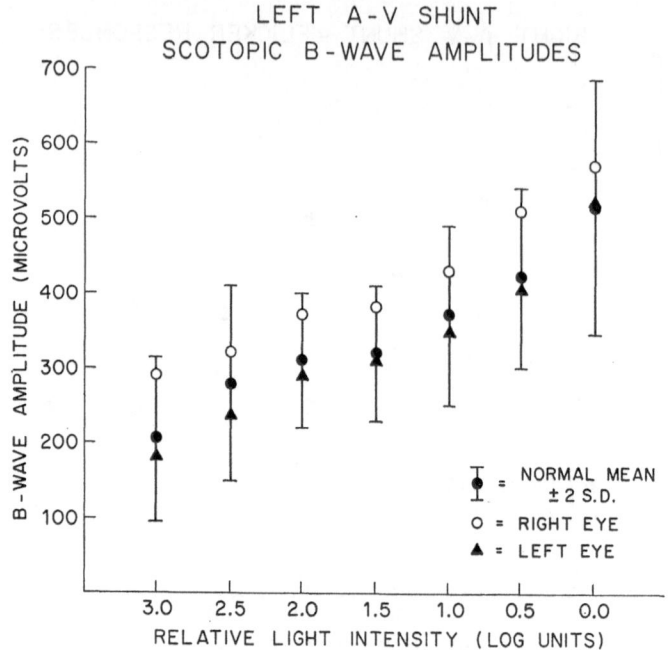

Fig. 11. Same type of plot as in Fig. 10 from both eyes of Case 5. Amplitudes are smaller from involved left eye.

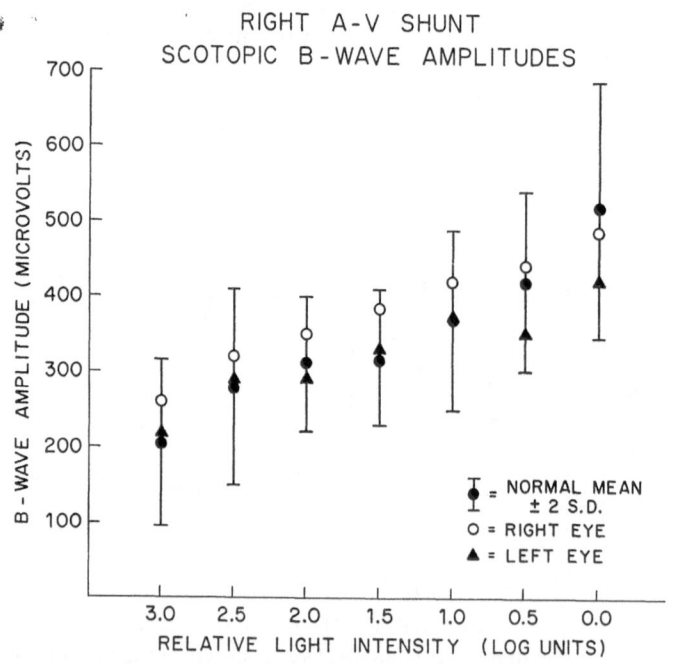

Fig. 12. Same type of plot as in Fig. 10 from both eyes of Case 2. Amplitudes are smaller from right eye with normal eyegrounds.

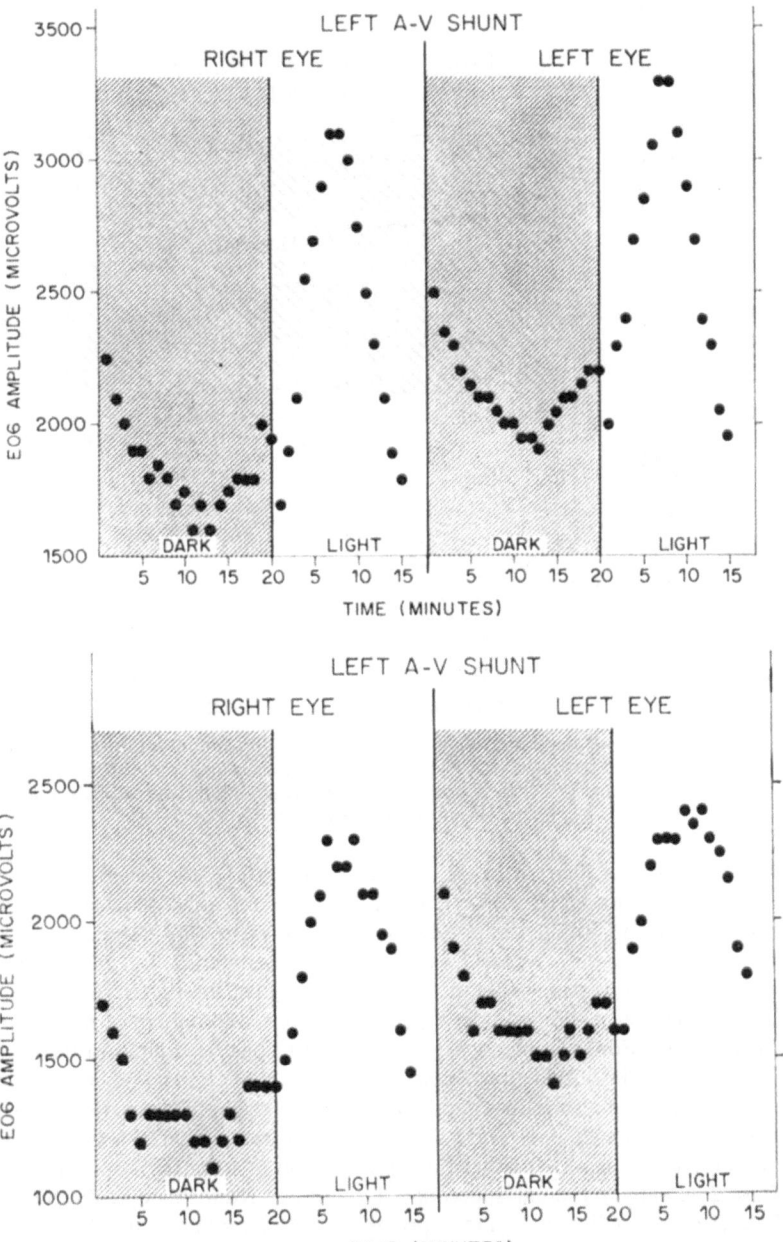

Figs. 13A and B. A plot of the average amplitudes for both eyes from the EOG of Cases 3(A) and 4(B). Both patients show a smaller amplitude increase during light adaptation in the involved left eye.

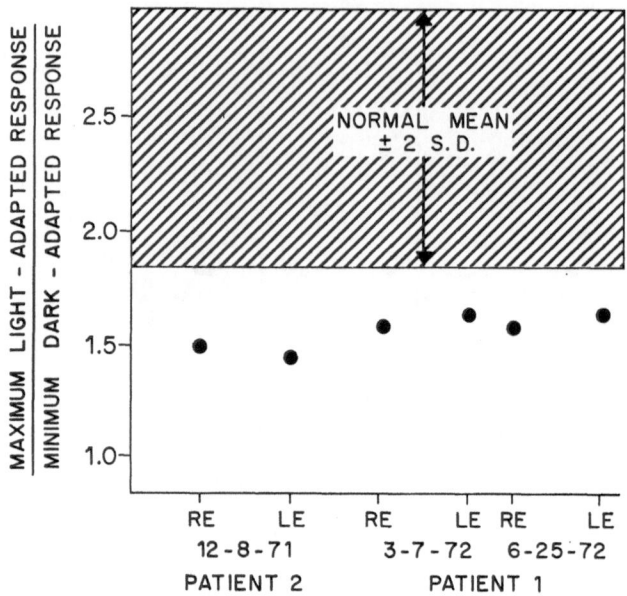

Fig. 14. Plot of maximum light-adapted response to minimum dark-adapted response from both eyes of Cases 1 (on two test occasions) and 2 (on one test occasion) compared with a normal control group. Note that ratios are abnormal from both eyes of each patient.

in which there is ligation of the central retinal artery, the b-wave completely disappears (FUJINO & HAMASAKI, 1965). Ligation or compression of the carotid artery results in initial disappearance of the b-wave with subsequent disappearance of the a-wave as well (WULFING, 1963; HORSTEN & WINKLEMAN, 1957).

In less severe vascular alterations, abnormalities of the ERG are more subtle and may be detected only under certain conditions, and only in certain portions of the ERG. For example, a supernormal ERG has been cited in incomplete and branch vein obstructions, vascular congestion secondary to narrow angle glaucoma, commotio-retinae, and some cases with papilledema (KRILL, 1959; KARPE & UCHERMANN, 1955; KARPE & GERMANIS, 1962; VANNAS, 1960; HENKES, 1957). It may be that the larger responses from the abnormal eye of Case 2 actually represent supernormal responses from this eye. On the other hand, the possibility of a more proximal vascular abnormality (e.g. in the ophthalmic artery) in the eye with normal eyegrounds must be considered, as it is well known that arterio-venous communications in the retina can be associated with arterio-venous communications elsewhere in the central nervous system (ARCHER et al.). Indeed, the Wyburn-Mason syndrome has been applied to this association (WYBURN-MASON, 1943).

38

Flicker responses may be a more sensitive way of detecting less severe vascular abnormalities and this was true for two of our patients (Cases 3 and 4). Some workers emphasize a disappearance of the oscillatory potential (the two or three positive wavelets on the ascending limb of the b-wave) as an initial abnormality in certain disorders with vascular alterations (ALGVERE, 1968). However, we were not able to detect any difference in oscillatory potentials from the involved and normal eyes in our patients.

In a study of carotid artery disease (KRILL et al., 1962), it was noted that low-intensity responses during the first portion of dark adaptation after recovery from fairly bright preadaptation were likely to show differences between involved and uninvolved sides in patients with unilateral partial carotid obstruction. We did not find more pronounced differences in this portion of the test.

An abnormal EOG from only the involved eye was noted in the two patients (Cases 3 and 4) who also had a reduced flicker ERG in this eye. Both of these patients showed less of an amplitude increase in the EOG from the affected eye during light adaptation ('light rise') compared to the normal eye.

It is well known, on the basis of both animal experimentation (BROWN & WIESEL, 1958; NOELL, 1953) and clinical material (KRILL, 1970), that the EOG reflects function of the pigment epithelium. However, the notion that a portion of the light rise of the EOG originates from the internal retina, or at least relates to the blood supply of this portion of the retina, was first suggested by experimental data in monkeys (GOURAS & CARR, 1965). GOURAS showed that ligation of the central retinal artery in monkeys caused a decrease in the light-rise portion of the EOG. However, this relationship is not completely clear in humans as both normal and abnormal electrooculograms have been obtained from eyes with fresh as well as from eyes with old central retinal artery occlusions (ASHWORTH, 1966; NAGAYA, 1969; FRANCOIS et al., 1957; CARR & SIEGEL, 1969; IMAIZUMI, 1966; HECHT & PABST, 1957). Furthermore, a normal EOG has been obtained from eyes with glaucoma (KRILL, 1959). In addition, cutting off the blood supply at more proximal sites (for example, at the carotid artery) does not seem to affect the EOG (ASHWORTH, 1966). The data from the two patients in this study suggest a definite relationship of a portion of the light rise of the EOG to retinal vascular integrity.

On the other hand, an alternate explanation for the data in these two patients (Cases 3 and 4) must also be considered. It may be that arterio-venous abnormalities exist in the ophthalmic artery of each patient. The possibillity of associated arterio-venous communications elsewhere in the central nervous system must be again emphasized (ARCHER et al.). This would, of course, affect the choroidal blood supply and, therefore, the integrity of the pigment epithelium. An abnormality of the pigment epithelium could then explain the abnormal EOG.

Indeed, it becomes difficult to explain the bilateral abnormality of the EOG in Cases 1 and 2 unless we also assume that existence of a more proximal arterio-venous communication, particularly on the side of the eye with normal eyegrounds. Obviously, then, our data only suggest, but do not confirm a relationship of the retinal vasculature to the light rise of the EOG.

39

SUMMARY AND CONCLUSIONS

Electrophysiological data were obtained from five patients with arterio-venous communications of the retina.

High-intensity photopic flicker responses on the ERG were the most sensitive way of demonstrating a difference between a normal eye and an eye with a shunt. In some patients scotopic b-waves were also smaller from the involved eye.

A decreased light rise of the EOG was noted from the involved eye in four patients and may reflect a dependence of this portion of the record on retinal *vascular* integrity. On the other hand, the possibility that associated arterio-venous communications exist at a more proximal level in the central nervous system is also a possibility to be considered. If this is true, an abnormality of the choroidal blood supply, affecting function of the pigment epithelium, would explain the abnormal EOG both from the abnormal eye and from the normal eye in two of our patients.

REFERENCES

ALGVERE, P. Studies on the oscillatory potentials of the clinical electroretinogram. *Acta Ophth. Supp.* 96 (1968).

ARCHER, D. B., KRILL, A. E. & NEWELL, F. W. Fluorescein studies of the normal choroidal circulation. *Amer. J. Ophth.* 69:543 (1970).

ARCHER, D. B., DEUTMAN, A. F., ERNEST, J. T. & KRILL, A. E. Arterio-venous communications of the retina. *Amer. J. Ophth.* 75:224 (1973).

ASHWORTH, B. The electrooculogram in disorders of the retinal circulation. *Amer. J. Ophth.* 61:505 (1966).

BROWN, K. T. & WIESEL, T. Intraretinal recording in the unopened cat eye. *Amer. J. Ophth.* 46:91 (1958).

CARR, R. E. & SIEGEL, I. M. Electrophysiological aspects of several retinal diseases. *Amer. J. Ophth.* 58:95 (1964).

FRANCOIS, J., VERRIEST, G. & DeROUCK, A. Electrooculographie en tant qu'examen functionel de la retine. *Progr. Ophtal.* 7:1 (1957).

FUJINO, T. & HAMASAKI, T. I. The effect of occluding the retina and choroidal circulations on the electroretinogram of monkeys. *J. Physiol.* 180:837 (1965).

GOURAS, P. & CARR, R. E. Light induced D-C responses of monkey retina before and after central artery interruption. *Invest. Ophth.* 4:310 (1965).

HECHT, J. & PABST, W. Ueber den Ursprung des corneoretinalen Ruhepotentials. *Electroretinographie Bibl. Ophth.* 48:96 (1957).

HENKES, H. E. Electroretinogram in circulatory disturbances of retina: Electroretinogram in cases of retinal and choroidal hypertension in arteriolar sclerosis. *Arch. Ophth.* 52:30 (1954).

HENKES, H. E. Electroretinography: An evaluation of the influence of the retina in general metabolic condition on the electrical response of the eye. *Amer. J. Ophth.* 43:67 (1957).

HENKES, H. E. Electroretinogram in circulatory disturbances of retina: Electroretinogram in cases of occlusions of central retinal artery or one of its branches. *Arch. Ophth.* 51:4 (1954).

HORSTEN, G. P. M. & WINKLEMAN, J. E. Effect of temporary occlusion of aorta on electroretinogram. *Arch. Ophth.* 57:557 (1957).

IMAIZUMI, K. Clinical application of electrooculography in BURIAN, H. M. & JACOBSON, J. H. editors: Clinical Electroretinography, Visual Res. (Supp.) London, Pergamon Press, pp. 311–326, (1966).

KARPE, G. & UCHERMANN, A. The clinical electroretinogram. VII. The electroretinogram in circulatory disturbances of the retina. *Acta Ophth.* 33:493 (1955).

KARPE, G. & GERMANIS, M. The prognostic value of the electroretinogram in thrombosis of the retinal veins. *Acta Ophth. Supp.* 70:202 (1962).

KRILL, A. E. Clinical electroretinography in Hughes, W. F., editor: Year Book of Ophthalmology, Chicago, Year Book Medical Publishers, Inc. (1959).

KRILL, A. E., DIAMOND, M. & ISER, G. The electroretinogram in carotid artery disease. *Arch. Ophth.* 68:42 (1962).

KRILL, A. E. The electroretinographic and electrooculographic findings in patients with macular lesions. *Trans. Amer. Acad. Ophth. Otol.* 70:1063 (1966).

KRILL, A. E. The electretinogram and electrooculogram: Clinical applications. *Invest. Ophth.* 9:*600* (1970).

KRILL, A. E., POTTS, A. M. & JOHANSON, C. E. Advanced chloroquine retinopathy. Investigation of a discrepancy between dark adaptation and the electroretinogram. *Amer. J. Ophth.* 71:*530* (1971).

KRILL, A. E. & MARTIN, D. Photopic abnormalities in congenital stationary nightblindness *Invest. Ophth.* 10:*625* (1971).

NAGAYA, T. Standing potential of the eye in vascular and degenerative disease of the retina. *Bull. Yamaguchi Med. Sch.* 11:*187* (1964).

NOELL, W. K. Experimentally induced toxic effects on structure and function of visual cells and pigment epithelium. *Amer. J. Ophth.* 36:*103* (1953).

VANNAS, S. Electroretinographic observations in central retinal vein occlusion. *Acta Ophth.* 38:*312* (1960).

WULFING, B. Clinical electroretino-dynamography. *Acta Ophthalmologica*, Supp. 73 (1963).

WYBURN-MASON, R. Arterio-venous aneurysm of mid-brain and retina, facial naevi and mental changes. *Brain* 66:*163* (1943).

41

ELECTROPHYSIOLOGICAL ASPECTS IN RETINAL VENOUS THROMBOSIS*

J. FRANÇOIS, A. De ROUCK & E. CAMBIE

(Ghent)

Electrophysiological examinations, including EOG and ERG, were performed in 19 cases of retinal venous obstruction (8 branch occlusions, 11 total occlusions of the central retinal vein). A few were examined during the first week, others more than 6 months after the onset.

METHODS

The ERG was performed with a Xenon discharge tube (Van Gogh). The flash intensities were modified by neutral density filters. Stimulus intensities from $\overline{3},0$ (minimal flash) to $\overline{0},0$ (maximal flash), stepwise increased by 0.50 log. unit, were used. The examinations were performed in dark adapted as well as in light adapted state. The pupil was fully dilated by mydriaticum 0.5 % (mydriacyl) and phenylephrine 10 %. The electrical potentials were registered by a corneal contact lens electrode (Karpe) and a silver frontal electrode. They were recorded by a preamplifier E, connected to an ink jet recorder (Mingograph Elema) and a CAT 900 B for the response summation.

The recordings were made at different levels of background illumination, using a perimeter cupola (diameter 90 cm). This cupola was illuminated by four argenta bulbs of 100 W (P_2E_5 Philips) connected to a rheostat. This was calibrated to give a stepwise increase of the illumination from 0 (darkness) to 3.000 lux, measured by a luxmeter at the level of the patient's eye. Background illuminations of 10, 30, 100, 300, 1,000 and 3,000 lux were used.

In the centre of the dome was an opening of 15 cm, where the flash light was placed at a distance of 33 cm from the subject.

For each level of illumination, the complete range of flash intensities was used. After the room adaptation, the patients were fully adapted to the background illumination for 3 minutes before examination. We always started with a 10 lux illumination. For the maximal flash intensity ($\overline{0},0$), not only single flashes, but also low flicker flashes (1.5/sec.) were used.

I. ELECTRORETINOGRAPHY

1. Dark adapted ERG

When the flash intensities are increased from $\overline{3},0$ to $\overline{0},0$ the ERG shows a gradual change. We first obtain a scotopic response (flash I $\overline{3},0$, no a-wave, large b_2-wave), then a mixed response (flash I $\overline{2},0$, a_1- and a_2-waves, b_1- and b_2-waves) and finally a photopic response (flash I $\overline{1},0$ till $\overline{0},0$, a_1- and b_1-waves, early and late oscillatory potentials).

* From de ophthalmological Clinic of the University of Ghent. Director: Prof. JULES FRANÇOIS, De Pintelaan 135, B-9000, Ghent (Belgium).

4

The following characteristics are taken into consideration: the amplitude curves of the a- and b-waves, the peak-time of the a- and b-waves, the number and the frequency of the oscillatory potentials (4 or 5 at $\bar{0},0$).

2. Light adapted ERG (300 lux)

At $\bar{3},0$ log. units, a small photopic b-wave is seen, which increases gradually at higher flash intensities. At $\bar{2},0$ the late photopic oscillation becomes visible as 2 oscillation peaks with a peak-time of respectively 55–60 msec and 80–85 msec. Early oscillatory potentials appear between $\bar{1},0$ and $\bar{0},0$. Normally, three distinct peaks appear in the photopic b- or b_1-wave and the two late oscillatory potentials. The maximal amplitude of the b-wave is mostly obtained at $\bar{1},0$ or $\bar{1},25$. At the maximal intensity ($\bar{0},0$) the response is mainly characterized by an enlargement of the b-wave with increased peak-time and by the disappearance of the first photopic late potential. The photopic b-wave is always the principal component of the photopic response, the late oscillations having always a lower amplitude.

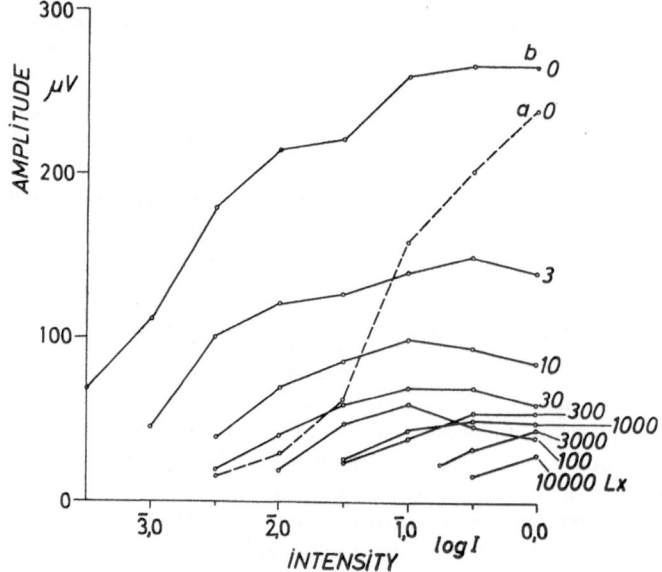

Fig. 1. Amplitude curves of the b-wave in relation to the stimulus intensity and an increasing background adaptation. Normal case.

3. ERG at different levels of background illumination

When the background illumination is increased, there is a gradual but rapid change in the amplitude, as well as in the peak-time of the response, as a result of the progressive inhibition of the scotopic activity.

Fig. 1 shows the amplitude curves of the a- and b-waves at increasing levels of light adaptation. These curves show a downwards shift with decreasing slope till about 30 lux. From 30 till 300 lux, there is also a shift at the onset of the response,

44

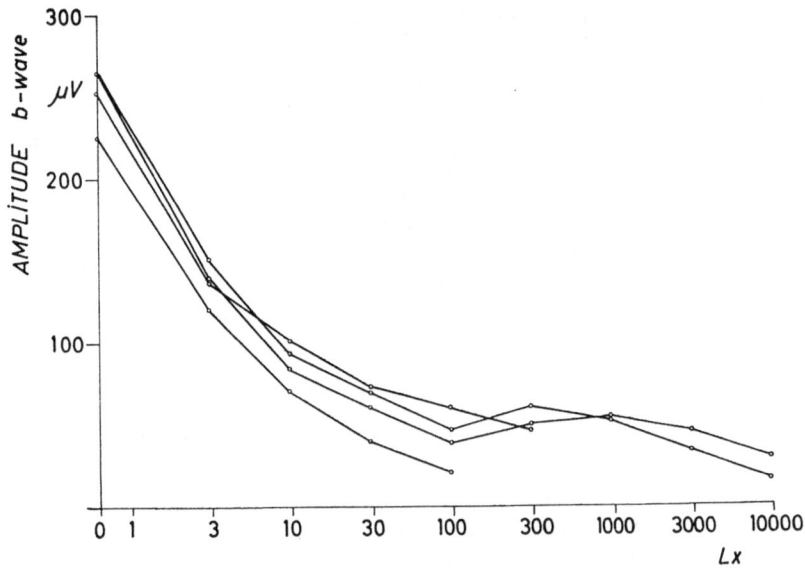

Fig. 2. Amplitude of the *b*-wave in relation to the background adaptation and 4 stimulus intensities, ($\overline{2}$,5; $\overline{1}$,0; $\overline{1}$,5; $\overline{0}$,0).

but the maximal amplitude remains unchanged. When the amplitude of the *b*-wave is plotted against the background illumination, the curve corresponding with the maximal intensity response ($\overline{0}$,0–$\overline{1}$,0) shows a distinct break at about 30 lux (Fig. 2). A scotopic (darkness), a mesopic (from 0 to 30 lux) and a photopic part (from 100 to 3,000 lux) can be distinguished in the curve.

Table I gives the mean values, in 40 normal subjects, of the amplitude of the *a*- and *b*-waves in darkness and in light adaptation at 300 lux.

II. ELECTRO-OCULOGRAPHY

For the EOG we used the technique described by us (FRANÇOIS et al., 1966). The following parameters were taken into account:

M: base value (amplitude of the EOG after room light adaptation).

m_2: maximal amplitude after light adaptation.

Table I

	I	m	m + 2S	m − 2S	real observed minimum value
Darkness	$\overline{3}$,0 *b*	95	125	65	70
	$\overline{0}$,0 *a*	220	290	150	170
	b	320	440	200	210
300 lux	$\overline{0}$,0 *a*	50	72	28	30
	max *b*	100	136	66	70

45

m_3: minimal amplitude after the second period of dark adaptation.

t: dark-light ratio, measure by $\dfrac{m^2}{m^3} \cdot 100$.

Table II gives the mean values in 40 normal subjects.
A value lower than 175 was only found in three cases (162, 164, 174), so that we may conclude that values below 160 are definitely abnormal.

III. Review of the Literature

1. *Electroretinography.*

Retinal vascular disturbances were studied by many authors since KARPE in 1945. Mostly, the behaviour of the scotopic ERG was analyzed. The most im-

Table II

	m	m + 2S	m − 2S	real minimal value observed
M	470	712	228	260
m_2	655	970	340	390
m_3	370	445	165	165
t	210	272	148	162

portant contributions are these of HENKES (1953, 63 cases), KARPE & UCHERMAN (1955, 35 cases), KARPE (1958, 73 cases), KARPE & GERMANIS (1966, 141 cases) and PONTE (1966, 122 cases).

The characteristics of the dark adapted ERG can be summarized as follows:

1. The *a*-wave remains normal for a long time. It may even be supranormal in the initial stage.

2. The amplitude of the *b*-wave tends to increase during the initial stage and to decrease in the cicatricial stage. Some authors insisted on the increase of the peak-time of the *b*-wave (MULLER & HAASE, 1967; KUBOTA, 1970).

3. The oscillatory potentials disappear very rapidly, as they are very sensitive to circulatory disturbances. They are generally affected before any other component of the ERG (USAMI, 1965; ALGVERE, 1968), although they may be present in the initial stage (YONEMURA et al., 1962).

4. Several types of pathological ERG's can be distinguished according to the relative interaction of *a*- and *b*-waves (HENKES, 1953; KARPE, 1958). The pathological ERG can be negative plus, negative minus or extinguished.

5. There is a correlation between the type of ERG and the prognosis of the disease (HENKES, 1953) or the duration of the occlusion (PONTE, 1966).

6. Pathological alterations of the photopic ERG (CARR & SIEGEL, 1964) as well as of the scotopic ERG (PONTE, 1966) were reported.

The alterations of the ERG are less severe in retinal venous branch occlusions. The same types of pathological ERG are reported as in total occlusions, but they are less frequent and less pronounced (HENKES, 1953; PONTE, 1966).

On the other hand, STRAUB (1966) did not find any significant difference between 15 eyes with retinal venous branch occlusion and 15 normal eyes.

46

2. *Electro-oculography*.

Pathological EOG's in venous occlusions were already published in 1957 by FRANÇOIS, VERRIEST and DE ROUCK. This was confirmed by ARDEN et al. (1962), KELSEY (1966), HEILEMAN & SPINDLER (1967). GLIEM (1970), reporting 12 cases of venous occlusion, stated that the EOG showed pathological alterations, but less regularly than in arterial occlusions. Sometimes these alterations were severe, sometimes slight. There seemed to be a correlation between the EOG and the prognosis of the disease, as well as between the behaviour of the EOG and the *b*-wave of the ERG.

IV. PERSONAL OBSERVATIONS
A. RETINAL VENOUS BRANCH OCCLUSIONS

Eight cases, of which 4 recent occlusions examined within one week after the onset (Cases 1 to 4) and 4 old cases seen more than 6 months after the onset Cases 5 to 8).

Table III. *EOG and ERG of the affected eye, EOG of the fellow-eye.*

case	EOG				ERG			EOG fellow-eye			
	M	m_2	m_3	t	3,0	0,0	photop. *b*-wave	M	m_2	m_3	t
1	410	590	370	160	140	430	125	400	550	250	220
	275	405	270	170	120	340	130	410	670	330	203
A.L.	275	375	226	166	100	310	125	305	420	190	215
2	610	740	580	127	80	220	80	775	1005	645	155
A.L.	550	655	500	130	75	220	70	690	780	460	169
	400	500	350	143	85	240	85	500	710	390	182
3	395	640	250	245	80	320	120	530	640	260	245
	480	500	230	213	80	260	95	330	410	190	215
4	810	1150	740	155	140	430	110	690	820	520	160
	760	940	650	145	120	300	110	780	810	550	148
5	436	705	320	129	60	130	25	505	950	350	271
6	570	590	460	129	45	280	70	600	608	360	185
7	460	465	375	124	55	305	66	690	760	330	205
8	580	740	330	220	10	155	165	460	735	340	215
mean values 1–4	496	649	417	165	102	307	105				
5–8	511	625	371	176	42	218	56				
1–8	500	643	403	168	85	281	91	550	709	369	201

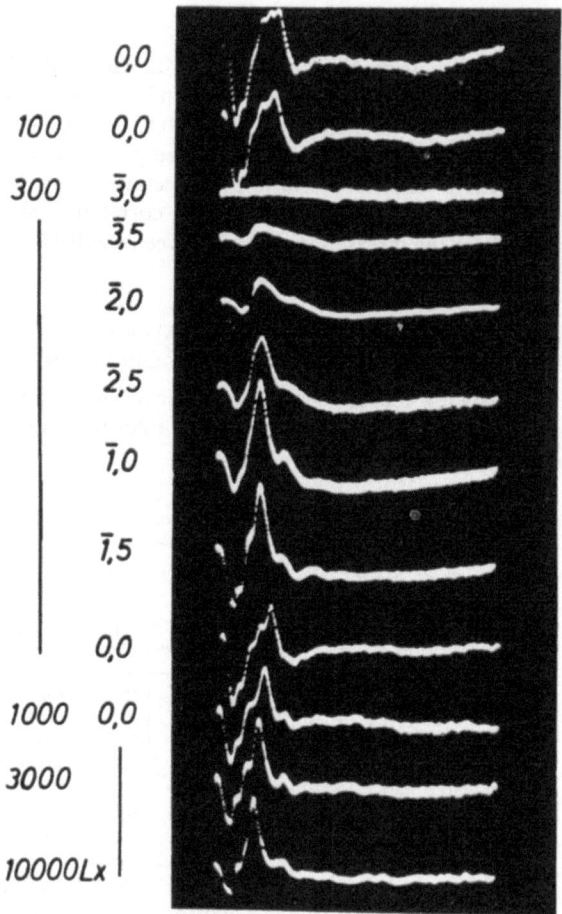

Fig. 3. Branch occlusion of the retinal vein. Case 1. Low flicker ERG (1,5 C/S).
The first column at the left indicates the background illumination. The second
column indicates the stimulus intensity. Normal recordings. The oscillatory
potentials and the late photopic potentials are present.

1. *Electroretinography* (Table III).

The ERG was normal in the recent cases (1–4), but definitely pathological in the
old cases (5–8). In all the recent cases the recordings were within normal limits
(Fig. 3). The oscillatory potentials were normally present during dark as well as
during light adaptation. In three of these cases, a very distinct c-wave was found
(Fig. 4), while in normal cases the c-wave is hardly to be seen. It was present for all
flash intensities. In one case, it lasted up to a background adaptation of 3,000
lux. In the two other cases, it persisted only till a 100 lux adaptation.

In the old cases the ERG characteristics can be summarized as follows: normal
amplitude curves of the a-wave, pathological amplitude curves of the b-wave in

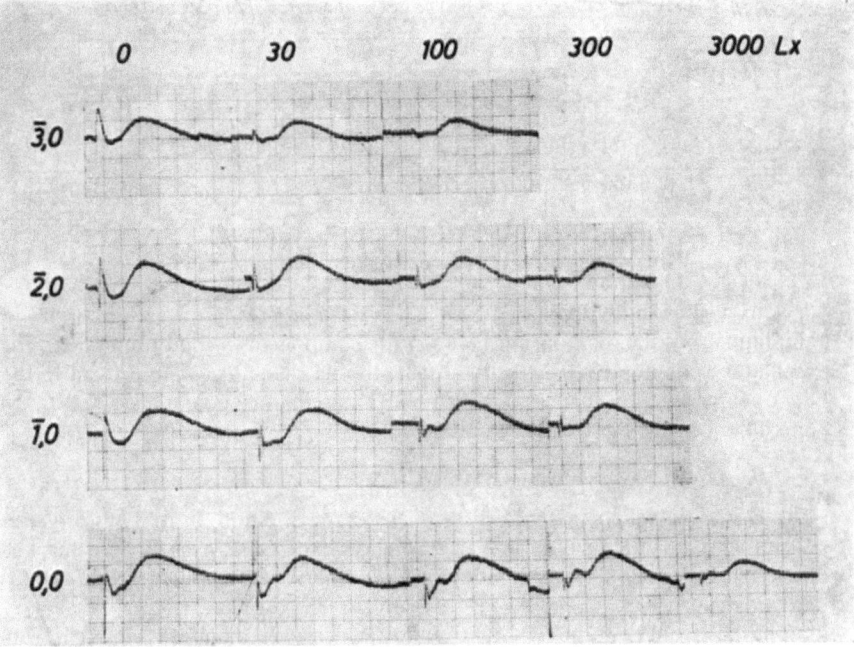

Fig. 4. Branch occlusion of the retinal vein. Case 2. Recordings of the ERG at various stimulus intensities and background adaptations. Low speed recording (2,5 mm/sec.). Large *c*-wave.

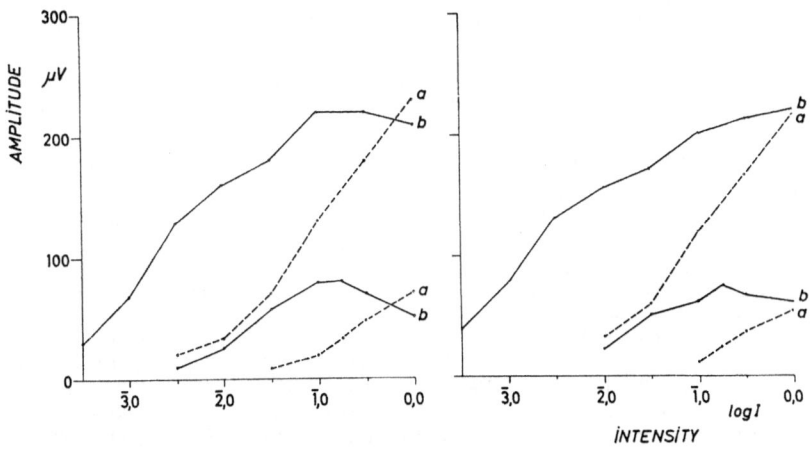

Fig. 5. Branch occlusion of the retinal vein. Case 2. Amplitude curves of *a*- and *b*-waves in dark and light adapted state, before and after argon laser photocoagulation.

Table IV. ERG and EOG in 3 recent cases of central retinal vein occlusion.

Case	EOG				ERG			EOG fellow-eye			
	M	m_2	m_3	t	$\bar{3},0$	$\bar{0},0$	phot. b-wave	M	m_2	m_3	t
9	310	500	310	165	120	360	75	360	650	340	192
10 RE	325	410	310	147	75	260	130				
11 LE	430	590	360	165	80	270	85				

dark as well as in light adapted eyes. The photopic response was subnormal in amplitude, but the relationship between the components was not modified. The oscillatory potentials were mostly absent. In one case, they were present in the dark adapted state (darkness intensity $\bar{0},0$; 4 oscillatory potentials 0, 0_2, 0_3, 0_4) and absent in the light adapted state.

2. Electro-oculography (Table III).

The EOG was subnormal in 5 cases (Cases 2, 4, 5, 6 and 7). In 2 cases (Cases 2 and 4) it was also subnormal in the fellow-eye. These eyes showed marked hypertensive and arteriosclerotic changes (narrow arteries, arterio-venous crossing sign).

The mean values of the EOG of the affected eye were manifestly different from these of the fellow-eye not only concerning the dark–light ratio, but also concerning the absolute amplitudes.

Two patients with a retinal venous branch occlusion were treated by argon laser photocoagulation.

Case 1. A 44 years old patient was seen for the first time one week after the occlusion of a macular vein, branch of the supero-temporal vein. The vision was 0,3. The visual field showed a fascicular defect in the infero-nasal quadrant. The ERG was completely normal. All the components were present with normal

Table V. EOG and ERG in central retinal vein occlusion with severe visual impairment.

Case	EOG				ERG			EOG fellow-eye			
	M	m_2	m_3	t	$\bar{3},0$	$\bar{0},0$	phot. b-wave	M	m_2	m_3	t
12	660	820	590	140	70	260	90	660	990	470	210
13	375	375	370	102	30	200	110	445	490	305	165
14	180	175	175	100	10	220	100	450	925	416	220
15	445	640	330	148	20	150	45	980	1000	615	170
16	530	530	435	122	10	115	55	930	960	630	157
17	300	410	280	144	25	200	80				
18	280	325	205	107	30	280	150				
19	540	540	375	140	5	100	20	430	590	365	163
m	414	477	361	129	25	190	79	649	804	466	180

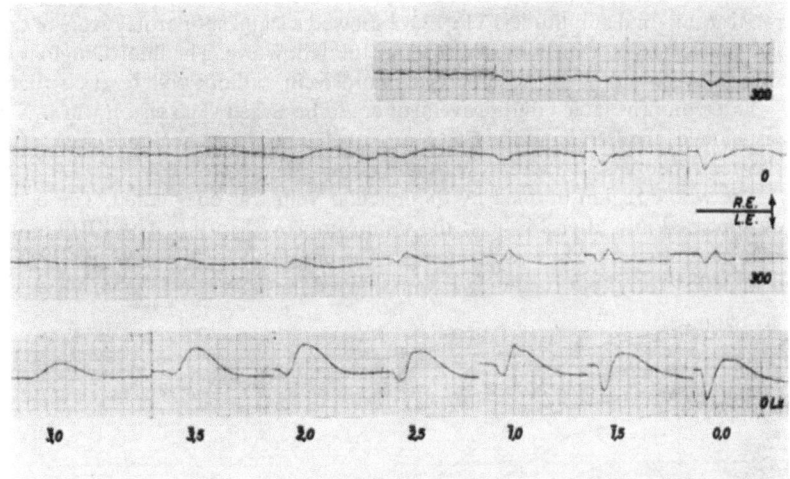

Fig. 6. Thrombosis of the central retinal vein (R.E.). Case 19. This is the only case with a reduction of both *a*- and *b*-waves. L.E. (fellow-eye): normal records but no oscillatory potentials.

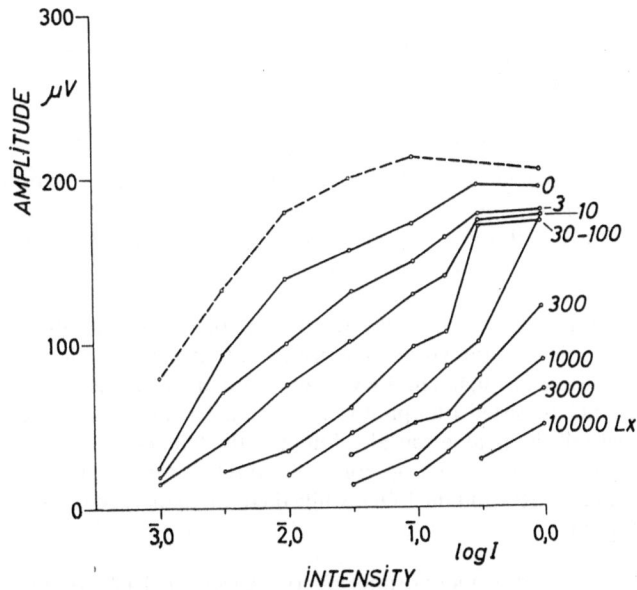

Fig. 7. Thrombosis of the central retinal vein. Case 13. Amplitude curves of the *b*-wave at increasing background adaptations. The maximal amplitude remains nearly unchanged for intensity $\overline{0},0$ till about 100 lux background illumination. Dotted line: amplitude curve of the *b*-wave of the dark-adapted fellow-eye.

relationship and amplitudes. The EOG showed a slight subnormal value of dark–light ratio (160), which was normal in the fellow-eye. The fluoro-angiography showed a slow flow in the supero-temporal vein without collateral circulation.

Three months later no improvement could be stated. The vision was 0,2. The visual field, the EOG and the ERG were unchanged, but the fluoro-angiography showed a neo-vascularization with late fluorescence.

The whole region drained by the macular vein was coagulated. The oedema disappeared and after 14 days, the vision improved to 0,6. The ERG and the EOG examinations showed no change. The amplitude of the scotopic ERG had dropped slightly, but remained within normal limits.

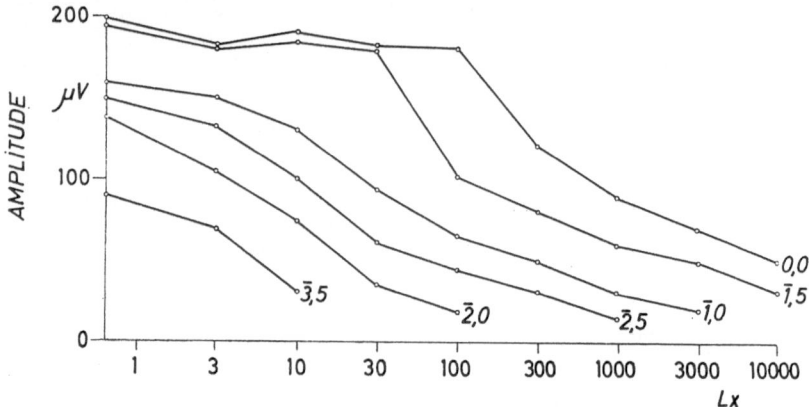

Fig. 8. Thrombosis of the central retinal vein. Case 13. Amplitude of the b-wave in relation to the background adaptations.

Case 2. This patient showed an occlusion of the supero-temporal vein. The vision was 1/100. One week after the onset the ERG amplitude was within normal limits. All the components were present, including the oscillatory potentials. The EOG was subnormal in both eyes: the dark–light ratio was 127 in the affected eye, 155 in the fellow-eye.

Two months later, the macular oedema and the haemorrhages persisted without improvement of the vision. We performed laser coagulations. Three weeks later, the vision was 0,4. The ERG showed no change. There was a very large c-wave, which persisted after photocoagulation. The EOG improved slightly, but the increase of the t value was also found in the fellow-eye.

In conclusion, although large zones of the retina were coagulated, no change was seen in the ERG and the EOG, while there was a marked subjective improvement (Fig. 5).

B. Total Occlusions of the Central Retinal Vein

Two patients, one with a bilateral vein occlusion, were examined in the first week after the onset (Cases 9, 10 and 11). The visual functions were rather well preserved. The visual field showed only an enlargement of the blind spot. The visual acuity remained between 0,8 and 1,0. The ERG was normal. In one case,

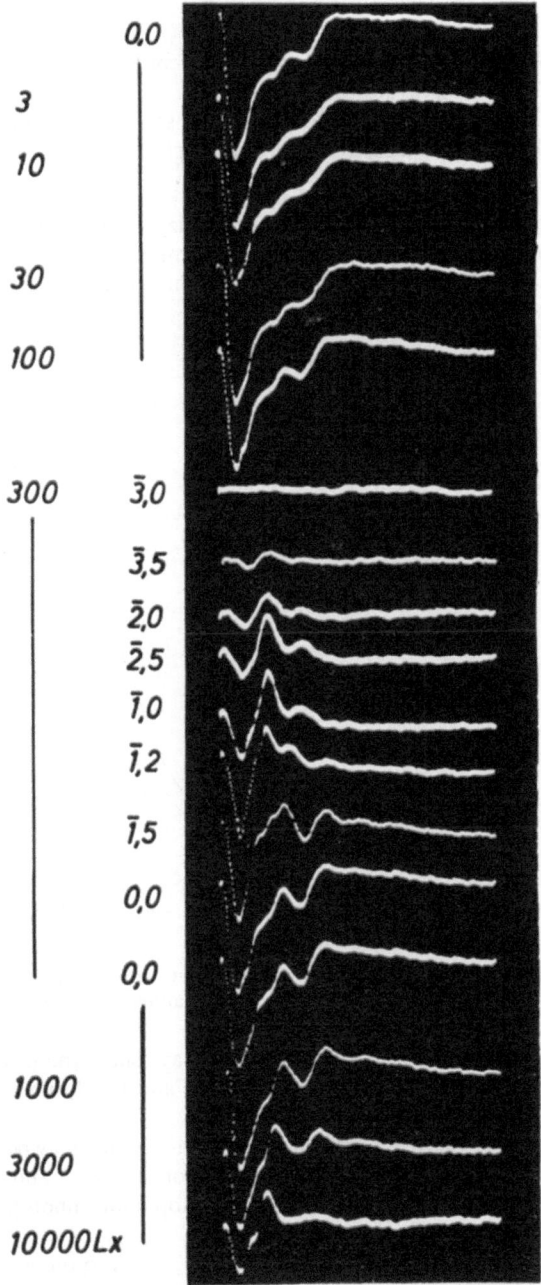

Fig. 9. Thrombosis of the central retinal vein. Case 13. First column at the left background illuminations. Second column stimulus intensities. Single flash ERG. Predominance of the photopic components (photopic *b*-wave and late photopic waves). The EOG was severely disturbed.

however, no oscillatory potentials could be recorded. The EOG was slightly subnormal (Table IV).

Seven patients, on the contrary, had a very severe visual impairment. In all these cases, both EOG and ERG were pathologic.

1. *Electroretinography.*

The characteristics of the ERG can be summarized as follows:

1. The amplitude of the *a*-wave is always normal. Its maximal amplitude was sometimes higher than in the fellow-eye. In one case only a reduced *a*-wave amplitude was observed (Fig. 6).

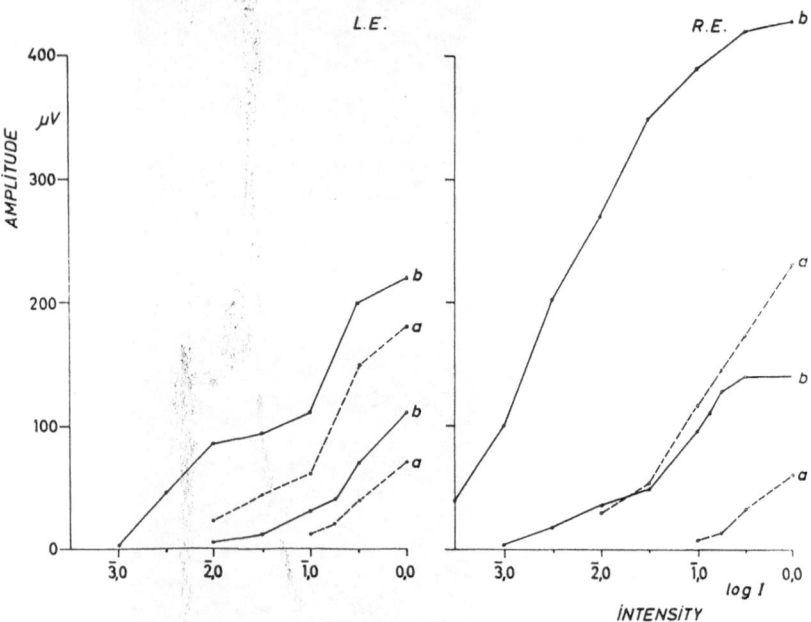

Fig. 10. Thrombosis of the central retinal vein. Case 14. Amplitude curves of the *a*- and *b*-waves in dark adapted and light adapted state. L.E.: affected eye. R.E.: fellow-eye.

2. The amplitude curve of the *b*-wave is always subnormal. Sometimes, the curve is much reduced at low intensity flashes and nearly normal at high intensity flashes (Fig. 7).

3. The amplitude curve of the photopic *b*-wave (300 lux) may be within normal limits, even when the scotopic *b*-curve is pathologic (Figs. 7 and 10).

4. The peak-times of the *b*-waves, both scotopic and photopic, are mostly longer than in normal eyes.

5. With increasing background illumination, the responses show marked differences at high intensity flashes, when they are compared with normal responses. The decrease in amplitude is delayed (Fig. 8).

6. The response in dark adapted state to high intensity flashes is mostly dominated by photopic components, namely the late photopic oscillations with

54

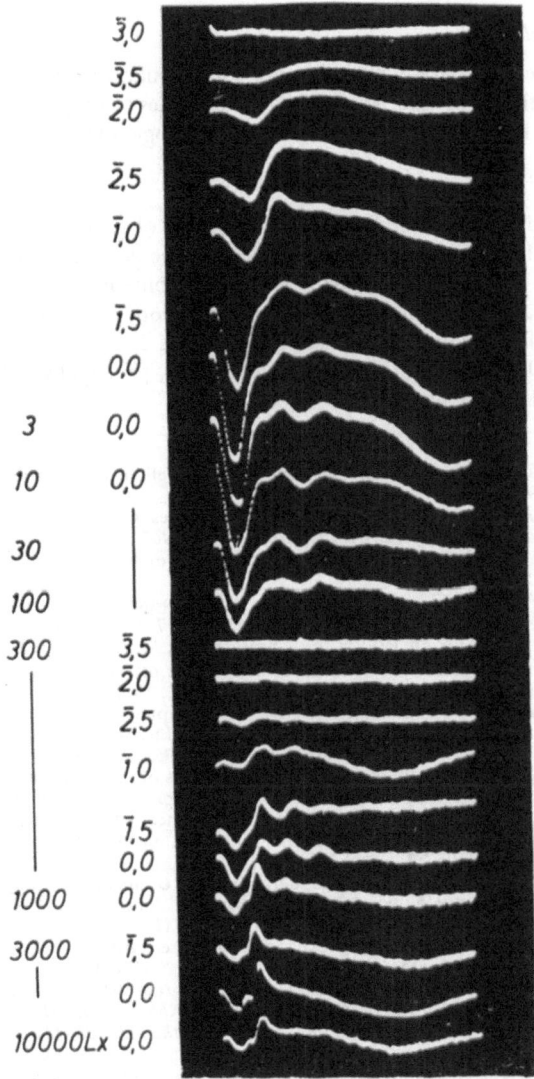

Fig. 11. Thrombosis of the central retinal vein. Case 14. First column at the left: background illuminations. Second column stimulus intensities. ERG: late photopic potentials. Analyzer time: 250 msec.

a peak-time of 60 and 90 msec., which in normal eyes are only visible in the light adapted ERG (Fig. 9 and 11).

With increasing background adaptation, the ERG response is not much modified, neither in amplitude nor in morphology. The late photopic oscillation remains the dominant component of the response at low illumination levels (from darkness to 100 lux) or even up to adaptations of 3,000 lux (Fig. 9 and 11).

55

2. Electro-oculography.

In all the cases the dark–light ratio was sub-normal (maximal value: 148) and lower than in the fellow-eye. The absolute amplitudes of M and m_2 were generally lower than in the fellow-eye and definitely pathologic (Table V).

SUMMARY

The ERG and the EOG were studied in 19 cases of retinal vein occlusions. In branch occlusion, abnormalities may sometimes be detected in only one examination, either EOG or ERG (usually EOG), but sometimes also, both EOG and ERG are impaired. In central retinal vein occlusion, both ERG and EOG are pathologic. The impairment is more pronounced in long standing cases. The morphological alteration of the ERG is discussed, principally with reference to the photopic late potentials.

REFERENCES

ALGVERE, P. Studies on the oscillatory potentials of the clinical electro-retinogram. Thesis, Stockholm (1968).

ARDEN, G. B., BARRADA, A. & KELSEY, J. H. New clinical test of retinal functions based on the standing potential of the eye. Brit. J. Ophthal. 46:449–467 (1962).

CARR, R. E. & SIEGEL, I. M. Electrophysiological aspects of several retinal diseases. Amer. J. Ophthal. 58:95–107 (1964).

FRANÇOIS, J., VERRIEST, G. & DE ROUCK, A. L'électro-oculographie en tant qu'examen fonctionnel de la rétine. Adv. Ophthal., Karger, Basel, 7:1–67 (1957).

FRANÇOIS, J., VERRIEST, G., DE ROUCK, A. & SZMIGIELSKI, M. An extended clinical test of the ocular standing potential and its results in some cases of retinal degeneration. Proc. IV. ISCERG Symp. Hakone, 1965, Jap. J. Ophthal., suppl., 10:257–268 (1966).

GLIEM, H. Das Elektro-okulogramm. Ed. G. Thieme, Leipzig (1971).

GLIEM, H., MOLLER, D. E. & KIETZMANN, G. Die bioelektrische Aktivität der Netzhaut bei der diabetischen Retinopathie. Acta Ophthal. Kbh. 49:353–363 (1971).

HEILEMANN, I. & BASTIAN, A. EOG in cases of thrombosis of the vena centralis retinae. Proc. VI. ISCERG Symp., Erfurt, 1967, Ed. G. Thieme, Leipzig, 83–87 (1968).

HENKES, H. Electroretinography in circulatory disturbances of the retina. I. Electroretinography in cases of occlusion of central retinal veins or of one of its branches. Arch. Ophthal., Chicago 49:190–201 (1953).

KARPE, G. The basis of clinical electroretinography. Acta Ophthal. Kbh. suppl. 24 (1945).

KARPE, G. Indications for clinical electroretinography. Amer. med. Ass., San Francisco, June 24, 1958, in Arch. Ophthal., Chicago, 60:889–896 (1958).

KARPE, G. & GERMANIS, M. The prognostic value of the electroretinogram in thrombosis of the retinal veins. Acta Ophthal., Kbh., suppl. 70:202–229 (1962).

KARPE, G. & UCHERMANN, A. The clinical electroretinogram. VII. The electroretinogram in circulatory disturbances of the retina. Acta Ophthal., Kbh., 33:493–516 (1955).

KELSEY, J. H. Clinical Electro-oculography. Brit. J. Ophthal. 50:438–439 (1966).

KUBOTA, Y. The peak latency time of the a-wave, the b-wave and the oscillatory potentials of the ERG in various retinal diseases. Proc. XXI Conc. Ophthal. Mexico (1970), II, 1767–1771 (1971).

MÜLLER, W. & HAASE, E. Measuring of peak times in patients with thrombosis of vena centralis retina. Proc. VI. ISCERG Symp. Erfurt, 1967, Ed. G. Thieme, Leipzig, 351–354 (1968).

PONTE, F. ERG and vascular disturbances. The clinical value of electroretinography. Proc. V. ISCERG Symp. Ghent, 1966, Ed. Karger, Basel, 300–311, (1968).

STRAUB, W. Das Elektroretinogramm. Experimentelle und klinische Beobachtungen. Ed. F. Henke, Stuttgart (1961).

USAMI, E. Studies on oscillatory potentials in the cases of occlusion of the retinal artery and thrombosis of the retinal veins. Proc. IV. ISCERG Symp., Hakone, 1965, Jap. J. Ophthal., suppl., 10:110–119 (1966).

YONEMURA, D., TSUZUKI, K. & AOKI T. Clinical importance of the oscillatory potentials in the human ERG. Proc. I. ISCERG Symp., Acta Ophthal., Kbh., Suppl., 70:115–120 (1962).

TOLERANCE OF MAMMALIAN RETINA TO CIRCULATORY ARREST

MARY HOFF, M.S. & PETER GOURAS,* M.D.

(*Bethesda, Maryland*)

INTRODUCTION

How long the mammalian retina tolerates total stoppage of its circulation is not completely clear. In the rat SMITH & BAIRD (1953) found that ischemic periods of longer than 15 minutes produced irreversible histological damage to the retina. In the rabbit both BORNSCHEIN & ZWIAUER (1952) and POPP (1955) found that the electroretinogram (ERG) recovered completely after 15 minutes of total ischemia but only incompletely after longer periods. Similar periods of tolerance were also observed in the superfused rabbit retina by AMES & GURIAN (1963) and WEBSTER & AMES (1965). In man WEGNER (1928) reported that normal visual function could recover after 22 minutes of total circulatory arrest, and BOCK, BORNSCHEIN & HOMMER (1963) observed complete recovery of the ERG and visual function after 60 minutes of such ischemia. In the cat REINECKE, KUWABARA, COGAN & WEIS (1962) found complete histological recovery up to 90 minutes of total ischemia.

These results in man and cat seem much longer than one might expect for such an actively metabolizing tissue as the retina. In these studies circulatory arrest was achieved almost entirely by raising the intraocular pressure above systemic blood pressure and there is a possibility that this technique does not always produce complete retinal ischemia. We have attempted to examine this problem in the isolated perfused cat eye where the circulation to the entire eye can be unquestionably interrupted and where function can be continuously monitored at both the input (receptors) and the output (optic nerve) of the retina.

METHODS

A more complete account of the methods used in the isolated, perfused cat eye preparation have appeared (GOURAS & HOFF, 1970; NIEMEYER, 1973; NIEMEYER & GOURAS, 1973). The perfusate in these experiments was tissue culture media 199 with 40% calf serum. This solution was saturated with 95% O_2 and 5% CO_2 and driven into the ophthalmociliary artery under a hydrostatic pressure of 160 mm of mercury. The perfusion could be started or stopped by a valve located proximal to a drop flow meter. The eye was maintained in the range of 35–37°C at all times. The ERG and optic nerve response to light stimulation was continuously monitored. Fig. 1 shows schematically the entire system.

* From the Section of Neurophysiology, Laboratory of Vision Research, National Eye Institute, National Institutes of Health, U.S. Department of Health, Education, and Welfare, Bethesda, Maryland 20014.

57

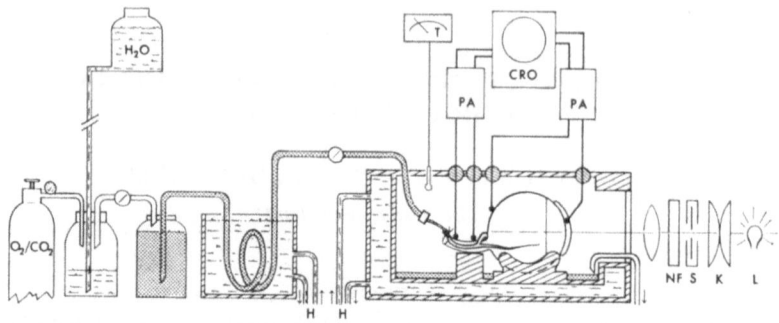

Fig. 1. Schematic diagram of the perfusion, testing and recording system for studying the isolated cat eye. CRO, cathode ray oscilloscope; H, heating device; K, condenser; L ribbon filament light source; NF, neutral density filters; PA, preamplifier; S, shutter; T, thermometer; H_2O, water solution with a pressure head of 160 mm Hg.

RESULTS

Fig. 2, 3 and 4 show the changes with time of the retinal responses of perfused eyes subjected to different periods of total circulatory arrest: 5 min. (Fig. 2); 1 hour (Fig. 3) and 2 hours (Fig. 4). When the eye is deprived of perfusate electrical responses to light disappear rapidly. The b-wave of the ERG and the optic nerve response disappear within seconds followed by the a-wave which lingers for several minutes (GOURAS & HOFF, 1970). When the perfusion is restarted responses reappear gradually, reaching their maximum amplitude more slowly when the period of circulatory arrest is relatively long (Fig. 3 and 4). The a-wave recovers first, indicating by its presence the return of photoreceptor activity. Shortly afterwards the b-wave appears suggesting that synaptic transmission is beginning in the external plexiform layer. Optic nerve activity usually appears later indicating that not only are impulses propagating along the axons of ganglion cells, but synaptic transmission from the receptor cells through the bipolars to the retinal ganglion cells must be occurring. This entire chain of events can recover even after the circulation to the eye has been completely stopped for 2 hours. What is remarkable is that the recovery from such an insult can take as long as 6 to 8 hours. We should add here that the perfused eye preparation usually begins to deteriorate slowly after 8 to 10 hours and sometimes earlier under current conditions, so that it is still unclear whether some retinas might require even longer periods before maximal recovery is attained.

Fig. 5 shows actual ERG and optic nerve responses recorded from perfused cat eyes. The responses on the left are from an eye which was perfused 5 minutes after enucleation; those on the right are from an eye which was first perfused 2 hours after enucleation. These responses are comparable with one another and the ERG's are within the range of those recorded from the intact cat (GOURAS & HOFF, 1970).

Fig. 6 shows the distribution of maximum response amplitudes obtained from eyes subjected to 5 minutes, 1 hour or 2 hours of circulatory arrest. Responses

58

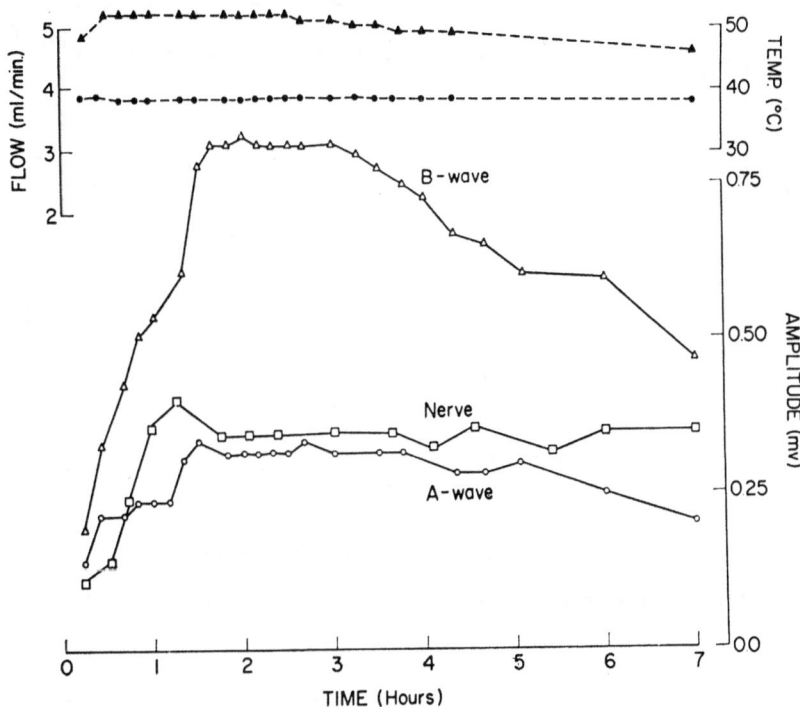

Fig. 2. Time course of the changes in maximum amplitude for the a-wave (○) and b-wave (△) of the ERG and the optic nerve potential (□) during a control perfusion. Temperature (●) and flow rate (▲) are indicated above.

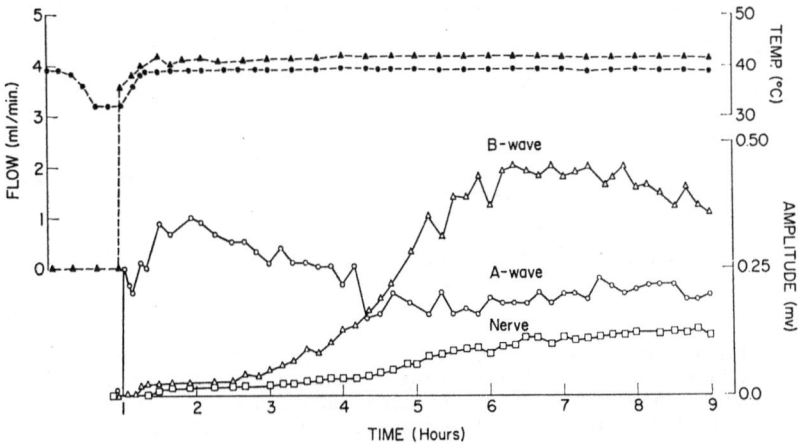

Fig. 3. Time course of the changes in maximum amplitude for the ERG a-wave and b-wave and the optic nerve response during the following one hour of circulatory arrest. Temperature and flow rate are indicated above.

59

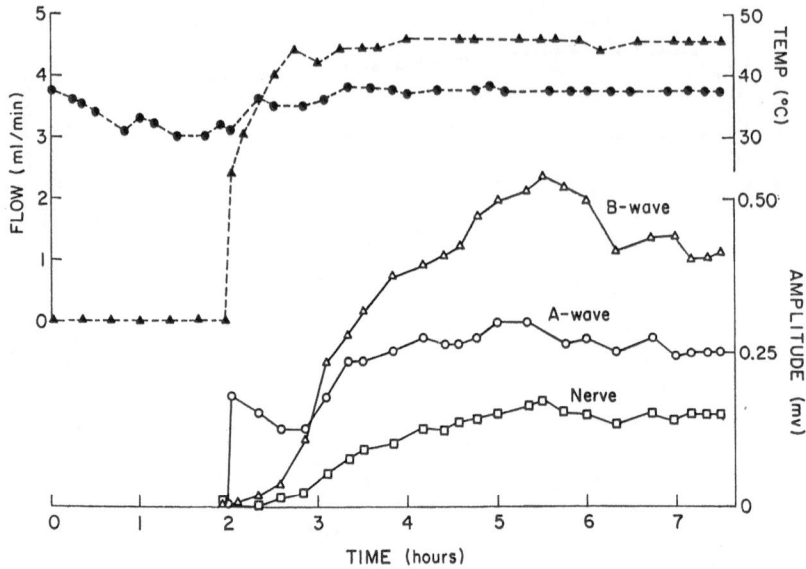

Fig. 4. Time course of the changes in maximum amplitude for the ERG a-wave and b-wave and the optic nerve response during and following two hours of circulatory arrest. Temperature and flow rate are indicated above.

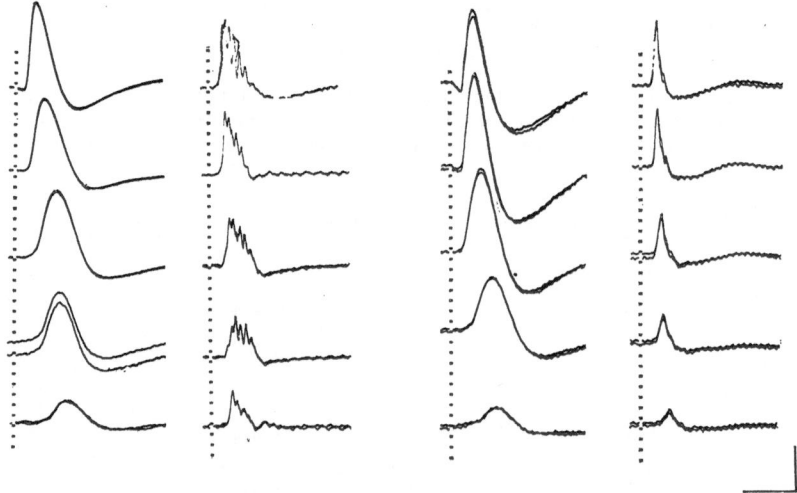

Fig. 5. Pairs of ERG's and optic nerve responses recorded from the perfused cat eye. The responses in the left two columns were recorded after 5 minutes anoxia; those in the right columns were recorded following a two hour period of total circulatory arrest. Two responses to the same stimulus are superimposed in each trace. The energy of the stimuli is the same for each horizontal row of responses and is decreased from above downwards. The calibration signifies 150 msec horizontally and, vertically, 200 μv for the traces of columns 1 and 3 and 100 μv for those of columns 2 and 4.

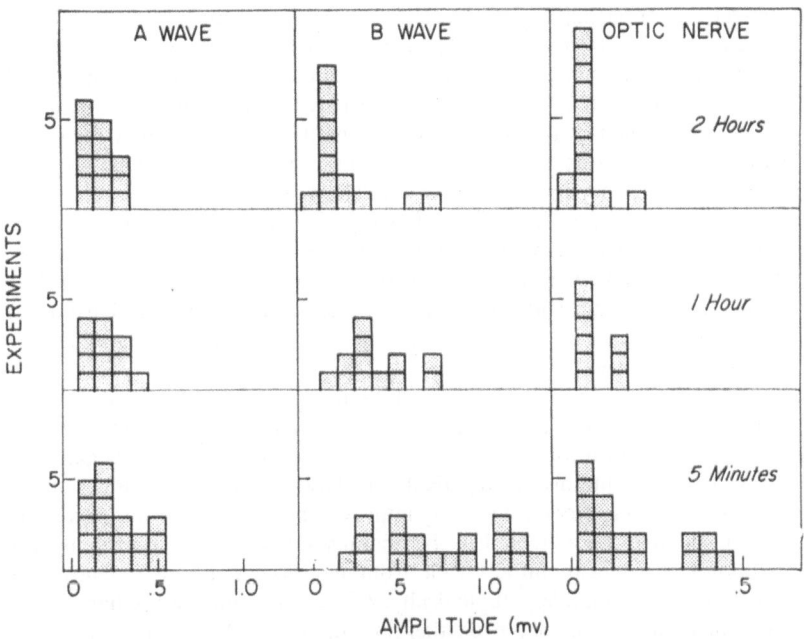

Fig. 6. A comparison of the amplitudes of the a- and b-waves of the ERG and the optic nerve potential following 5 minutes (below), 1 hour (middle), and 2 hours (above) of circulatory arrest.

tend to be smaller when the period of arrest is long but in all cases some recovery is apparent. Even after two hours ischemia some retinas manage to generate responses within or close to the normal range. The optic nerve response is the most and the a-wave the least vulnerable to this insult.

DISCUSSION

The results tend to agree with those of REINECKE et al. (1962) who used elevated intraocular pressure to occlude the circulation in the intact cat eye and studied recovery in an entirely different way, i.e. histologically. The cat retina appears capable of recovering considerably after 1 or 2 hours of complete circulatory stoppage, sometimes even reaching the range of normal function. These results also support the observations of BOCK et al. (1963) that retinal function in man can recover fully after complete ischemia of 1 hour in duration. The results differ somewhat from those in the rabbit where complete recovery has never been seen after ischemic periods longer than 15 minutes, although both POPP (1955) and AMES & GURIAN (1963) did detect considerable recovery after longer periods of ischemia. What seems to be important here is that the retina, a very

61

actively metabolizing part of the central nervous system, can undergo considerable recovery following relatively long periods of circulatory arrest. This contrasts with the brain which becomes irreversibly damaged by ischemic periods of 8 to 10 minutes at 37°C. This difference between retina and brain seems most likely due to the fact that the brain contains the control circuitry for the entire circulation while the retina does not. The brain itself might be much more tolerant of ischemia if its circulation could be maintained long enough during the post-ischemic period for these relatively slow recovery processes to occur. Recent experiments along these lines (HOSSMANN & SATO, 1970) suggest that this hypothesis may be correct. It would seem more reasonable to expect that the retina and the brain show a similar tolerance to ischemia and that both these tissues despite their high metabolic rate are much more tolerant to ischemia than is generally believed.

We believe our results are important in another respect. They show that artificial perfusion can allow the retina to recover considerably after it has been without circulation for as long as 2 hours. They imply that the quality of the retina in an eye obtained from patients who have been dead for this period of time and possibly longer could be vastly improved by perfusing them for a sufficient period of time. Eyes treated in this manner may be much more suited for the fixation techniques required for electronmicroscopy and consequently may be much more informative pathologically. At the same time an eye handled in this way might also be amenable to either physiological or biochemical studies which would be impossible to do with the eye in situ. For certain unique retinal or possibly choroidal diseases this approach might prove useful.

Several papers dealing with the tolerance of the mammalian retina to ischemia have come to our attention since this symposium. In the rat SCHMIDT shows complete recovery after 35 minutes of ischemia at 35°C, while longer periods of ischemia at this temperature result in incomplete recovery. This sensitivity of the retina to ischemia is temperature dependent so that recovery is complete after 60 minutes of ischemia at 27°C and 13 minutes at 40°C. (SCHMIDT J. G. H. Revival time of the b-wave of the electroretinogram following retinal and choroidal ischemia as related to various body and eye temperatures. Seventh ISCERG Symposium, Istanbul, 1969).

In support of the findings of BOCK et al., FUJINO & HAMASAKI report complete recovery of squirrel and owl monkey retina after one hour periods of ischemia produced by raising the intraocular pressure. Longer periods result in permanent ERG and histological changes. (FUJINO, T. & HAMASAKI, D. I.: Effect of intraocular pressure on the electroretinogram. *Arch. Ophthal.* 78:*757–765*, 1967).

HAMASAKI & KROLL report even greater tolerance of the squirrel monkey retina to ischemia after occlusion of the central retinal artery. They show that from 2 to 3.5 hours of ischemia are required to produce irreversible changes in the electrical activity of the retina and optic tract. (HAMASAKI, D.I. & KROLL, J.: Experimental central retinal artery occlusion. *Arch. Ophthal.* 80:*243–248*, 1968).

We feel that all of these data support the conclusion that the central nervous system is more tolerant to ischemia than has been previously assumed.

62

J. G. H. Schmidt (*Cologne*)

In earlier experiments (J. G. H. Schmidt, VIIth ISCERG-Symposium, Istanbul 1969) I measured the revival time of the b-wave of the electroretinogram (Wistar rats) following retinal and choroidal ischemia as related to various body and eye temperatures. Under urethane anesthesia (1 g/kg body weight) the permissible occlusion time ran up to 35 minutes at 35°C body temperature, whereas under halothan anesthesia at the same temperature a complete recovery could not be obtained after a duration of ischemia longer than 25 minutes.

ACKNOWLEDGEMENTS

We would like to express our thanks to Drs. Ralph Gunkel, Gunter Niemeyer, Astrid von Lützow-Kafka, Dan Finkelstein for the assistance and suggestions they have given us during the course of these studies.

REFERENCES

Ames, A. III & Gurian, G. S. Effects of glucose and oxygen deprivation on function of isolated mammalian retina. *J. Neurophysiol.* 26:*617–634* (1963).

Bock, J., Bornschein, H. & Hommer, K. Die Wiederbelebungszeit der menschlichen Netzhaut. *Graefes Archiv f. Ophthal.* 165:*437–451* (1963).

Bornschein, H. & Zwiauer, A. Das Elektroretinogramm des Kaninchens bei experimenteller Erhohung des intraocularen Druckes. *Graefes Archiv f. Ophthal.* 152:*527–531* (1952).

Gouras, P. & Hoff, M. Retinal function in an isolated perfused mammalian eye. *Invest. Ophthal.* 9:*388–399* (1970).

Hossmann, K. A. & Sato, K. Recovery of nueronal function after prolonged cerebral ischemia. *Science* 168:*375–376* (1970).

Niemeyer, G. Intraretinal ERG and single cell responses from an isolated perfused mammalian eye. *Vis. Res.* (in press).

Niemeyer, G. & Gouras, P. Rod and cone signals in S-potentials of the isolated perfused cat eye. *Vis. Res.* (in press).

Popp, C. Die retinafunktion nach intraocular Ischamie. *Graefes Archiv f. Ophthal.* 156:*395–403* (1955).

Reinecke, R. D., Kuwabara, T., Cogan, D. G. & Weis, D. R. Retinal vascular patterns. Part V: Experimental ischemia of the cat eye. *Arch. Ophthal.* 67:*470–475* (1962).

Smith, G. C. & Baird, C. D. Survival time of retinal cells when deprived of their blood supply by increased intraocular pressure. *Am. J. Ophthal.* 35:*133–135* (1952).

Webster, H. DeF. & Ames, A. III. Reversible and irreversible changes in the fine structure of nervous tissue during oxygen and glucose deprivation. *J. Cell Biol.* 26:*885*–909 (1965).

Wegner, W. Die Funktion der menschlichen Netzhaut bei experimenteller Ischaemia retinae. *Archiv f. Augenheilk.* 98:*514–564* (1928).

THE ERG AND ITS CORRELATION WITH DAMAGE CAUSED BY CHRONIC EXPOSURE TO LIGHT

THEODORE LAWWILL,* M.D.

(*Louisville*)

Light damage to the retina can occur under at least two conditions. The first, and possibly better known to the clinical ophthalmologist might be called short pulse small spot damage. This type is produced in photocoagulation. It is also the type caused by Q-switched lasers, and in most cases of solar burns. The second type of damage is that caused by long term (hours or days) exposure to moderate or high illumination over a wide field. Interest in the mechanisms and parameters of this second type was initiated by NOELL's discovery in the rat (NOELL et al., 1966). It is becoming apparent that the mechanism of damage under these two conditions is totally different and that the response in the second type is in some manner different in animals which are not nocturnal.

The author has in the past established the threshold for detectable damage for four hour exposure for white light and argon laser light in the rabbit eye (LAWWILL, 1971). He uses as criteria for damage ERG amplitude reduction, ophthalmoscopic findings, and histopathology. In the rabbit, the ratio of damage thresholds between broadband white light and single line laser light was equal to the ratio in sensitivity of the ERG response to the two sources.

In this paper I shall show some of the effects of superthreshold four hour exposures in rhesus monkeys on ERG, fundus appearance and histopathology, and present early threshold data for broad spectrum white and argon laser light in the rhesus monkey.

Before and after exposure, data were collected including repeated ERG's, fundus photographs and opthalmoscopic examinations. One to three months after the eye was exposed, the animal was killed and light and electron microscopic examinations performed on the retina.

PROCEDURE

In our exposure system, the monkey is placed in a primate chair and given intravenous barbiturate anesthesia. The eye is held in place by temporary sutures. The white light is presented by the optical system shown in Fig. 1. The laser uses the same system without the filters. The laser beam is diverged and collimated and passed through the same final lens. The final lens is very close to the eye and allows a field of exposure of more than 180 degrees. The position of

* From the Department of Ophthalmology, The University of Louisville, School of Medicine, Louisville, Kentucky 40202. This work was supported in part by Army Contract #DADA17-68-C-8105 and US PHS Grant #EY00412. Reprint requests to THEODORE LAWWILL, M.D., 301 E. Walnut Street, Louisville, Kentucky 40202.

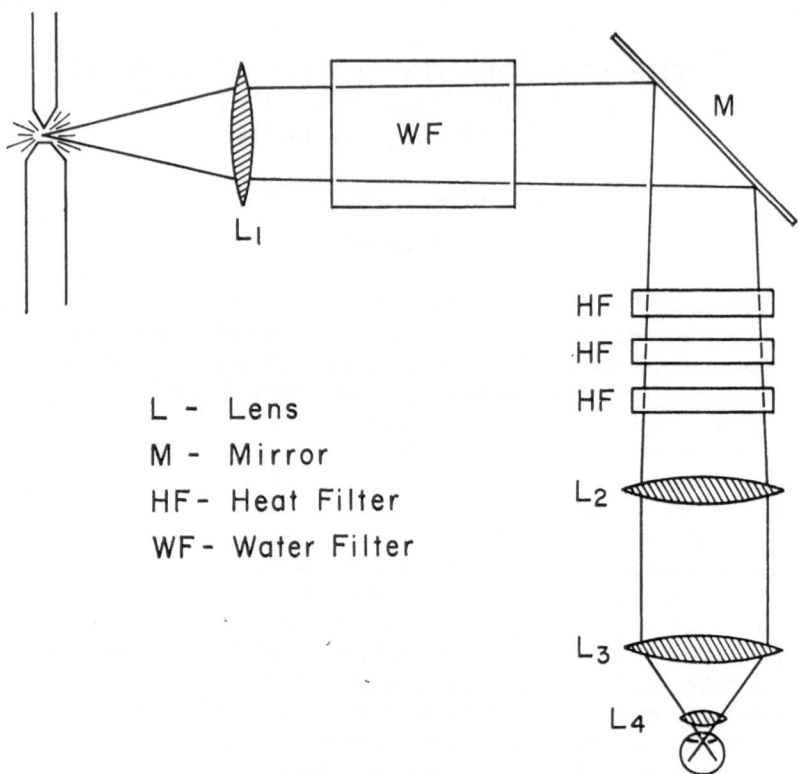

L - Lens
M - Mirror
HF- Heat Filter
WF- Water Filter

Fig. 1. Schematic representation of the light system by which the eyes are exposed to wide field illumination.

the entering beam in the pupil is monitored on closed-circuit TV to avoid exposure of the technician and to allow her to monitor respiration simultaneously.

Power measurements are made with a spectroradiometer. The reported values are taken as the total power entering the cornea divided by the total area of retina exposed. The white light source is fairly flat in the visible spectrum, but has a small peak in the far red (Fig. 2). The laser source provides a very narrow chromatic line at 514.5 nanometers, using a Littrow prism for line separation.

The monkey ERG procedure employs bipolar contact lens electrodes. The signals are amplified and displayed on a storage oscilloscope from which they are measured and the amplitudes are recorded.

Preadaptation of 400 ft-L is supplied by an indirectly lighted hemisphere painted flat white on the inside. The stimulus is supplied by a xenon flash tube which indirectly lights the same hemisphere.

Preadaptation is carried out for 2 minutes and ERG's are recorded every three minutes thereafter for 30 minutes. The a- and b-wave amplitudes are then graphed. Figures 3 and 4 show the mean and standard deviation of the a- and b-wave amplitudes for 11 examinations over a 55 day period in a normal eye.

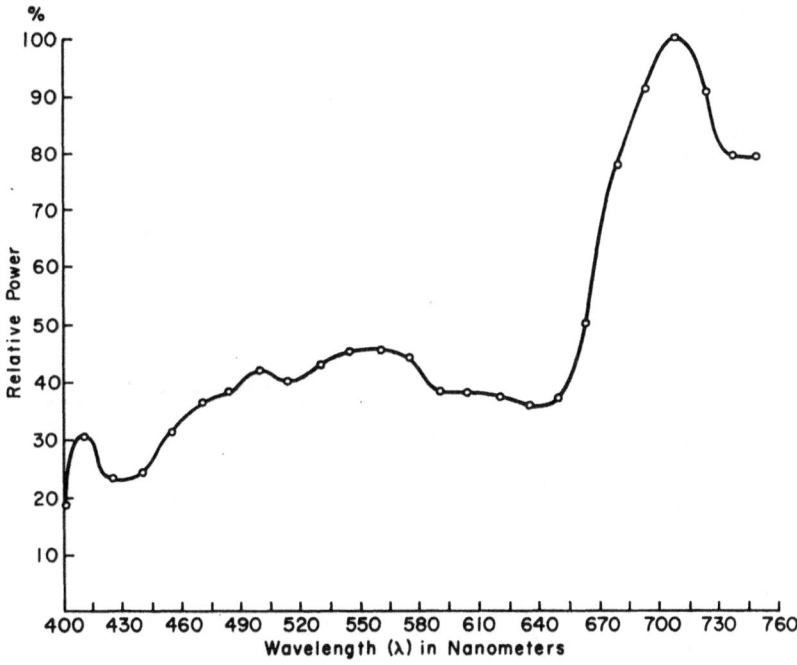

Fig. 2. Power spectrum curve for the white light source. Measurements of power excluded any energy outside of the bounds of this curve. Therefore, there was some infrared energy which was not included in the measurement.

RESULTS

Damage was graded on a ∅ to 4 + scale for ERG, ophthalmoscopy and histopathology, and the three were combined to give an overall grading for each of the eyes exposed. The appearance of one eye which was graded 3 + fundus, 3 + histology, and 4 + ERG is shown. The macular pigment was disturbed and previous photographs had shown some retinal edema. (Fig. 5.) The histopathology of this eye showed a loss of pigment in the pigment epithelium with preservation of the pigment epithelium cells, and loss of a large portion of the outer segments with phagocytosis of the outer segments and of the pigment which was formerly in the pigment epithelium. Vacuolization was prominent in the areas of destruction. Figure 6 shows 3 + histological damage and Fig. 7 shows an area of less damage. Figures 8a, b, c, and d show the a- and b-wave amplitudes before and after exposure resulting in 4 + ERG changes.

Our initial data showed a four hour threshold very close to that in the rabbit eye for white light. Indications also are that the laser threshold will be slightly less than the white light threshold. Figure 9 shows the combined effect on the ∅–4 grading scale for each eye at the level of retinal exposure in milliwatts/cm^2.

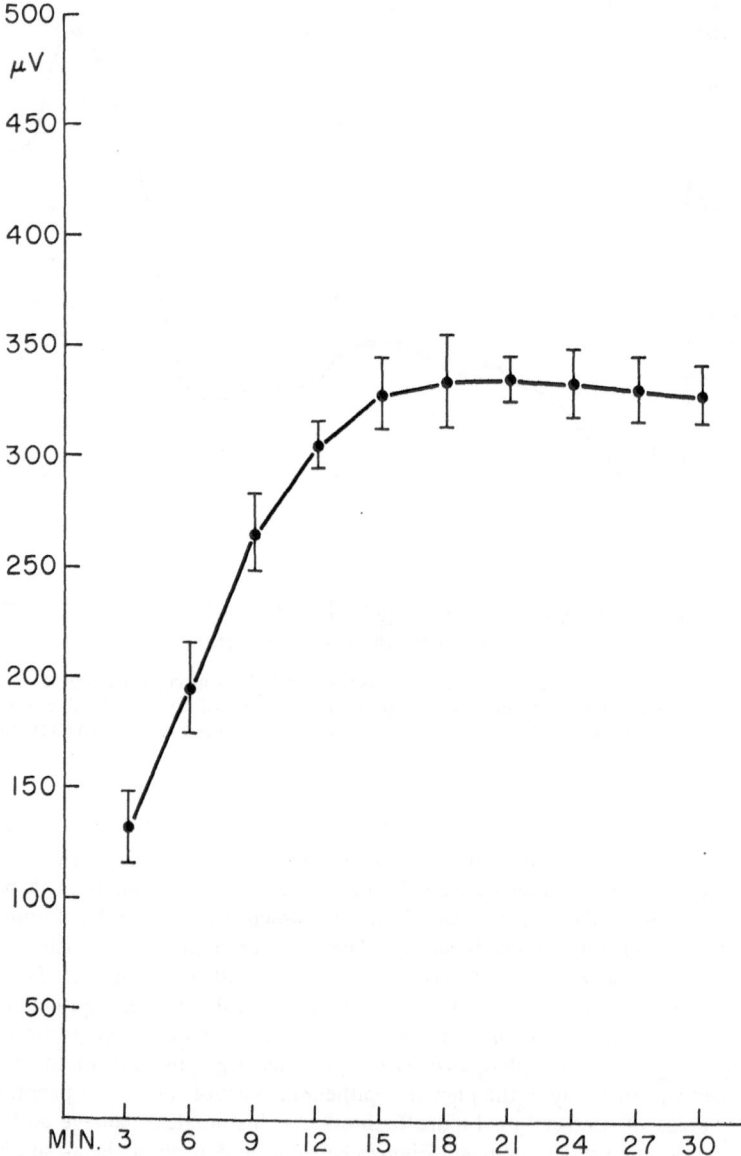

Figs. 3 and 4. The a- and b-wave amplitudes taken every three minutes for 30 minutes during dark adaptation after 2 minutes preadaptation. These results show the mean and standard deviation for 11 examinations in a normal animal over 55 days.

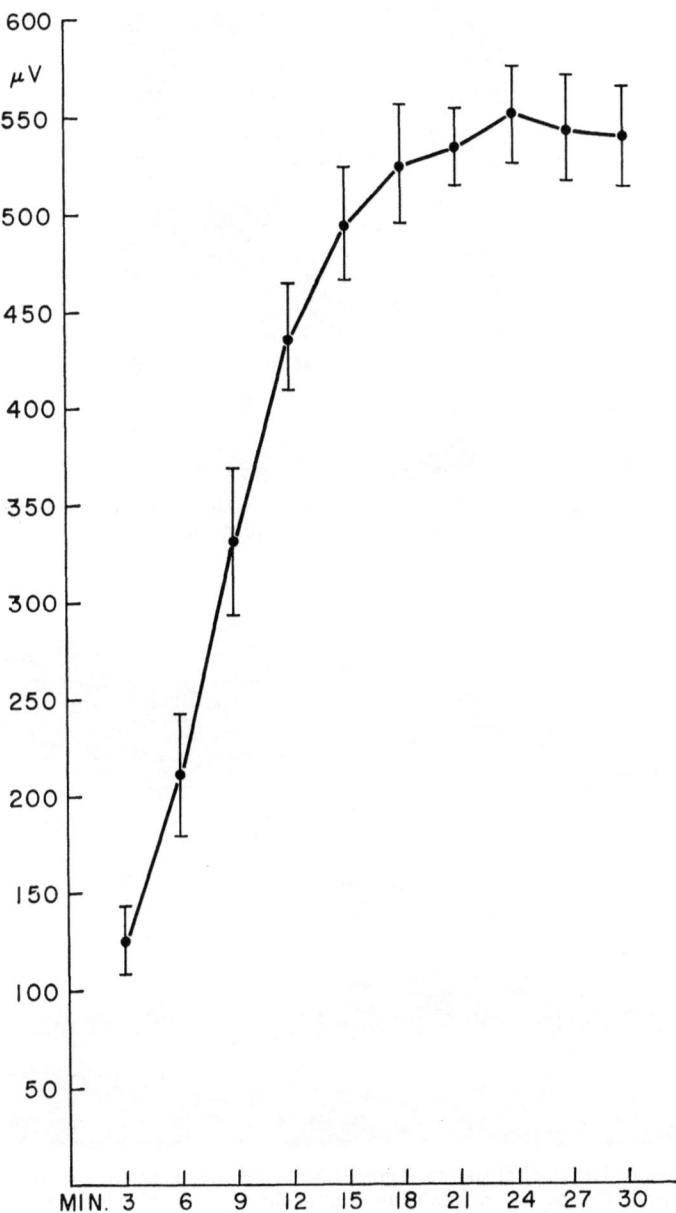

69

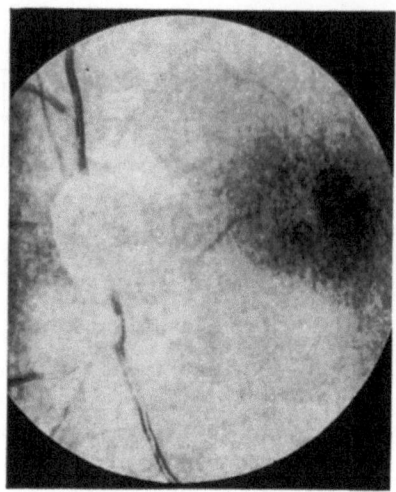

Fig. 5. Fundus photograph of monkey eye with 3+ fundus changes. Note changes in macular pigment.

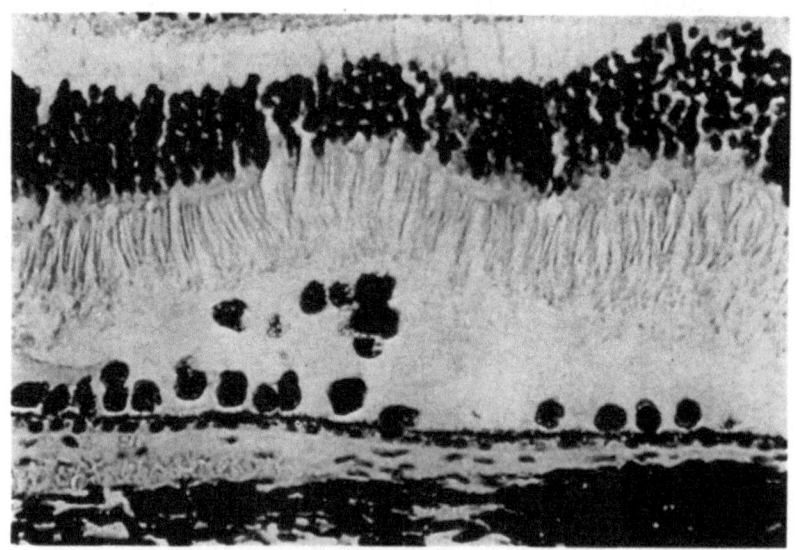

Fig. 6. Histological specimen graded 3+. There is destruction of outer segments. Phagocytes are located in front of the pigment epithelium and contain pigment from the pigment epithelial cells. The pigment epithelial cells lack their normal pigment but are intact. (H & E ×400).

For several reasons, it appears that the damage in these eyes is proportional to the amount of energy absorbed in the area of the outer segments, and that the pigment epithelial changes are usually secondary to tissue destruction of the receptors. In contrast to this, in higher level exposures, there are scattered areas where the pigment epithelium appears to be directly affected. Some of these reasons will be enumerated.

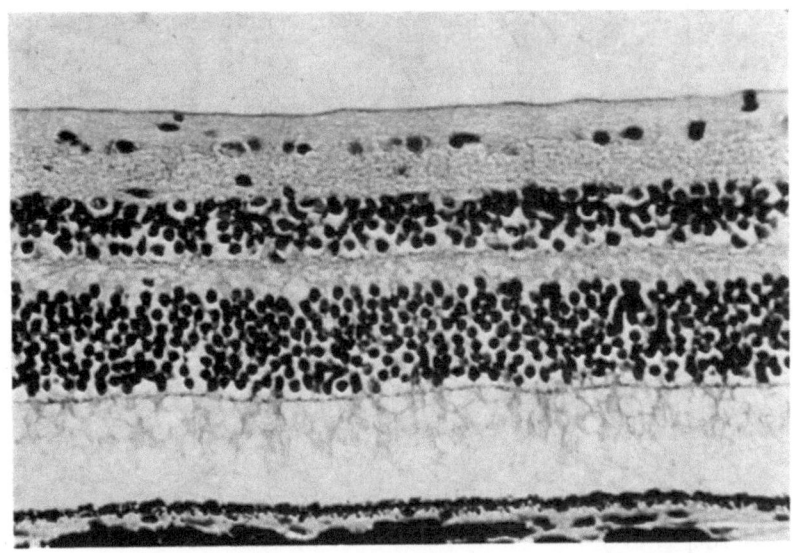

Fig. 7. Histological specimen graded 1–2+. There is vacuolization in the area of the outer segments with little disruption of the pigment epithelium. (H & E ×400).

Electron microscopic examination shows areas where the pigment epithelium appears perfectly healthy but the overlying outer segments are obviously damaged. A pigment epithelial cell can show severe degenerative changes when the adjacent cell appears normal. The damage to the pigment epithelium is quite patchy while the outer segment destruction is uniform over larger areas.

There are some eyes where the fundus appears normal, the ERG is slightly reduced and there is vacuolization and distortion of the outer segments without apparent involvement of the pigment epithelium.

The greater susceptibility to the monochromatic green light which is also more visually efficient also suggests a receptor mechanism.

I do not know whether pure destruction of tissue calls forth the histocyte reaction or whether mild changes in the protein or mucopolysaccharide structure causes a type of immune response in the area, but the data do indicate that the primary damage is in the outer segments.

71

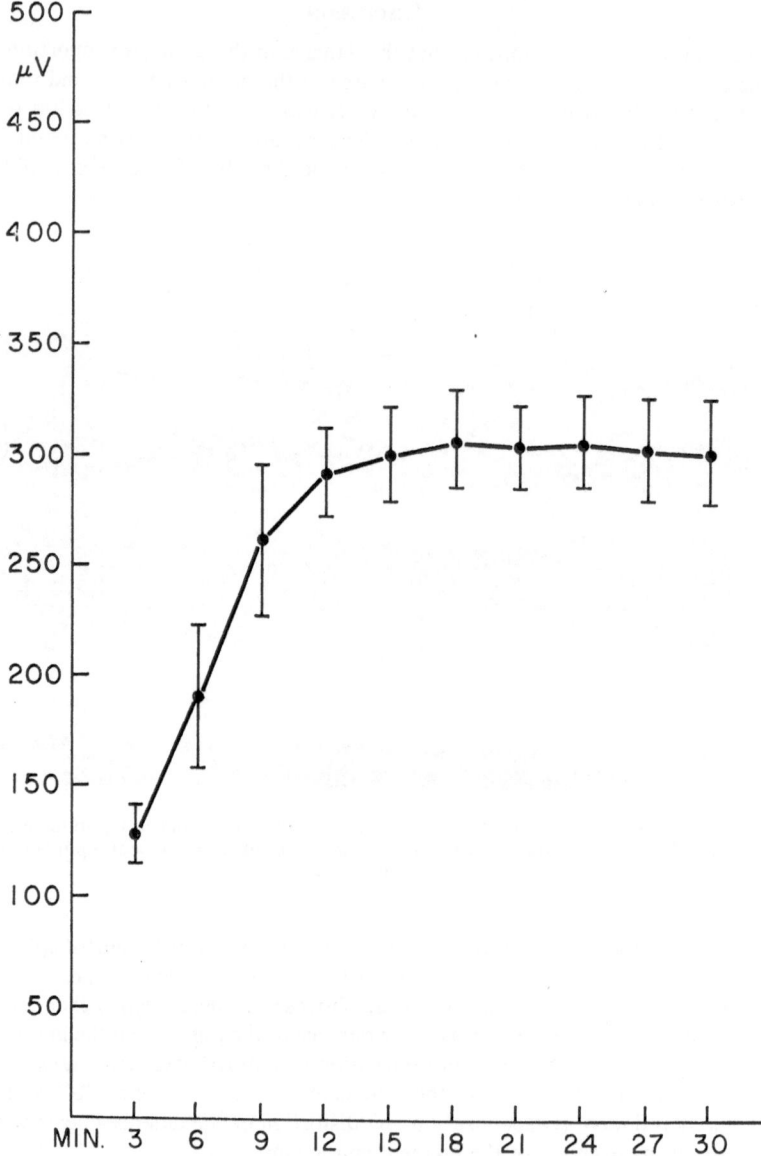

Fig. 8a. The a-wave amplitude and standard deviation prior to exposure.

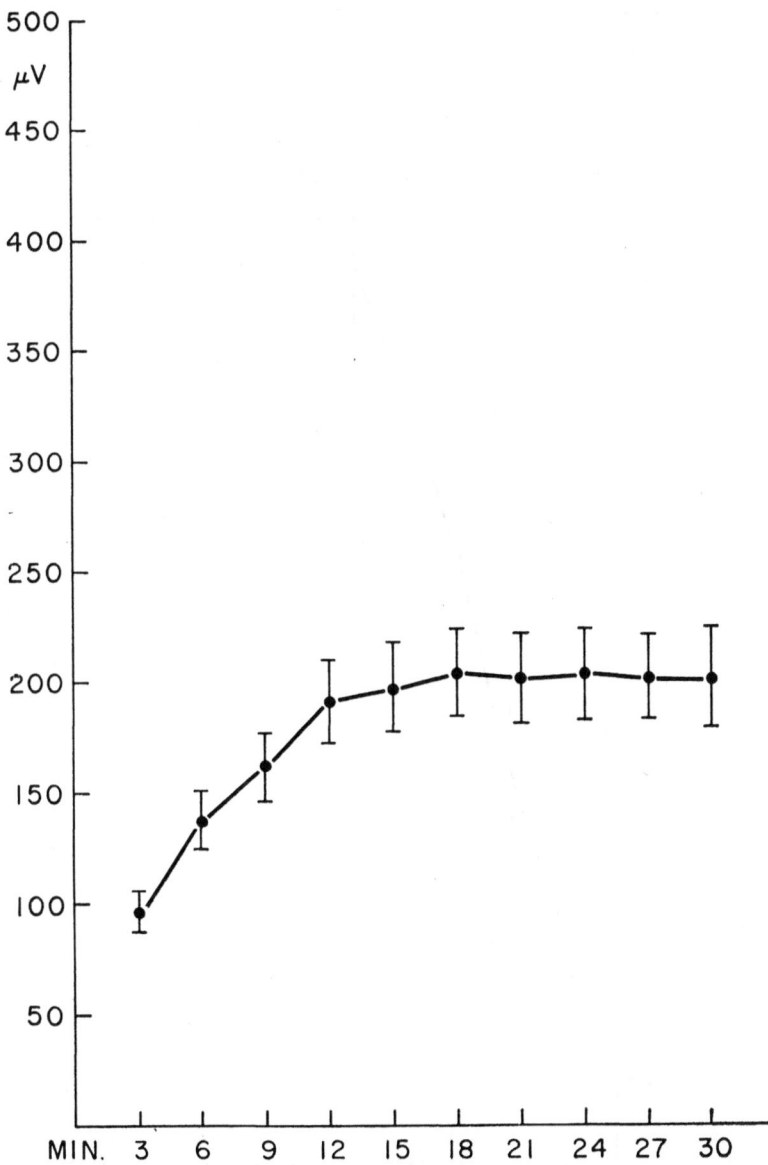

Fig. 8b. The a-wave amplitude and standard deviation for 32 days after exposure, 4+ effect.

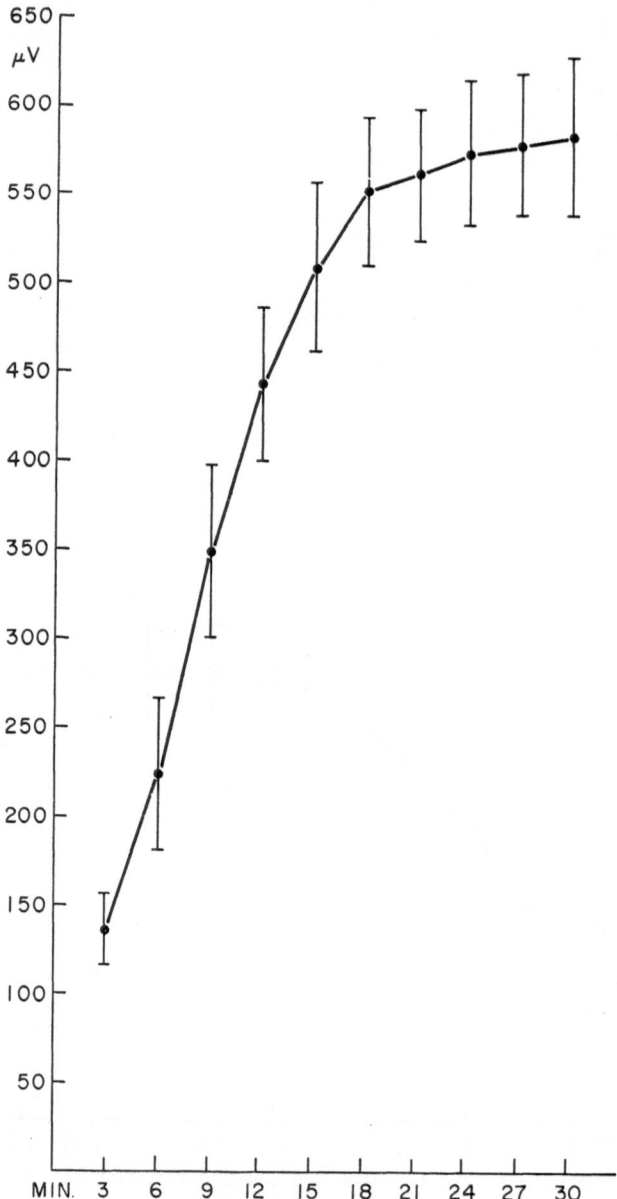

Fig. 8c. The b-wave amplitude and standard deviation prior to exposure.

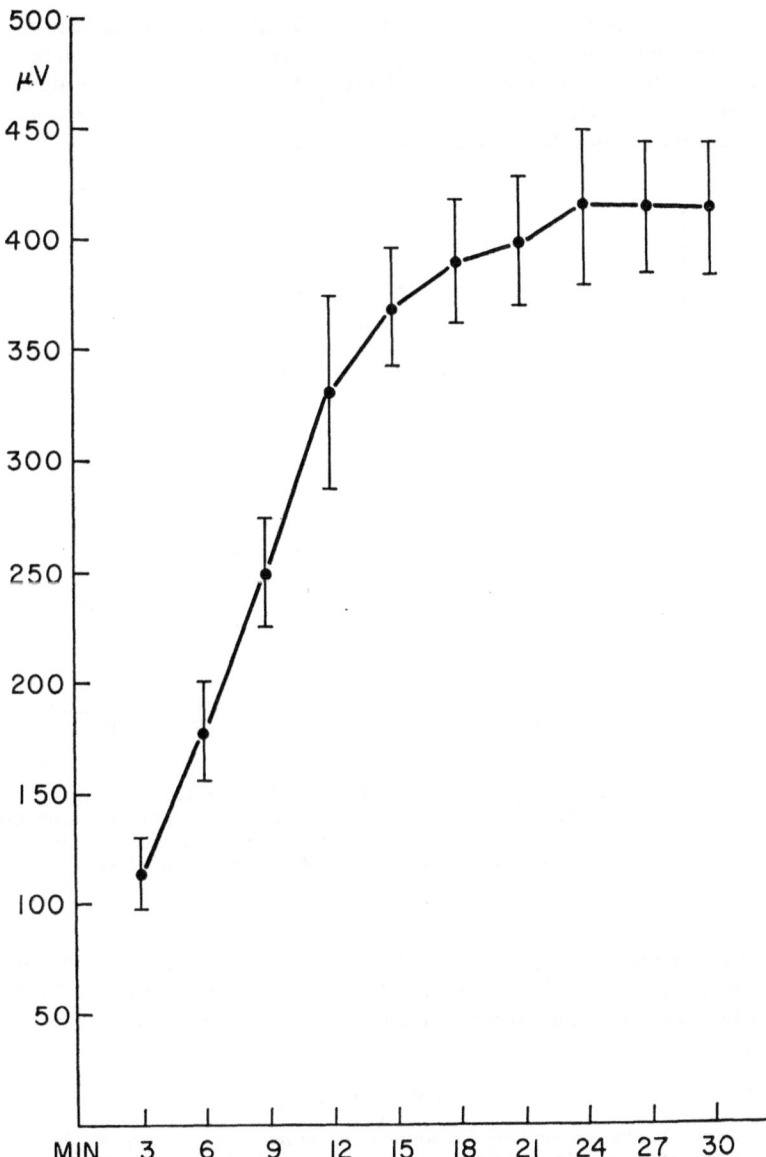

Fig. 8d. The b-wave amplitude and standard deviation for 32 days after exposure, 4+ effect.

It is also noted that the area damaged is in all cases smaller than the area exposed. In the monkey the area of greater damage is central, while in the rabbit it follows the visual streak. A possibility is that damage occurs in the area of highest concentration of receptor cells or that there is a receptor orientation effect which spares the more peripheral receptors.

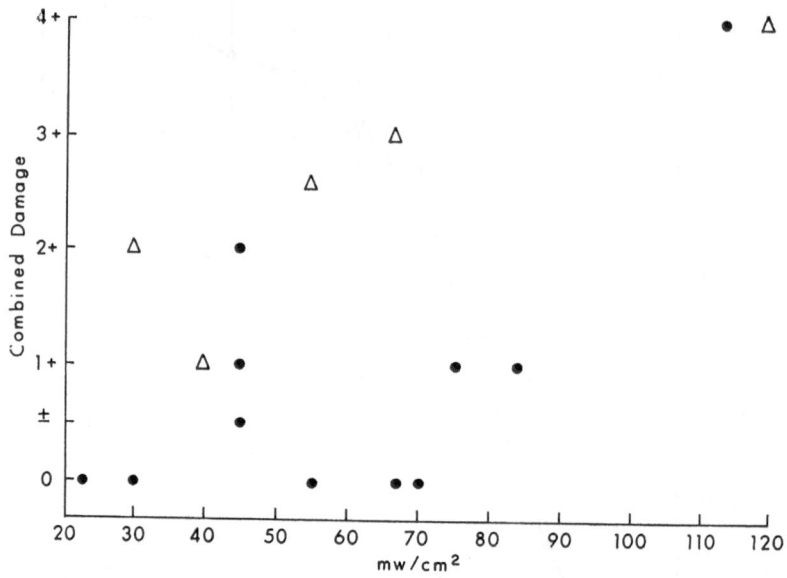

Fig. 9. Initial results of threshold studies. The dots represent white light exposures and the triangles laser exposures. The exposure scale represents the power in milliwatts per cm² of retina and the damage scale represents the combined indicators of ERG, ophthalmoscopy and histology.

SUMMARY

Rhesus monkey eyes were exposed for four hours to various levels of white and laser light and the damage produced was evaluated by electroretinography, ophthalmoscopy, and histopathology. Initial data for threshold values are presented.

REFERENCES

LAWWILL, T. Effects of prolonged exposure of rabbit retina to low intensity light. Presented AAOO and Assoc. Res. Ophthal. Las Vegas, Nev., Sept. 1971. In press Investigative Ophthalmology.
NOELL, W. K., WALKER, V. S., KANG, B. S. & BERMAN, S. Retinal damage by light in rats. Invest. Ophthal. 5:450–473 (1966).

THE SUPERNORMAL EOG: EVIDENCE OF LIGHT-INDUCED RETINAL DAMAGE?

GEORGE W. WEINSTEIN, M.D., BRIAN WARD, Ph.D. &
ROBERT R. HOBSON*

The electro-oculogram (EOG) is a useful electrophysiological test of retinal function. We have previously described (REESER, WEINSTEIN et al., 1970) our experience with this measurement, and have noted that abnormally high light : dark ratios (>4.0) had been recorded in certain individuals. These individuals were some of those studied with aniridia (congenital absence of the iris) or albinism (generalized or ocular).

In both aniridia and albinism, the possibility exists for chronic exposure to excessive amounts of light entering the eye of the subject. In no other conditions have supernormal EOG ratios been recorded to date. Therefore, it was supposed that this EOG abnormality might somehow reflect retinal damage due to excessive light exposure over long periods of time. The possibility of short term retinal effects had been excluded in our earlier investigations. Studies with normal subjects showed that the EOG ratio was not influenced by pupillary dilation.

DOWLING (1954) showed that darkness protects the rat with inherited retinal dystrophy from developing degeneration as quickly as animals exposed daily to light. NOELL et al. (1966) studied the harmful effects of chronic light exposure on the retina of the normal rat. However, rats were deemed an unsuitable experimental animal subject for these experiments, since the EOG did not show much of a light rise.

METHODS

Three adult rhesus monkeys were studied. EOG recordings were made under anesthesia obtained with Nembutal given intraperitoneally. With the animal's head fixated, the right globe was rotated over a 30° arc by means of a pulley arrangement and winter weights attached with sutures at the medial and at the lateral limbus (Fig. 1). A bank of fluorescent bulbs covered by a diffusing screen was placed 30 centimeters before the animal. Luminance at the screen was 800 foot-candles. Skin electrodes were attached at the medial and lateral canthi of the right eye. DC amplification was utilized and the EOG recording was displayed on a cathode ray oscilloscope with storage tube using a slow sweep speed. After an initial test period used to determine the adequacy of recording, dark adaptation was instituted and carried on for 12 minutes. Then the fluorescent light panel was illuminated and light adaptation was carried out for 15 minutes. Throughout the test period, 30° rotations of the animal's eye were carried out each minute in order to elicit an EOG response. The responses were photographed from the oscilloscope tube using a Polaroid camera.

* From the Division of Ophthalmology, The University of Texas Medical School at San Antonio, San Antonio, Texas, U.S.A.

Recordings were made from each animal prior to a 3 day exposure to continuous light. The light was delivered by 2 panels of fluorescent bulbs, each containing 4 lamps housed in a ceiling type fluorescent fixture, and covered with a plastic diffusing panel. Luminance of each panel was 1,000 foot-candles.

The animal was allowed to remain unrestrained in its cage. Metal foil was wrapped around all sides of the cage in order to maximize the light exposure.

For each animal, EOG's were repeated after 3 days of exposure. For animal

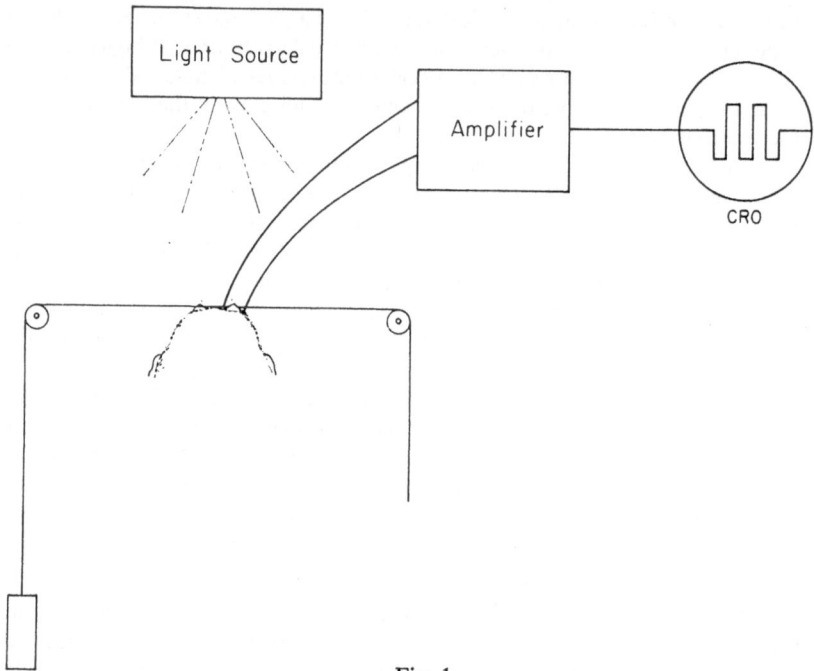

Fig. 1.

No. 1 the EOG was repeated again one week later, although no additional light exposure has been given.

A third animal was used as a control, and not subjected to the light exposures described above.

RESULTS

The EOG record is plotted for monkey No. 1 in Fig. 2. The graph illustrates both a dark trough and a light peak. An EOG ratio of 2.3 was obtained.

On the third day of a three day exposure to light, the EOG was repeated. The EOG ratio at this time was 2.1 (Fig. 3). One week later the EOG was repeated and a ratio of 2.0 was obtained (Fig. 4).

For monkey No. 2 the pre-exposure EOG is shown in Fig. 5. The ratio was 2.0. On the third day of a three day exposure the EOG ratio remained 2.0 (Fig. 6).

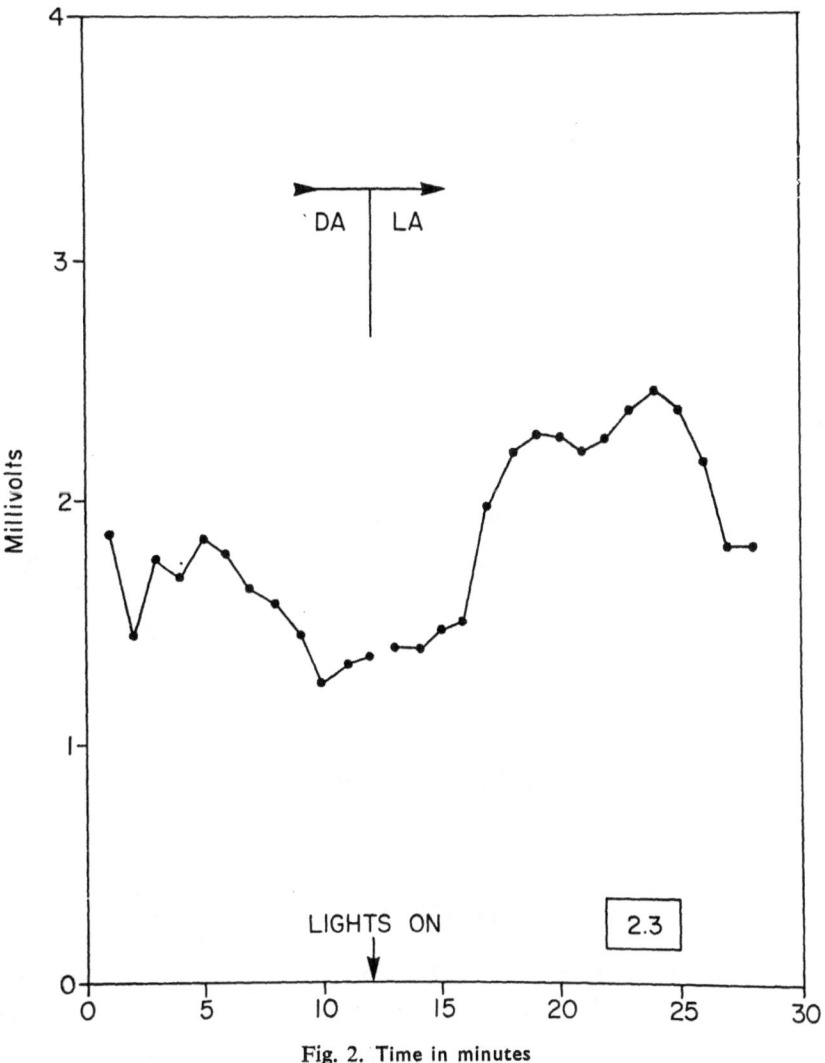

PRE-EXPOSURE
MONKEY NO. 1

Fig. 2. Time in minutes

The control animal showed no changes in the EOG ratio as recorded on several occasions throughout the course of the experiments.

DISCUSSION

In the 2 animals studied, no significant changes could be produced in the EOG ratio after three day exposures to light. Light of this intensity and duration was

79

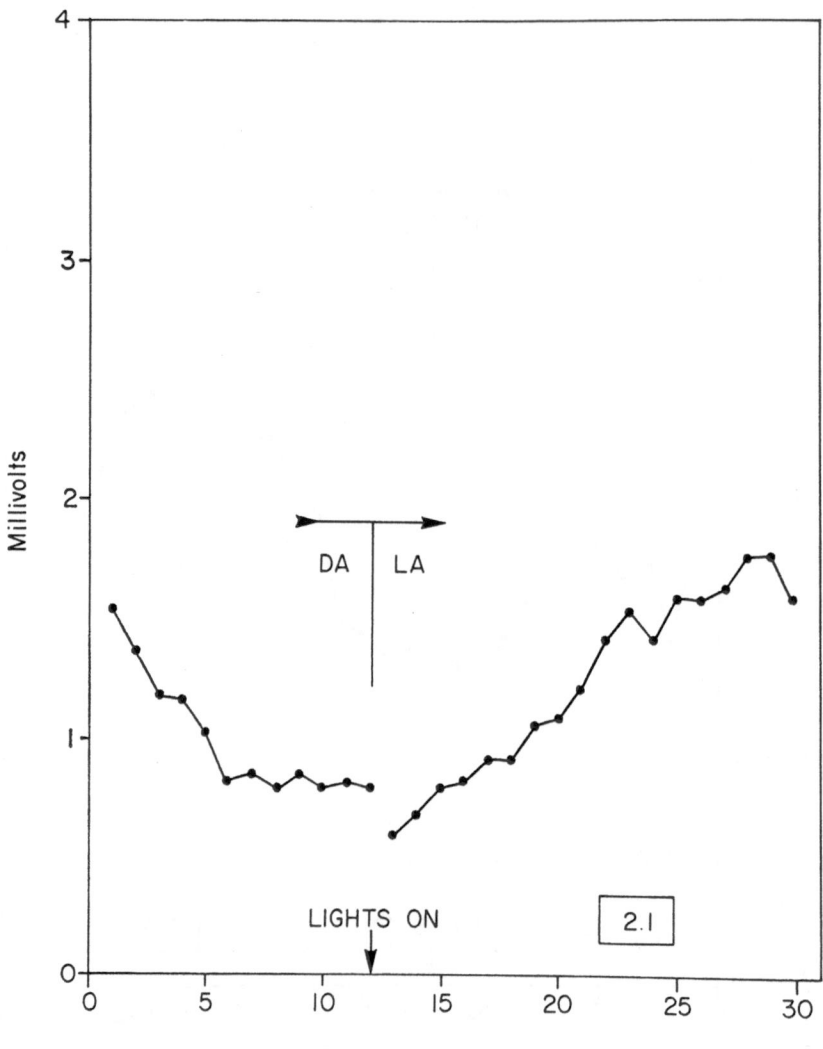

Fig. 3. Time in minutes

sufficient to produce retinal degeneration in normal albino rats. There are several possibilities to explain why a supernormal EOG ratio was not observed in the present experiment:

1. The rhesus monkey eye differs significantly from the albino rat in its vulnerability to the degree of light exposure.

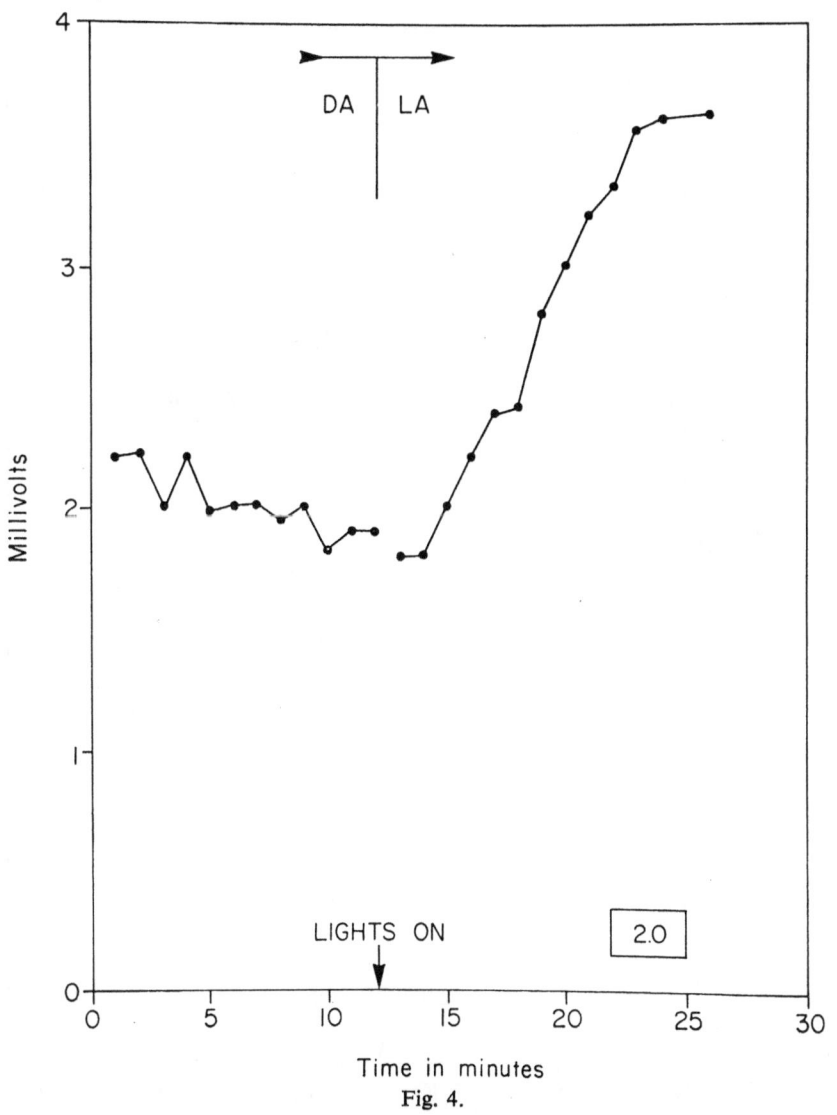

ONE WEEK LATER – NO ADDITIONAL EXPOSURE
MONKEY NO. I

DA | LA

LIGHTS ON

2.0

Millivolts

Time in minutes
Fig. 4.

2. The EOG is not sensitive to early changes in light induced retinal damage.
3. The assumption that a supernormal EOG resulted from light-induced retinal damage in subjects with aniridia and albinism is incorrect.

Regarding the first of these assumptions, higher levels of illumination or longer test periods could be attempted in order to confirm this. It should be

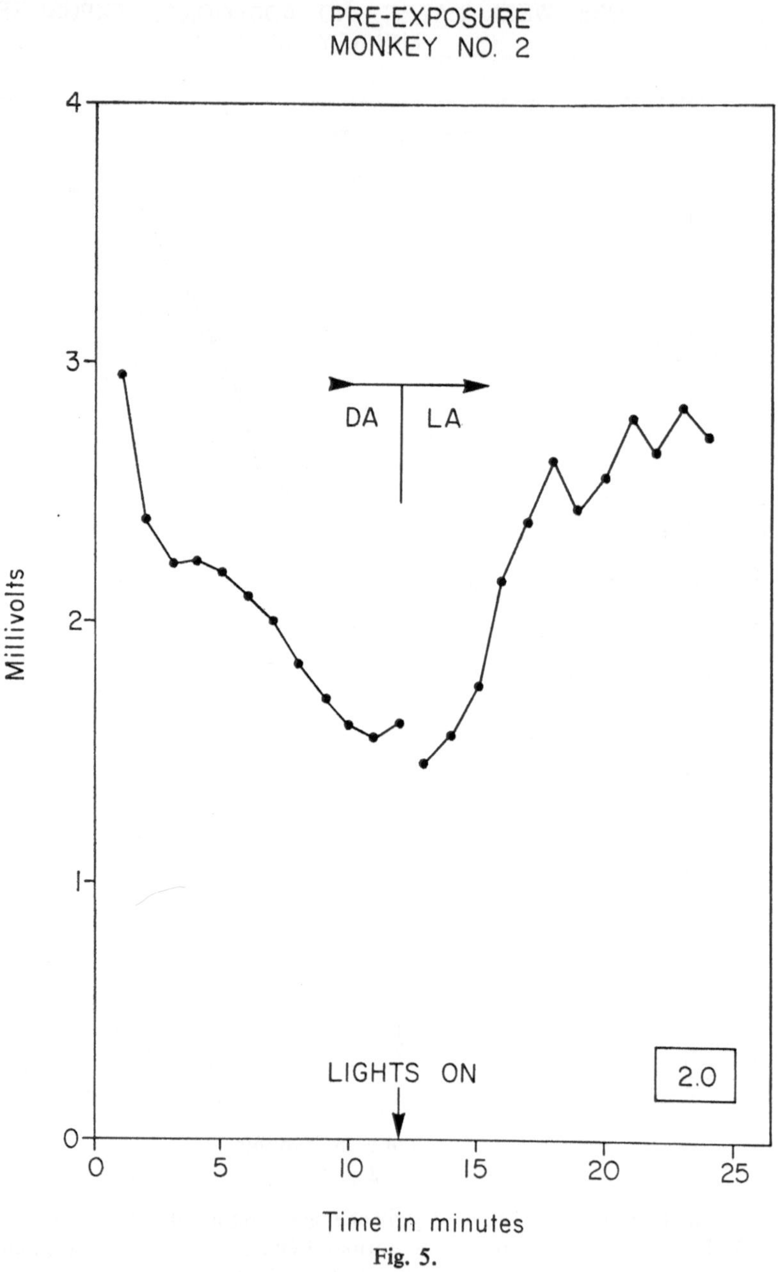

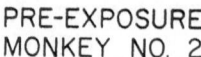

PRE-EXPOSURE
MONKEY NO. 2
4
3
2
1
0
Millivolts
DA
LA
LIGHTS ON
2.0
0
5
10
15
20
25
Time in minutes

Fig. 5.

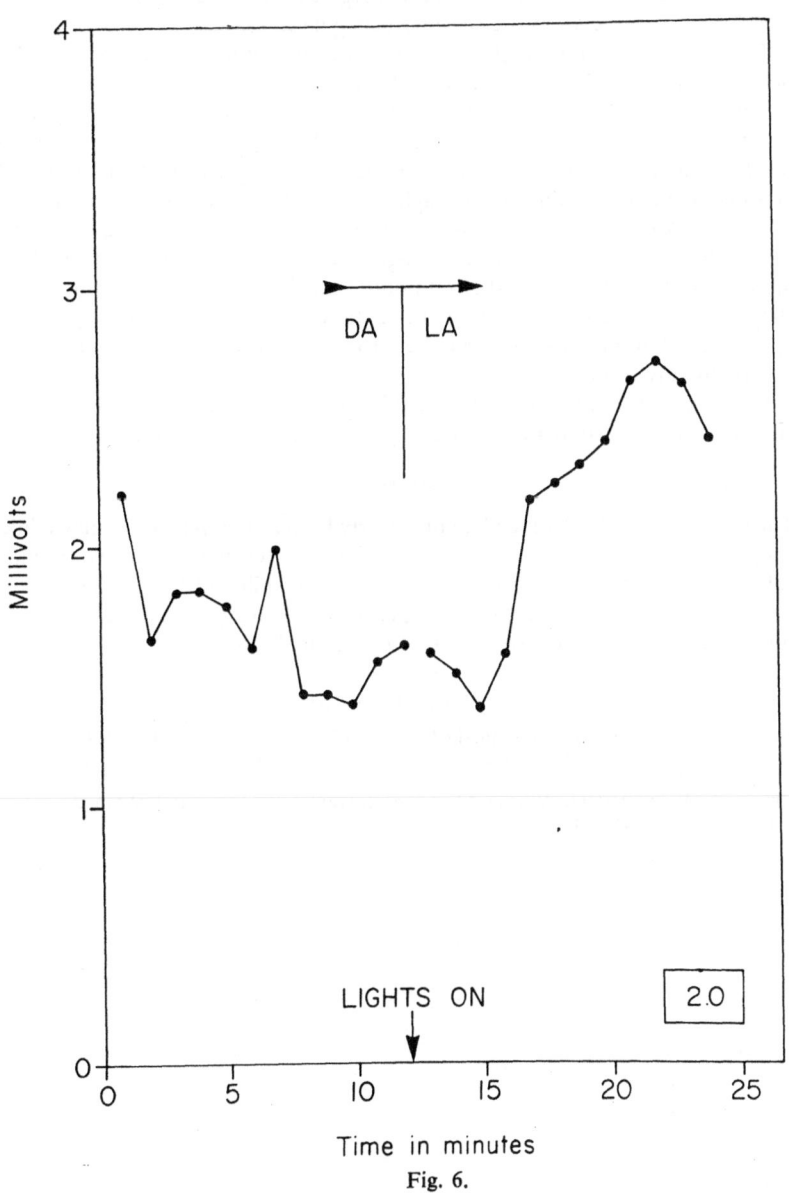

THIRD DAY OF 3-DAY EXPOSURE
MONKEY NO. 2

Millivolts

DA | LA

LIGHTS ON

2.0

Time in minutes

Fig. 6.

83

emphasized that the amounts of light irradiation involved are considerably below that utilized in photocoagulation of the retina. It yet remains to be proven definitively that light-induced retinal damage can be produced in primate (and therefore, human) eyes at the sub-photocoagulation levels.

The second possibility might be resolved by intraretinal recordings of the DC-potential linked to detailed histological investigation.

The final possibility would leave the explanation for the clinically observed supernormal EOG still open to question. The EOG presumably develops as the result of metabolic processes between the retinal pigment epithelium and the neuroepithelium. An abnormally high value might imply that these processes have been accelerated. It is conceivable that this could occur as a result of chronic light exposure. Perhaps the phagocytic activity of the pigment epithelium upon the outer segments of the rod photoreceptors is being accelerated to destructive levels during constant light adaptation. If so, this might explain why light-induced retinal damage can be produced more easily in animals with predominantly rod retinas.

It is hoped that extensions of the studies reported here will obtain more conclusive answers to some of the clinically significant questions raised.

SUMMARY

The supernormal EOG which had previously been found in some human clinical subjects with aniridia and albinism could not be reproduced in two monkeys subjected to three day exposure to light. The possibility of light-induced retinal damage being responsible for the supernormal EOG is discussed, as are the possible explanations for the failure of this animal model.

REFERENCES

DOWLING, J. E. Nutritional and inherited blindness in the rat. Exp. Eye Res. 3:*348* (1954).
NOELL, W. K., WALKER, V. S., KANG, B. S. & BERMAN, S. Retinal damage by light in rats. *Invest. Ophth.* 5:*450* (1966).
REESER, F., WEINSTEIN, G. W. et al. Electro-oculography as a test of retinal function. *Am. J. Ophthal.* 70:*505* (1970).

ELECTRORETINOGRAM AND OPHTHALMOSCOPIC FINDINGS IN INTRA-VITREOUS IRON, COPPER AND LEAD PARTICLES*

J. G. H. SCHMIDT & A. STUTE

(*Cologne*)

Perforating injuries inflicted by non-magnetic intra-ocular foreign bodies are of a much more serious character than those caused by magnetic particles. Apart from the higher operative standard required, it is especially the danger of metal intoxication (metallosis bulbi, KARPE) that poses special problems.

Nearly two thirds of 152 non-magnetic intra-ocular splinters which were removed by NEUBAUER at the University Eye Hospital in Cologne contained copper. The other third included mostly iron alloys, and in a few cases lead particles.

The varying degree of mechanical damage as well as size, surface, location, chemical composition and the time lapse before surgery introduce such a large variation of factors that the influence of the individual parameters can be assessed only with difficulty. It is here that experiments with animals can be much more instructive by varying one parameter at a time under controlled conditions. A number of investigations have been performed by STRAUB, SUGITA et al., SETO, KNAVE, BABEL, SCHMIDT & WEBER.

In our last experiments (SCHMIDT, STUTE & WEBER) we introduced wire particles of copper, iron and lead (purity 99.999%) in to the eyes of Wistar rats applying Halothan® anaesthesia. The ERG and ophthalmoscopy were carried out at regular intervals both on the injured and sound eye. In this way we demonstrated the dependence of the ERG on the chemical nature of the metal. In the case of copper particles with an active surface of 1.32 mm², generally no b-wave was detectable at the end of the first day and no a-wave after the second day. The peak times of the a-wave increased somewhat during the first day and markedly during the second. These results differed considerably from those for iron or lead. Initially, the b-wave amplitudes decreased for both metals, however, to varying degrees. After two weeks the amplitudes were down to 30%, a value which then remained constant until the end of the experiment (i.e. for 126 days). The peak times, in contrast, were much less affected and did not change after the first days.

In our experience (SCHMIDT & WEBER) small additions of other metals reduced greatly the toxic effect of copper on the ERG (LOSEVA). This may account for the slightly different findings reported by KNAVE who used copper of not quite such degree of purity (99.8%) as contrasted to our metal which has a specified purity of 99.999%. Another explanation for the differences between the two sets of data may be derived from the fact that the ratios of the surface of the

* This research was supported by Deutsche Forschungsgemeinschaft, Bonn/Bad Godesberg.

foreign bodies and the volume of the eyes was different, amounting to a higher concentration of the toxic material in the smaller eyes of rats.

The influence of the lead intoxication upon the ERG can be seen from Fig. 1. The first column—showing the ERG before injury—gives the a- and b-waves as a function of light stimulus intensity. Initially, a fourfold increase of intensity causes a doubling in a-wave amplitude. A saturation becomes apparent only for the last two intensity levels. The clear constant level of the b-wave amplitude actually also increases when one is measuring the amplitude from the (negative) peak of the a-wave rather than from the zero level.

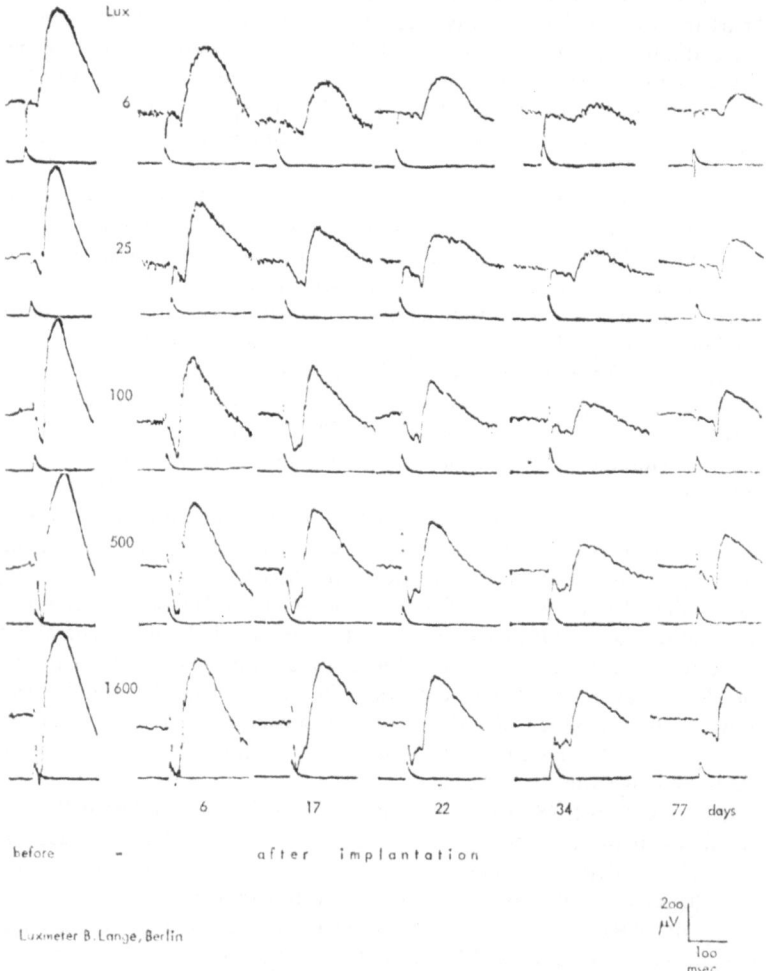

Fig. 1. The effect of intra-vitreous lead particles on the ERG.

86

Regarding the peak times of the normal ERG one finds a reduction of the a-wave from 40 to 20 msec for an increasing light stimulus, whereas those of the b-wave remain almost constant.

The following columns show the effect resulting from implantation of lead particles. In each column ERG recordings are reproduced as obtained at the test-days indicated to stimuli of increasing intensities. Five such tests have been taken over the course of 11 weeks, and the sample recording reproduced exhibits the general character of the consequences of the procedure.

The lead intoxication caused a noticeable splitting of the a-wave within a few days after implantation. We call the two potentials a_1- and a_2-wave. We found this change in such a distinct and constant manner only in cases of lead particles. But this phenomenon is not specific for this metal. We also observed the appearance of a second negative potential in some animals with intra-vitreous iron splinters, weakly marked between the 2nd and 12th day.

One can see a prolongation of the latency period of the b-wave which is of smaller size, but has approximately the same rise time. It might be supposed that under the influence of the intoxication the trigger of the b-wave is delayed.

From this point of view we have to ask the question whether we are right to call the second negative potential an a-wave. It is doubtful that this part of the ERG is analogous to a_1.

In detail, we can see that the lead intoxication caused a noticeable decay of the a_1- and b-wave within a few days after implantation. For a subsequent period of 77 days these potentials showed a further decline, whereas the amplitude of the a_2-wave remained constant. It became more prominent as the a_1-level was reduced. Similarly, it was found that the reactions of the a_1- and b-waves with respect to light stimulus intensity were more pronounced than the reactions of the a_2-wave.

At this point I would like to refer to some ophthalmoscopic findings which we have reported on in part several months ago. (SCHMIDT, STUTE & WEBER). Table I summarizes the types of complications which may develop after implantation of iron, copper or lead splinters into the vitreous body. It should be emphasized that after a few days both iron and copper particles became encapsulated, whereas this is generally not the case for lead splinters. The formation of a foggy cloud around an iron particle began within 24 hours after implantation increasing in density with time. This phenomenon was not observed with copper particles on the first day; the surrounding vitreous body remained clear. However, we always noticed some opacity right in front of the optic disc. On the second day this picture changed drastically: The copper splinter was encapsulated by a massive cloud, enlarging in size during the following days. As an hypothesis, one might explain this by a migration of copper ions toward the optic disc and later on to the retina, as was shown for healthy eyes of man and rabbit for iron particles by ULRICH, BERENS, POSNER and others. It is an open question as to whether the earlier pathway of a. hyaloidea has been used by the ions. At any rate, the diffusion of copper ions toward the posterior pole has been proved by observation of copper precipitation in the macular region. An ion migration in the opposite direction also takes place as shown by copper

Table 1

Appearance of clinical symptoms

after implantation of metal particles into the vitreous body of rats

Fe: 12 eyes   Cu: 32 eyes   Pb: 13 eyes

	Month 1	Month 2	Month 3	Month 4	Month 5
Cataracta complicata	Fe Fe ___ __ 8 x Cu __ __	Fe ____ 7 x Cu _____		Fe	Fe
Migration of the particles	___ __ 3 x Cu __ __	_ _ 3 x Cu _ _			
Encapsulation	12 x Fe 29 x Cu				
Retina — Tortuosity of the vessels	12 x Fe _____ 30 x Cu _____				
Hemorrhages	Fe Pb 21 x Cu _ _ _ _ Pb Pb _ Pb _	Pb			
Cysts		Pb Pb Pb Pb Pb Pb Pb		Pb	
Detachment	Pb	Pb Pb Pb Pb Pb		Pb	Fe

months after implantation

precipitation at the layers of the lens and the Descemet's membrane (JESS, VOGT). The experimental work of ITOI and MIELKE showed that electrolytic dissociation may play a large part both in the solution of the metal and its dissemination in the eye. If copper wires were placed in the vitreous of an enucleated eye and a current passed in the same direction as the resting potential, MIELKE (1940) found a similar localization of the metal in the lens and cornea as is known from clinical experience.

Several weeks after the implantation of lead particles, we found, ophthalmoscopically, retinal cysts, which promoted the development of holes thereafter. Frequently, we could observe a subsequent detachment of the retina. In a few cases the splinter slipped through such a perforation behind the retina. Intravitreous iron particles seldom produced a retinal detachment. In cases of copper splinters it was difficult to examine the fundus because of the intensity of the opacities of the vitreous body. Histological examination is in progress.

METHODS

Albino rats (Wistar), ranging in weight between 140 and 220 grams, were anesthetized with Halothan 'Hoechst': O_2: N_2O as 1:3 1/min containing 2.5% Halothan at the beginning; O_2: N_2O as 0.4:0.8 1/min containing 1% Halothan during the following 10–20 min.

88

The foreign bodies were slid through a cannula near the ora serrata into the center of the vitreous body. Leukomycin® ointment was applied to the cornea. *Iron* > 99.999%. Koch & Light Laboratories LTD, Colnbrook, Bucks, England, Nr. 8954 h.

Copper > 99.999%. DEGUSSA, 6450 Hanau, West Germany
Contamination (ppm): Pb, Fe, Ag, Bi, each <1, 0;
Sb, As, Ni, Sn, each <0, 5.

Lead > 99.999%. DEGUSSA.
Contamination (ppm): Bi < 5, 0; Cd < 2, 0; Tl < 2, 0; Ag < 1, 0; Cu < 1, 0.

The ERG was recorded by placing one electrode into the lid, another one into the skin between the ears and a cotton electrode on the cornea (SCHMIDT, 1969). The fast components of the ERG were recorded with a push-pull amplifier (Dr. ING. J. F. TÖNNIES, 78 Freiburg/Breisgau, West Germany, Nr. 0-353), having a time constant of 2 seconds, and photographed from the oscilloscope. The light source was a set of fluorescent tubes (Osram-L 20 W 15) which produced an intensity up to 1600 lux at the cornea. It was triggered for flash duration of 5 msec.

SUMMARY

Following the intravitreous implantation of metal particles, the toxic effects were studied using both ERG and ophthalmoscopy. Aside from quantitative differences, specific effects of iron, copper and lead, respectively, could be discriminated. Thus, electroretinography would offer the possibility of being put to use in recognizing the nature of foreign particles of unknown origin.

REFERENCES

BABEL, J. Experimental Siderosis. Proceedings XXI Intern. Congress, Mexico, D.F. Excerpta Medica Congr. Series No. 222 (1970).
BERENS, C. & POSNER, A. The circulation of the intra-ocular fluid. I. The importance of the optic nerve. *Amer. J. Ophthal.* 16:*19–28* (1932).
ITOI, M. Über das Wesen der Verrostung des Eisens im Augeninneren. *Acta Soc. Ophth. Jap.* suppl. 41:*669* (1937).
JESS, A. Die Verkupferung des Auges. *Dtsch. Med. Wschr.* 4:*118–120* (1922).
———. Linsentrübungen bei Kupfer- und Messingsplittern im Auge. *Klin. Mbl. Augenheilk.* 62:*964* (1919).
KARPE, G. Das Elektroretinogramm bei Siderosis bulbi. *Bibl. Ophth.* 48:*182–190* (1959).
KNAVE, B. The ERG and ophthalmological changes in experimental metallosis in the rabbit. I. Effects of iron particles. *Acta ophthalmologica* 48:*136–158* (1970).
———. Effects of steel, copper and aluminium particles. *Acta ophthalmologica* 48:*159–173* (1970).
LEBER, TH. Die Entstehung der Entzündung und die Wirkung der entzündungserregenden Schädlichkeiten nach vorzugsweise am Auge angestellten Untersuchungen. Verlag Wilhelm Engelmann, Leipzig (1891).
LOSEVA, E. K. Electroretinogram and Electric Sensitivity of the Eye in the Dynamic Course of Chalcosis and Siderosis of the Retina. Vestn. Oftal. (Moscow 52–57 (1971).
MIELKE, S. Die Rolle elektrochemischer Vorgänge bei der Entstehung der Linsen- und Hornhautverkupferung. *A. v. Graefes Arch. Ophth.* 141:*644–654* (1940).
NEUBAUER, H. Les corps étranger non magnétiques. Bull. Soc. Ophtalm. France, in press.
SCHMIDT, J. G. H. Revival time of the b-wave of the electroretinogram following retinal and choroidal ischemia as related to various body and eye temperatures, p. 293–298. VIIth ISCERG Symposium Istambul (1969).
SCHMIDT, J. G. H. & WEBER, E. The effect of intra-ocular copper-alloys on the ERG of human and rat retinas, p. 102–107. VIIIth ISCERG-Symposium, Pisa (1970).

89

Schmidt, J. G. H., Stute, A. & Weber, E. Elektroretinographische und ophthalmoskopische Befunde bei intraocularen Metallfremdkörpern der Ratte. Ber. Dtsch. Ophthal. Ges. Heidelberg 71:*391–396* (1972).

Seto, Y. The influence of intraocular iron pieces on the electroretinogram (ERG). *Acta Soc. Ophth. Jap.* 64:*1420–1426* (1960).

Straub, W. Das Elektroretinogramm. Bücherei des Augenarztes. Ferdinand Enke, Stuttgart (1961).

Sugita, Y. Yodokawa, M. & Tanabe, T. Electroretinographic studies in experimental siderosis. *Acta Soc. Ophth. Jap.* 64:*1427–1437* (1960).

Ulrich, R. Studien über die Pathogenese des Glaucoms. *A. v. Graefes Arch. Ophth.* 30:*4–10* (1884).

Vogt, A. Kupferveränderungen (Chalcosis) von Linse und Glaskörper. *Klin. Mbl. Augenheilk.* 66:*277–285* (1921).

90

THE APPEARANCE OF RHYTHMIC WAVELETS
ON THE ERG OF ALPHA-CHYMOTRYPSIN
POISONED MAMMALIAN RETINAS*

YOSHIHITO HONDA & JAY M. ENOCH

(St. Louis)

ABSTRACT

The effects of alpha-chymotrypsin (chym) of 0.1–40 units/ml on the *in vitro* preparation of rabbit retinas were studied. Chym (perfused from the ganglion cell side of the retina) was shown to abolish, at first, the P II component of the ERG, isolating the P III component. In succession, rhythmic wavelets having three or four peaks (about 10 Hz) were observed to appear. Some characteristics of these wavelets (named chym-wavelets) were studied. Chym-wavelets were about ten to twenty times slower in frequency than similar appearing potentials superimposed on the b-wave of the usual ERGs. They were still present even after the retina was re-immersed in the chym-free medium. Thus, the wavelets were the results of irreversible change. Chym-wavelets were recordable from the retinas of albino and pigmented rabbits and guinea pigs. They were recordable even from retinas affected by trypsin, if a higher dose than that of chym was applied. Chym-wavelets were shown to be sensitive to oxygen deprivation and their peak to peak time was prolonged in media having reduced temperatures. The appearance of chym-wavelets was affected by altering stimulus magnitude and frequency. Sodium-aspartate which isolates the P III component could not extinguish these wavelets. These characteristics of chym-wavelets have been considered in some detail.

INTRODUCTION

Since BARRAQUER (1958) introduced alpha-chymotrypsin (chym) in 1958, this enzyme has become well known and is frequently used for enzymatic zonulo-lysis. Indeed, it has been helpful for cataract extraction. However, chym has been observed to cause postoperative glaucoma (KIRSCH, 1964) and to be toxic to ocular tissues other than the zonules (cornea (RADNOT & PAJOR, 1959, 1961; LEMBECK & HOFFMANN, 1959; LANDOLT & HEINZEN, 1960), uveal tract (THOMANN, 1960; O'MALLEY et al., 1961; LESSELL & KUWABARA, 1969), vitreous body (O'MALLEY et al., 1961) and retina (MAUMENEE, 1960; RADNOT & PAJOR, 1960; O'MALLEY et al., 1961; HAMASAKI & ELLERMAN, 1965) even in relatively low concentrations. These effects of chym have been investigated mainly by injecting it into the anterior or the posterior chamber or the vitreous body of the *in vivo* eye of mammals. In this investigation, the acute effects of chym on some physiological properties of retinas were investigated in detail by utilizing perfused, excised retinas of mammals.

---

* This research has been supported in part by Research Grants, No. EY-00233, EY-00004 and EY-00204 of the National Eye Institute, National Institutes of Health, Bethesda, Maryland, and, in part, by a Research Manpower Grant of Research to Prevent Blindness, Inc.

Reprint request to: Dr. JAY M. ENOCH, Department of Ophthalmology Washington University School of Medicine, 660 South Euclid Avenue, St. Louis, Missouri 63110, U.S.A.

7

91

About forty eyes of albino rabbits weighing about 2 kg each and several eyes of pigmented rabbits and guinea pigs were used. The excision and perfusion methods for the retina were the same as those described in previous reports (HONDA, 1969, 1972). Ames solution was used as an incubating medium (AMES & GURIAN 1960; AMES et al., 1967). No blood plasma was added in this investigation. The medium was oxygenated by perfusing it continuously with a mixture of 95% O_2 and 5% CO_2 prior to and during use. The pH of the medium after equilibration with the mixture of gas remained at 7.3. Alpha-chymotrypsin from bovine pancreas, Type IV, 46 BTEE units/mg at pH 7.8 at 25°C; trypsin from bovine pancreas, Type III, 10,000 BAEE units/mg at pH 7.6 at 25°C; and trypsin inhibitor from soybean, Type I-S, 1 mg of which biochemically inhibits approximately 1.8 mg trypsin, (Sigma Chemical Co., St. Louis) were used. The enzymes were dissolved in Ames solution immediately before use and were administered to the incubating chamber. The temperature of the incubating medium was 36°C. The enzymes reached their active site by perfusion from the ganglion cell side of the retina.

The electroretinogram (ERG) was used as an indicator of retinal activity. Responses were amplified by cascaded differential AC amplifiers (Tektronix 122) providing a gain of 10,000 and having a passband of 8.0 to 1,000 Hz (0.8 to 1,000 Hz in Figs. 3, 4, 6 and 14). Such a narrow passband was employed in this study, because we were concerned mainly with rhythmic wavelets (see below). Responses to 32 stimuli were summed on an averaging computer (Nicolet 1072). The averaged responses were displayed on an oscilloscope (Tektronix 564B) and were photographed by a Polaroid camera (Tektronix C-12). In some cases responses were recorded by a polygraph (Grass M7). The positivity of the active electrode, placed on the ganglion cell side of the retina, was recorded as an upward deflection. The reference electrode was placed on the receptor side. Stimuli were provided by xenon flashtube (Grass SP 22) triggered by an electric stimulator (Grass S4DR). The light from the photostimulator was attenuated by 1.96 log units. Direct radiometric measures corrected by this factor indicated that approximately 2.5×10^{-2} ergs/flash/cm² of white light were falling at the position at which the perfused retinas were placed. The stimulus frequency was 1 flash/sec, except for Fig. 13.

In one experiment, the data of which are shown in Fig. 7, the ERGs were recorded from the rabbit eye *in vivo*. Chym (90 units/0.1 ml) was injected into the anterior portion of the vitreous by inserting a needle (26G) with a micro-syringe (Hamilton Co., Whittier, Calif.) through a small section in the sclera. The pupil was dilated maximally (approximately 10 mm) by the application of 5% euphthalmine. Photostimuli of approximately 2.7 ergs/flash/cm² in the plane at the entrance pupil were applied to this eye at a frequency of 1 flash/sec.

RESULTS

A series of ERGs in Fig. 1 illustrates typical effects of 40 BTEE units/ml alpha-chymotrypsin (chym) on the *in vitro* preparation of albino rabbit's retina. The P II component of Granit (GRANIT, 1963) decreased in amplitude after the administration of chym. Then, on the ascending phase of the P III component, there appeared rhythmic wavelets having three or four peaks (about 10 Hz). The same phenomenon was observed when a smaller dose (1 unit/ml chym) was added (Fig. 2). In Fig. 2, furthermore, these effects of chym were shown to be irreversible. No recovery of P II was observed and the wavelets did not disappear even after the retina was re-immersed in the chym-free medium. Almost the same phenomenon, that is the decrease of P II isolating P III and the appearance

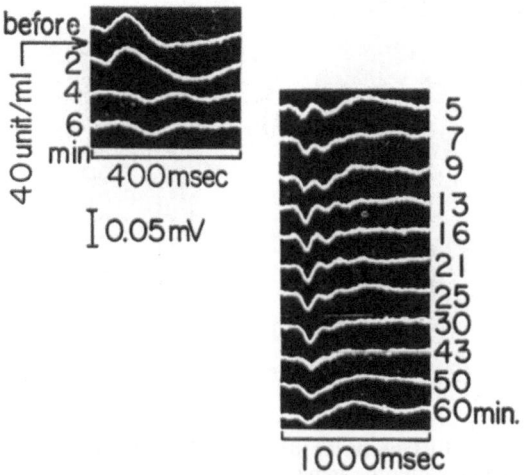

Fig. 1. The effect of 40 units/ml alpha-chymotrypsin (chym) was shown by a series of ERG recordings. Numbers on both sides indicate time elapsed after administration of chym. These times were measured at the final response of these averaged (1 response/sec). Responses were followed by a recording system having two sweep speeds.

of the rhythmic wavelets, was observed in the concentration of 0.1 units/ml, although the time course of the change was prolonged (Fig. 3).

Chym of 2.5 and 5 units/ml was administered to perfused retinas of pigmented rabbits and of guinea pigs (Fig. 4 and 5). The P II component was abolished and rhythmic wavelets also were observed as in the case of the albino rabbits. When sodium-aspartate (20 mM/1) was administered after chym, there was almost no change in P III and the wavelets were less distinct (Fig. 5). Chym, which had been heated in a water bath of 60°C for one hour, failed to affect the activity as shown in Fig. 6. Chym (90 units/0.1 ml) administered to the vitreous of a rabbit eye in vivo abolished the P II component, isolating the P III component. Then, on the ascending phase of P III, rhythmic wavelets were found although not so clear as those *in vitro* (Fig. 7).

Trypsin of 100 BAEE units/ml affected the excised retina of an albino rabbit in a manner similar to chym (Fig. 8). P II decreased in amplitude and the wavelets appeared on the ascending phase of P III about 45 minutes after the administration of 100 units/ml trypsin. In Fig. 9, 1 mg of trypsin-inhibitor derived from

93

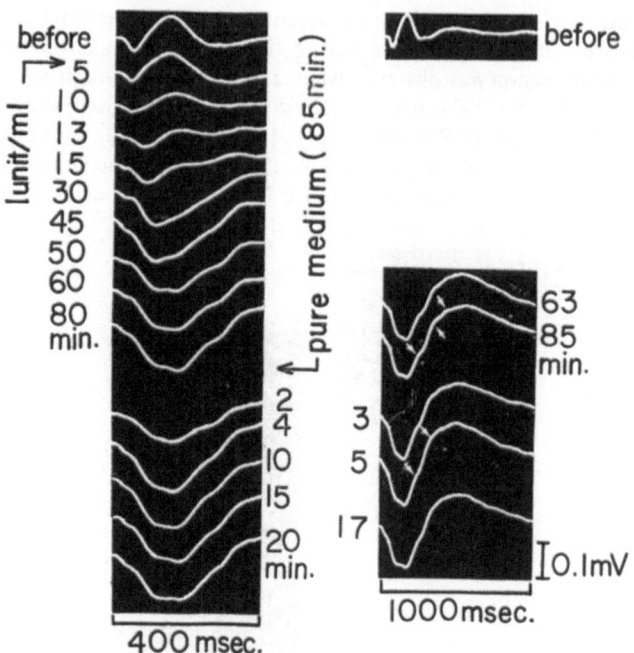

Fig. 2. A series of ERGs showing the effect of 1 unit/ml chym on a rabbit retina. Eighty five minutes after the administration of chym, the retina was immersed in the chym-free medium. The time elapsed after the substitution of the chym-free medium is shown in the middle.

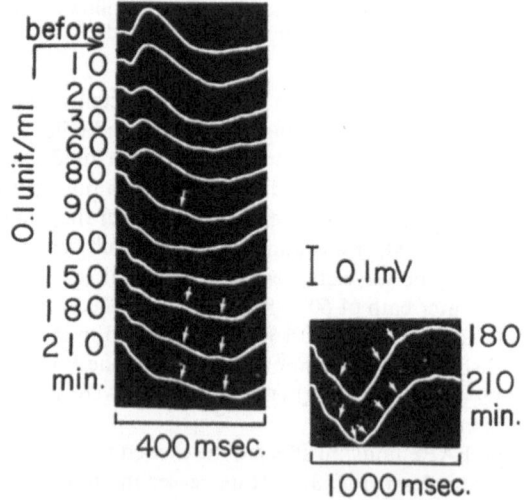

Fig. 3. A series of ERGs showing the effects of 0.1 units/ml chym on a rabbit retina. A passband of 0.8 to 1,000 Hz was employed in this figure.

94

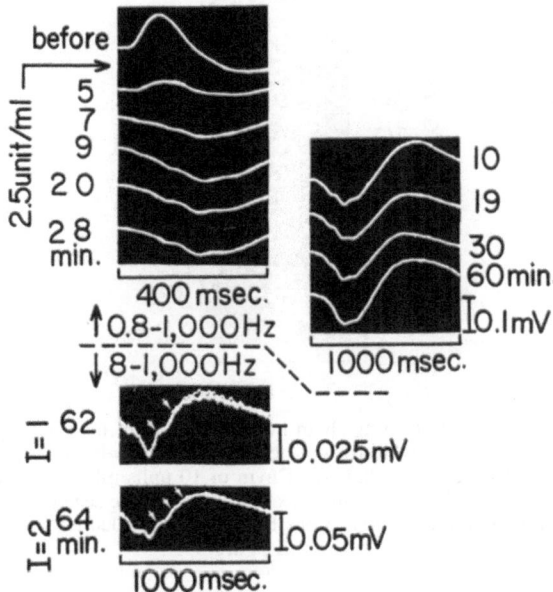

Fig. 4. A series of ERGs showing the effect of 2.5 units/ml chym on a pigmented rabbit retina. Two kinds of passband were used, 0.8–1,000 Hz (the upper portion of this figure) and 8–1,000 Hz (the lower portion of this figure). The lower-most response was evoked by stimuli of double magnitude (shown I = 2).

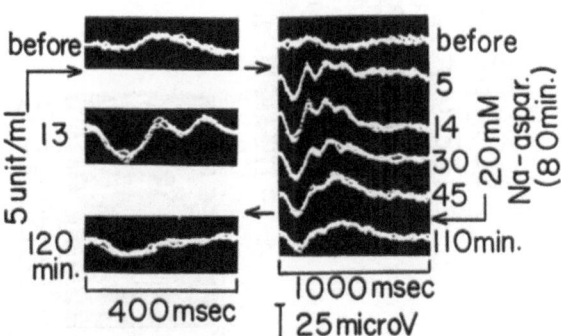

Fig. 5. A series of ERGs showing the effect of 5 units/ml chym on the guinea pig retina. Sodium-aspartate (20 mM/l) was administered 80 minutes after the administration of chym.

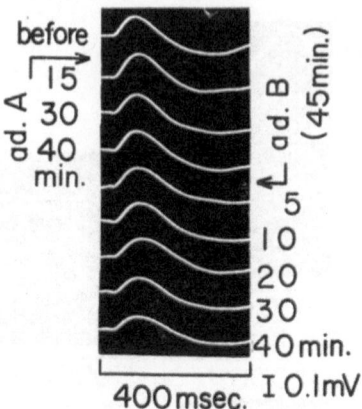

Fig. 6. The effect of heating chym in a water bath of 60°C for 60 minutes is shown. Chym of 1 unit/ml (before heating) was administered after heating at the point of time shown 'ad. A.' Chym of 10 units/ml (before heating) was administered at a later time after heating (ad. B). The second administration was 45 minutes after the first. A passband of 0.8 to 1,000 Hz was employed in this figure.

soybeans (1 mg inhibits biochemically 1.8 mg trypsin) resulted in no change in the ERG by itself, but inhibited the appearance of the effect of 1 mg trypsin administered at a later time. The addition of an excess amount of trypsin (5 mg) abolished the P II component and revealed the wavelets (Fig. 9), although they were not as clear as those in Fig. 8. No effect was observed when trypsin of 1 unit/ml or below was administered. In general, a proportionally higher dose of trypsin was needed in order to obtain the same magnitude of effect as that produced by chym.

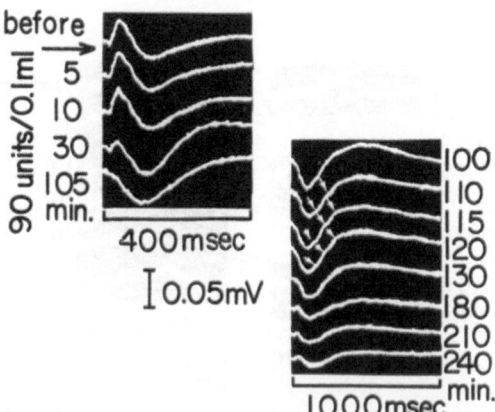

Fig. 7. Chym of 90 units/0.1 ml was administered to the *in vivo* eye of a rabbit.

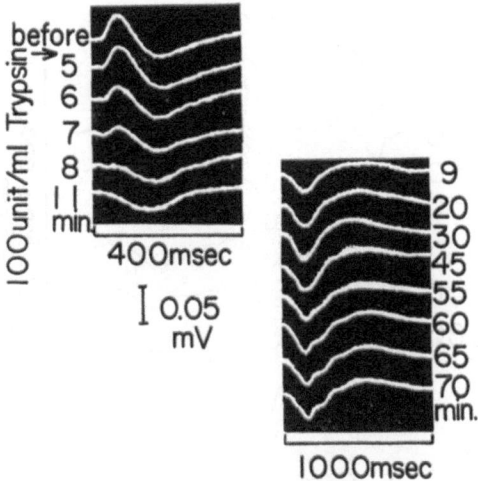

Fig. 8. The effect of 100 units/ml trypsin on a rabbit retina *in vitro* was shown by a series of ERG recordings.

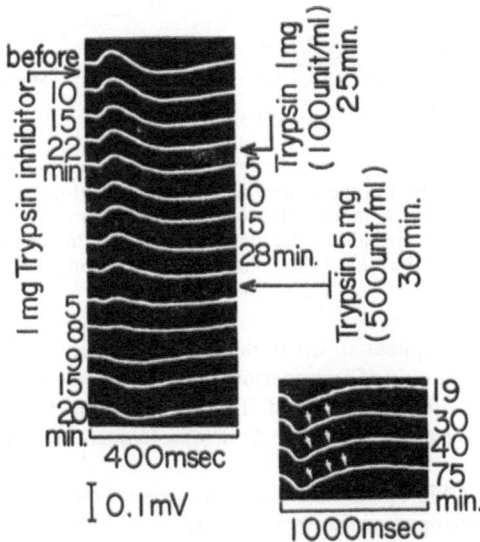

Fig. 9. Trypsin of 1 mg (100 units/ml) was administered 25 minutes after the administration of 1 mg trypsin-inhibitor (which theoretically inhibits the activity of 1.8 mg trypsin). Trypsin of 5 mg (500 units/ml) was further administered 30 minutes after the first administration of trypsin.

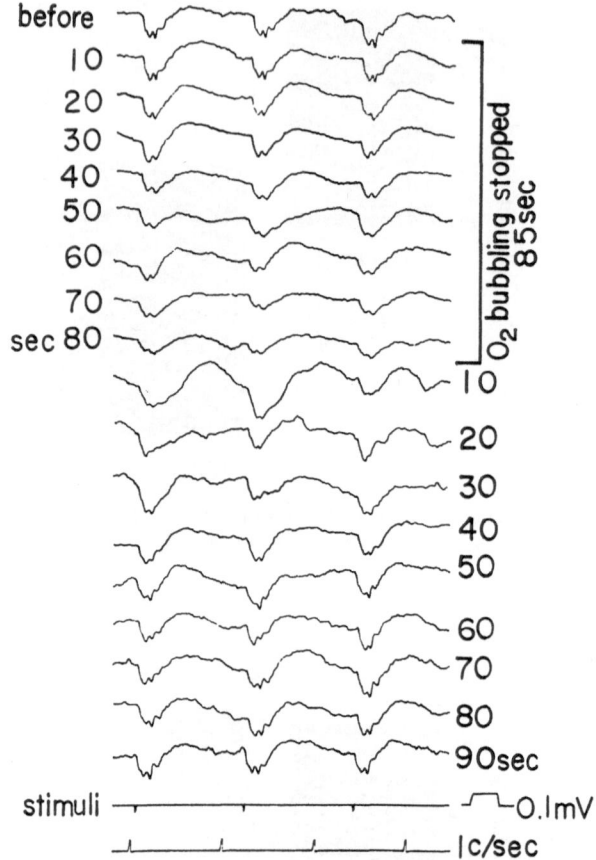

Fig. 10. Oxygenation in the incubating chamber was stopped for 85 seconds, 80 minutes after the administration of 1 unit/ml chym to the rabbit retina. Figures on the left side indicate the times elapsed after the cessation of oxygenation. Figures on the right side indicate the times elapsed after the start of oxygenation.

The wavelets disappeared when the oxygen supply was cut off and reappeared after beginning of oxygenation (Fig. 10). In Fig. 11, the temperature of the incubating medium was reduced. This resulted in a change in peak to peak time of the wavelets (prolonged). At lower temperatures the wavelets were retained.

A stimulus of a high magnitude failed to evoke these wavelets (Fig. 12). The wave form was changed as shown in Fig. 13 when high frequency stimuli were applied.

Sodium-aspartate (20 mM/1), which was sufficient to abolish permanently the P II component of the ERG (Fig. 14), slightly affected the appearance of these wavelets immediately after its administration but it did not extinguish these

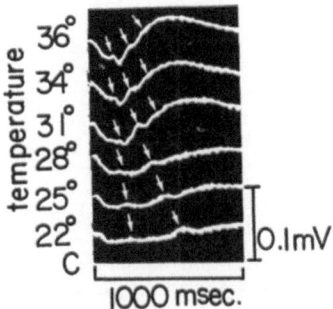

Fig. 11. Temperature of the incubating medium was changed. A retina, affected by 5 units/ml chym for 90 minutes, was used as an experimental material.

waves (Fig. 15). On the recordings taken 35 to 80 minutes after the administration of sodium-aspartate, the wavelets were still prominently observed (c.f. Fig. 5).

DISCUSSION

The mode of action of alpha-chymotrypsin on the ERG of mammals

The present study has established that alpha-chymotrypsin (chym) in concentrations ranging from 0.1 to 40 units/ml inhibits the appearance of P II of the ERG, isolating P III. This finding is essentially similar to that described by HAMASAKI & ELLERMAN (1965). They studied the effects of chym on the *in vivo* eye of owl and squirrel monkeys, and reported the high sensitivity of the retina to chym, especially that of the P II component of the ERG. The abolition of P II, which isolates P III, is not unique for chym but has been found for many toxic chemicals (NOELL, 1959; HONDA, 1972). The difference in time courses of the effects described in this study apparently depended on the concentration of the enzyme. However, even when high concentrations were used, a relatively long latent period was recognized.

In the present study, additional findings of significance were noted. The first is that rhythmic wavelets of about 10 Hz were recordable from the chym

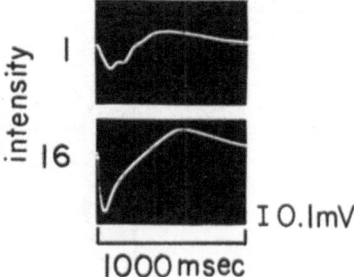

Fig. 12. The magnitude of the luminous stimuli usually used (shown I = 1) was increased by 16× in the lower recording (shown I = 16).

99

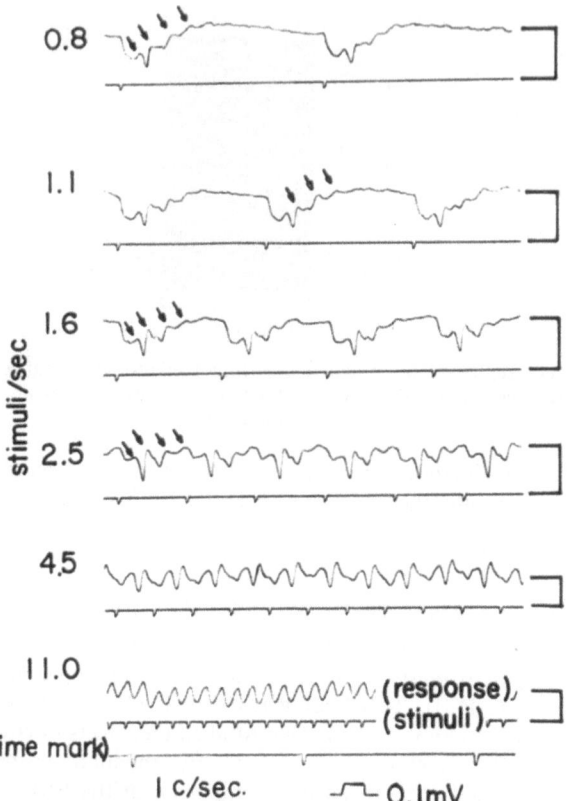

Fig. 13. The effects of changes in stimulus frequency are shown. The ERGs were recorded from a retina to which 1 unit/ml chym was administered, 80 minutes previously.

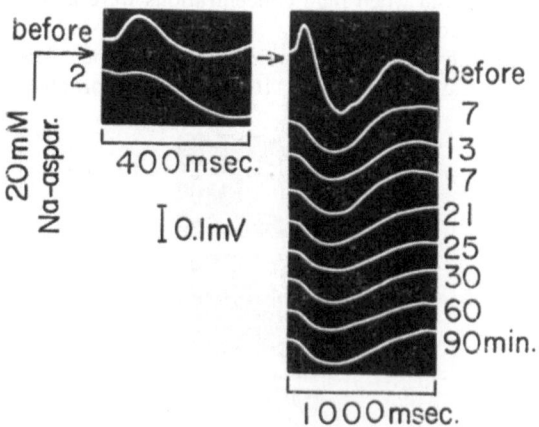

Fig. 14. The effect of 20 mM/l sodium-aspartate on an *in vitro* preparation of a rabbit retina is shown by a series of ERG recordings.

poisoned retina *in vitro*, employing an amplifying system having a short time constant. The second is that chym of a very low concentration, 0.1 units/ml, was shown to be toxic to the retina. This fact may be important clinically and should be further evaluated. In the case of enzymatic zonulolysis by chym, the contamination of, or perfusion of chym from the posterior chamber to the retina must be avoided by every means. In this study the retinal preparations were immersed in a medium made of inorganic ions and compounds (except for glucose). No

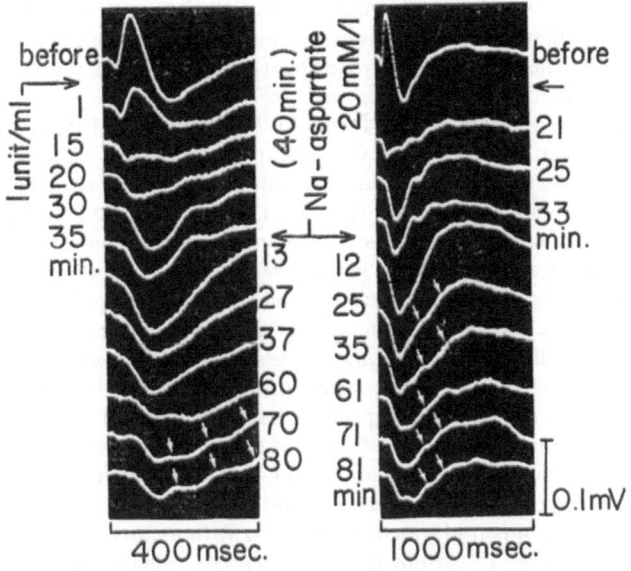

Fig. 15. Sodium-aspartate of 20 mM/l was administered to a retina affected by 1 unit/ml chym for 40 minutes.

blood plasma was added to our incubating medium. Hence, it is possible that the effects of low concentrations of chym are cancelled *in vitro* by chym-inhibitors which have been shown to exist in the aqueous humor (SCHEIE et al., 1965).

The appearance of the rhythmic wavelets superimposed on the P III component

It has been shown that on the ascending phase of the b-wave of the ERG oscillatory potentials of about 120 to 180 Hz are superimposed (COBB & MORTON, 1954; BORNSCHEIN & GOODMAN, 1957). They have been shown to be recordable even from *in vitro* preparations of mammalian retinas (HONDA, 1969). The rhythmic wavelets recorded in this study, however, were quite different from the oscillatory potentials superimposed on the b-wave of the usual ERG in several details. Some of the characteristics of the wavelets observed in this study will be summarized and discussed below.

The isolation of P III and the appearance of the wavelets (termed chymwavelets in this investigation) was an irreversible change as shown in Fig. 2.

101

This seems reasonable, because the mode of action of chym might be the digestion of the retina. These phenomena were observed over a wide range of concentrations, 0.1 to 40 units/ml. The wavelets were recordable from both pigmented and albino rabbits, and from guinea pigs.

Chym used in this investigation was a biological extract which was crystallized and lyophilized from bovine pancreas. We cannot completely overlook the possibility that these effects of chym come from some contaminated substances contained in the extract. Therefore, chym heated in 60°C for 60 minutes was added (Fig. 6). On the basis of this experiment, it can be clearly stated that changes were induced not by inorganic contaminating substances, but by the enzyme itself. The latter is sensitive to heat (NEURATH, 1961). Also consider Fig. 9, where enzymatic inhibition was tried.

Are the chym-wavelets unique for the *in vitro* retina? In Fig. 7, where chym was administered to the *in vivo* eye, similar wavelets were observed although they were proved to be not as prominent as those observed *in vitro*. On somewhat comparable recordings made by HAMASAKI (1964) and HAMASAKI and ELLERMAN (1965) no wavelets were found. This might depend on differences in administered doses and possibly the use of a very different time constant in the two recording systems or on stimulus magnitude difference (Fig. 12). In this study a very short time constant was employed. An amplifying system having a long time constant failed to reveal chym-wavelets, because fast waves of low amplitudes were concealed on the steep slope of a high amplitude P III component.

As shown in Figs. 8 and 9, trypsin of about 100 units/ml was shown to have fundamentally the same effects as those of chym. The effects of trypsin on the appearance of the ERG were quantitatively inhibited by an enzymatic trypsininhibitor. The active sites of chym and trypsin have been identified by differences in the side chains of peptide bonds (SCHWARTZ & SCHWARTZ, 1960; MCKENZIE, 1970). Peptide bonds formed by the carboxyl group of lysine or arginine and the amino group of the adjacent amino acid are hydrolysed by trypsin. Those formed by carboxyl group of tyrosine, phenylalanine or tryptophan and the amino group of the adjacent amino acid are hydrolysed by chym. The appearance of the wavelets, therefore, is believed to depend on the irreversible changes in some tissues closely related to these types of peptide bonds.

Some further characteristics of chym-wavelets

Chym-wavelets were shown to be sensitive to oxygen deprivation (Fig. 10). The peak to peak intervals were about ten to twenty times longer than those of the oscillatory potentials on the b-wave and were shown to be prolonged in media of low temperature (Fig. 11). These wavelets were eliminated by a certain magnitude of stimulus. It is interesting that intense stimuli failed to evoke the prominent wavelets (Fig. 12). Increasing stimulus frequency seemed to clarify the wavelets (Fig. 13), but no interaction between succeeding responses was observed. The findings mentioned above, the different time courses for the abolition of P III and the appearance of chym-wavelets, and the fact that sodium-aspartate could not extinguish these wavelets suggest that chym-wavelets might be independent of the P II component of the ERG.

What is the site of action of chym?

Chym is a proteolytic enzyme and is a protein itself (MCKENZIE, 1970; SCHWARTZ & SCHWARTZ, 1960; NIEMANN, 1964). The protein is not considered to be toxic itself to biological tissues except for its biological properties. Hence, the appearance of chym-wavelets might be related to the enzymatic hydrolysis of some peptide bonds by chym.

MAUMENEE (1960) stated that the supporting structure of the retina appeared to be more sensitive to this enzyme than the neural cells. If this proves to be the case, the P II component probably originating from Müller cells (DOWLING, 1970) (supporting structure) might be more severely affected by chym than the P III component originating from neural cells (BROWN, 1968).

On the contrary, HAMASAKI & ELLERMAN (1965) reported that photoreceptors were the retinal elements most damaged by the enzyme in the monkey retina, and that the outer segments appeared to be more affected than the inner segments. RADDING & WALD (1958) concluded that the digestion of rhodopsin by chym proceeded in two stages: an initial rapid hydrolysis which exposed about 30 amino groups per molecule, without bleaching, superimposed on a slower hydrolysis which exposed about 50 additional amino groups, with proportionate beaching. The appearance of chym-wavelets might possibly be related to a special process of hydrolysis of outer segments.

Histological analyses of retinas which are giving chym-wavelets are necessary in order to further discuss the origin of chym-wavelets. We are now engaged in this work and the results will be published at a later time.

REFERENCES

AMES, A. III & GURIAN, B. S. Measurement of function of an *in vitro* preparation of mammalian central nervous tissue. *J. Neurophysiol.* 23:676–691 (1960).

AMES, A. III, TSUKADA, Y. & NESBETT, F. B. Intracellular Cl, Na, K, Ca, Mg and P in nervous tissue. Response to glutamate and to changes in extracellular calcium. *J. Neurochem.* 14:145–159 (1967).

BARRAQUER, J. Totale Linsenextraktion nach Auflösung der Zonula durch alpha-Chymotrypsin = Enzymatische Zonulyse. *Klin. Mbl. Augenheilk.* 133:609–615 (1958).

BARRAQUER, J. Enzymatic zonulolysis: Contribution to surgery of the crystalline lens (preliminary note). *Acta Ophthal.* 36:803–806 (1958).

BORNSCHEIN, H. & GOODMAN, G. Studies of the a-wave in the human electroretinogram. *Arch. Ophthal.* 58:431–437 (1957).

BROWN, K. T. The electroretinogram: Its components and their origins. *Vision Res.* 8:633–677 (1968).

COBB, W. A. & MORTON, H. B. A new component of the human electroretinogram. *J. Physiol.* 123:36–37p (1954).

DOWLING, J. E. Organization of vertebrate retinas. *Invest. Ophthal.* 9:655–680 (1970).

FURUKAWA, T. & HANAWA, I. Effects of some common cations on electroretinogram of the toad. *Jap. J. Physiol.* 5:289–300 (1955).

GRANIT, R. Sensory mechanisms of the retina; Originally published by Oxford Univ. Press, 1947 and reprinted with new preface and corrections by Hafner Publishing Co., New York (1963).

HAMASAKI, D. I. Electroretinogram after application of various substances to isolated retina. *J. Physiol.* 173:449–458 (1964).

HAMASAKI, D. I. & ELLERMAN, N. Abolition of electroretinogram following injection of alpha-chymotrypsin into the vitreous and anterior chamber of monkey. *Arch. Ophthal.* 73:843–850 (1965).

HANAWA, I. & TATEISHI, T. The effect of aspartate on the electroretinogram of the vertebrate retina. *Experientia* 26:1311–1312 (1970).

HONDA, Y. Rhythmic wavelets recorded from an *in vitro* preparation of mammalian retina. *Experientia* 25:*551–553* (1969).

HONDA, Y. Quantitative analysis of some effects of ouabain upon the electrical activity of mammalian retinas., *Invest. Ophthal.* 11: *699–704* (1972).

KIRSCH, R. E. Glaucoma following cataract extraction associated with use of alpha-chymotrypsin. *Arch. Ophthal.* 72:*612–620* (1964).

LANDOLT, E. & HEINZEN, H. Pathologisch-anatomische Befunden an zwei mit Alpha-Chymotrypsin Cataract-operierten Augen. *Ophthalmologica* 139:*313–322* (1960).

LEMBECK, F. and HOFFMANN, H. Weitere experimentelle Untersuchungen zur enzymatischen Zonulolyse. *Klin. Mbl. Augenheilk.* 135:*232*–240 (1959).

LESSELL, S. & KUWABARA, T. Experimental alpha-chymotrypsin glaucoma. *Arch. Ophthal.* 81:*853–864* (1969).

MAUMENEE, A. E. Effect of alpha-chymotrypsin on the retina. *Trans. Amer. Acad. Ophthal. Otolaryngol.* 64:*33–36* (1960).

MCKENZIE, H. A. Amino acid, peptide and functional group analysis. In the Milk protein, (ed) McKenzie, H. A., Academic Press, New York and London, 181-218 (1970).

NEURATH, H. In the discussion of Sanger, F. The sequence of amino acid residues in proteins. *J. Polymer Science* 49:*3–29* (1961).

NIEMANN, C. Alpha-chymotrypsin and the nature of enzyme catalysis. *Science* 143:*1287–1296* (1964).

NOELL, W. K. The visual cell: Electric and metabolic manifestations of its life processes. *Amer. J. Ophthal.* 48:*347–370* (Series 3) (1959).

O'MALLEY, C., MOSKOVITZ, M. & STRAATSMA, B. R. Experimentally induced adverse effects of alpha-chymotrypsin. *Arch. Ophthal.* 66:*539–544* (1961).

RADDING, C. M. & WALD, G. The action of enzymes on rhodopsin. *J. Gen. Physiol.* 42:*371–383* (1958).

RADNOT, M. and PAJOR, R. Die Wirkung des Alpha-Chymotrypsins auf die Hornhaut., *Klin. Mbl. Augenheilk.* 135:*633–637* (1959).

RADNOT, M. & PAJOR, R. Histological investigations on the effect exerted by alpha-chymotrypsin on the retina. *Acta Ophthal.* 38:*583–586* (1960).

RADNOT, M. & PAJOR, R. Die Wirkung von alpha-Chymotrypsin auf die Netzhaut. *Klin. Mbl. Augenheilk.* 136:*370–376* (1960).

RADNOT, M. & PAJOR, R. Effect of alpha-chymotrypsin on the cornea. *Amer. J. Ophthal.* 51: *598–601* (1961).

SCHEIE, H. G., YANOFF, M. & TSOU, K. C. Inhibition of alpha-chymotrypsin by aqueous humor. *Arch. Ophthal.* 73:*399–401* (1965).

SCHWARTZ, B. & SCHWARTZ, J. B. A review of the biochemistry and pharmacology of alpha-chymotrypsin., *Trans. Amer. Acad. Ophthal. Otolaryngol.* 64:*17–24* (1960).

THOMANN, H. Klinische und experimentelle Beobachtungen zur Einwirkung von alpha-Chymotrypsin auf die Iris. *Klin. Mbl. Augenheilk.* 136:*376–379* (1960).

YONEMURA, D., MASUDA, Y. & HATTA, M. The oscillatory potential in the electroretinogram. *Jap. J. Physiol.* 13:*129–137* (1963).

Key words:
Alpha-chymotrypsin
Trypsin
Electroretinogram
P II component
P III component
Rhythmic wavelets (chym-wavelets)
Enzyme, Activity

ELECTROPHYSIOLOGICAL AND HISTOPATHOLOGICAL STUDIES ON THE RABBIT RETINA TREATED WITH SODIUM IODATE AND SODIUM L-GLUTAMATE

KITETSU IMAIZUMI, YUTAKA TAZAWA & HIDEJU KOBAYASHI

(*Morioka, Japan*)

INTRODUCTION

A series of experimental studies on retinopathy induced by the administration of sodium iodate (HAMATSU, 1964; YOSHIDA, 1965; IMAIZUMI et al., 1965, 1966, IMAIZUMI, 1969) or sodium 1-glutamate (HAMATSU, 1964; IMAIZUMI et al., 1965; OGAWA, 1967; KOBAYASHI, 1970; IMAIZUMI, 1970) have revealed that large dosage administration resulted in characteristic histological changes in the adult albino rabbit retina on light microscopic examination, and that these changes were reflected quite well in the electrophysiological responses.

The present study concerns the comparison of the effects of the single large dose administration with the effects of continuous small doses, and also the correlation between their electron microscopic findings and electrophysiological responses for the particular purpose of determining the effects of sodium iodate or 1-glutamate on the metabolism of the retina.

METHODS

Two per cent solution of sodium iodate was injected in the auricular vein of the rabbit. The iodate animals consisted of two groups: a single large dose group (30.0 mg/kg), and a group receiving continuous small doses (daily 1.0 mg/kg for 50 days).

The rabbits injected with intraperitoneal administration of 25% sodium 1-glutamate also consisted of a single large dose group (5.0 g/Kg) and a continuous small dose group (daily 0.1 g/Kg for 50 days).

The recording procedures for the ERG and the EOG were identical to those described by IMAIZUMI and others (1969). To elicit the scotopic ERG a xenon flash light of 80 joule was used, and the a- and b-wave amplitudes of the animals after injection were shown as percentage of the potentials before the injections. The EOG was recorded in light adaptation for 21 minutes at 3 minute interval after a 30 minute predark adaptation period. The amplitude at each 3 minute-recording point was shown as the percentage of the final amplitude at the predark adaptation.

Electron microscopic examinations were performed on the enucleated eyes of: (1) the iodate single large dose group two hours after the injection, (2) the glutamate single large dose group 4 days after the injection, and (3) the iodate or glutamate continuous small dose group on the 10th, 30th and 50th day after the injections. The examinations on synaptic bodies were limited to the presynaptic ones in the outer plexiform layer of the retina.

105

1. *Iodate single large dose group*

The amplitudes of a- and b-wave of the ERG increased by about 20% after 10 hours, above those recorded before the injection, but thereafter they gradually decreased and became non-recordable at the 96th hour after the administration of the iodate (Fig. 1).

The EOG time curve changed markedly after an hour showing an entirely different curve from that of a normal eye. The transient phenomenon (IMAIZUMI et al., 1968) usually observed at the begining of light adaptation was completely reversed in its polarity and showed a V-shape. The light rise on EOG became indistinct. This abnormal EOG curve remained for four days. The EOG base value decreased markedly with time (Fig. 3).

The electron microscopic examination 2 hours after the injection revealed changes in the Bruch's membrane, the pigment epithelium and the outer segment of the receptor cells; but in the inner segment of the visual cells the changes were not remarkable. However, 96 hours later, the degenerations of the outer layer, inner nuclear layer and the Müller cells were considerable (Fig. 5).

2. *Glutamate single large dose group*

A slight reduction in the a-wave amplitude of ERG was seen on the following day, while the b-wave amplitude was constant. Thereafter, the a- and b-wave amplitudes showed a parallel reduction and reached their lowest level on the 5th day, but on the sixth day they exhibited a tendency to return to their original values (Fig. 2).

The EOG time curve began to be affected on the 2nd day, showing a deterioration in the transient phenomenon and light rise amplitude. These amplitudes continued to decrease until finally they leveled off. It is interesting to note that unstable EOG values were observed during a period when the ERGs were most depressed, and the EOG of the 2nd day indicated that the reduction in the light rise of EOG was already noted, though the b-wave amplitude increased slightly and the transient phenomenon remained (Fig. 4).

In electron microscopic observations, the slight changes were observed by the 4th day in Bruch's membrane, the pigment epithelium, and the outer segment of the receptor cells. These changes were not greater than those observed in the iodate single large dose group. The light microscopic examination revealed changes on the 3rd day in the nuclei of the cells in the outer nuclear layers (Fig. 6).

3. *Iodate continuous small dose group*

The marked daily changes were observed in the amplitudes of both the a- and b-wave, but the a-wave amplitude was comparatively more inhibited. Two peaks, one on 14th day and another on 30th day, were recognized in the daily changes of both the a- and b-wave amplitudes (Fig. 7).

The daily transition of the EOG time curve is shown in Fig. 9. The daily changes in amplitude of the transient phenomena and the light rise were plotted

106

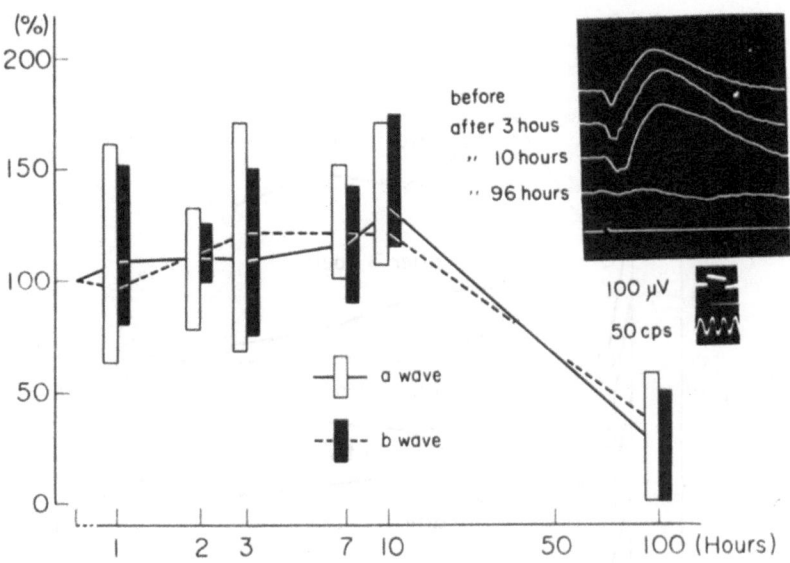

Fig. 1. The a- and b-wave amplitudes after an injection of single large dose of sodium iodate.

by per cent, compared with those of the control as shown in Fig. 10. The transition of amplitudes of the transient phenomena had 2 peaks, one on the 12th day and the another on 30th day. After 40 days, however, polarity of the transient phenomenon reversed. The daily fluctuation of the amplitudes of the light rise measured at 15 minute intervals showed itself as 3 distinct peaks and 2 troughs, but 45 days later the light rise amplitudes decreased gradually until they leveled off (Fig. 9 and 10).

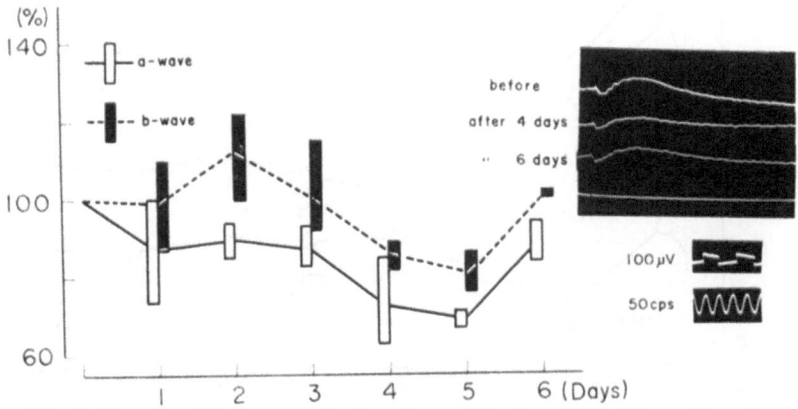

Fig. 2. The a- and b-wave amplitudes after an injection of single large dose of sodium 1-glutamate.

8

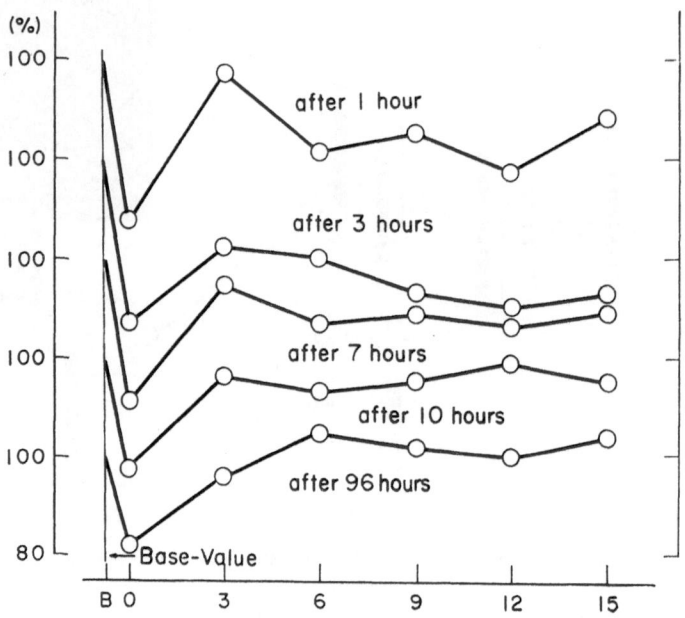

Fig. 3. The EOG time curve after an injection of single large dose of sodium iodate.

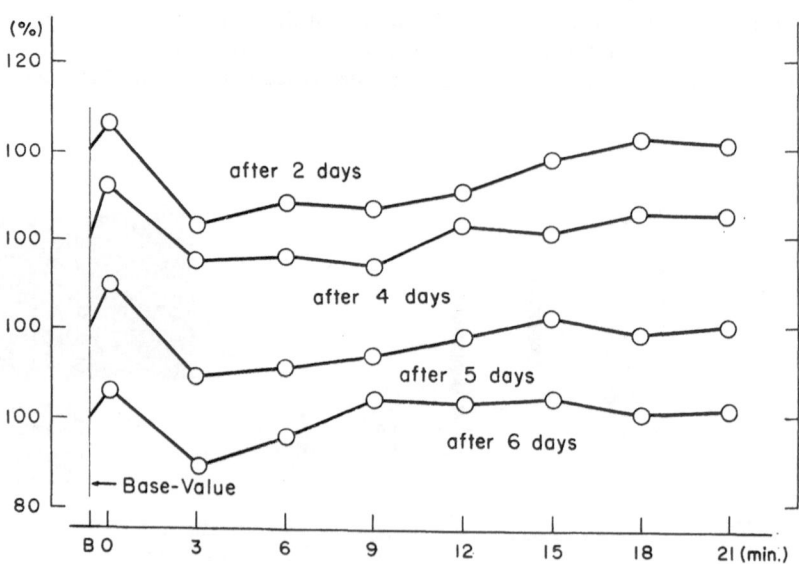

Fig. 4. The EOG time curve after an injection of single large dose of sodium 1-glutamate.

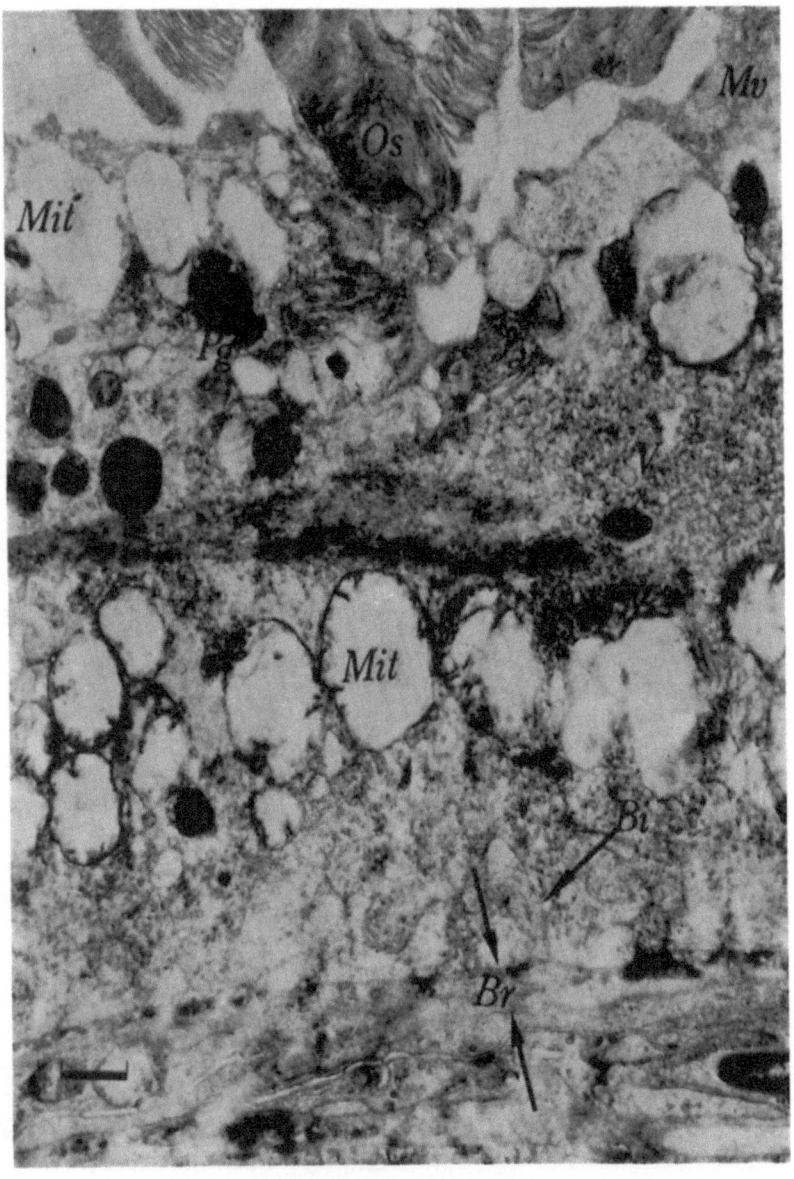

Fig. 5. An electron microscopic picture, 2 hours after an injection of single large dose of sodium iodate.

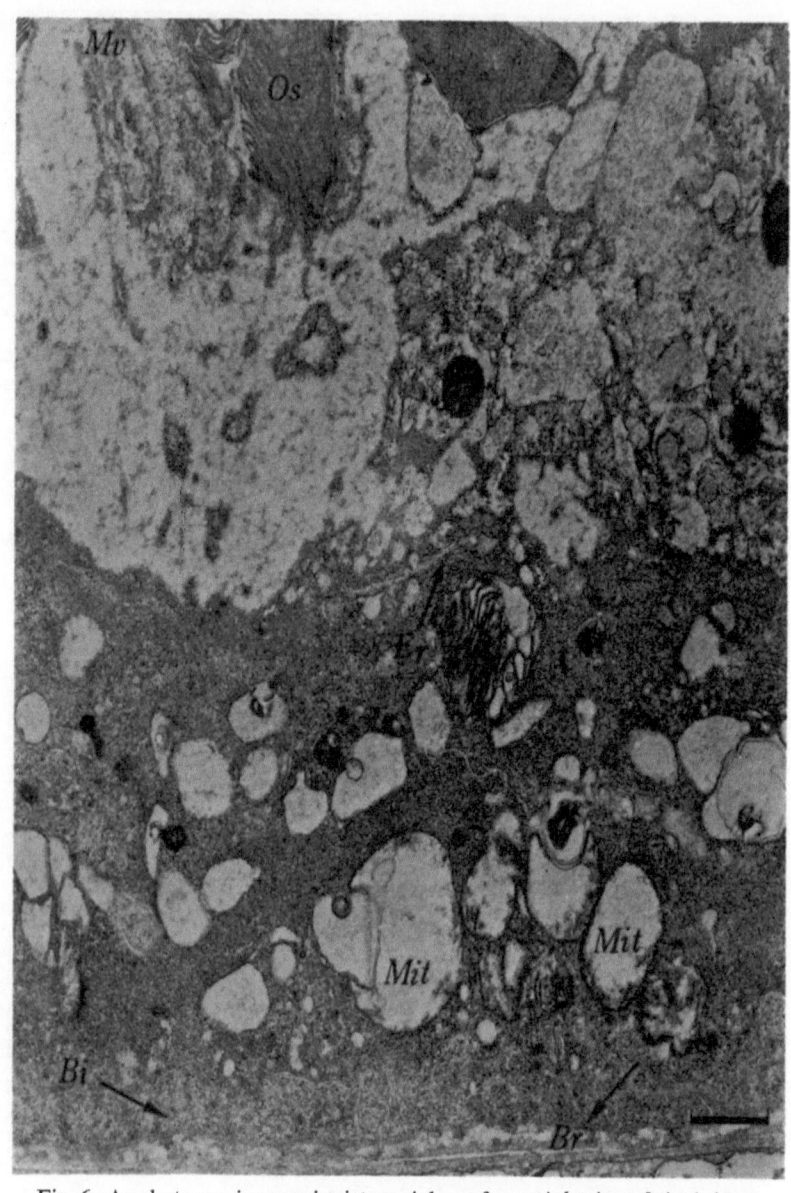

Fig. 6. An electron microscopic picture, 4 days after an injection of single large dose of sodium 1-glutamate.

The changes in Bruch's membrane and the pigment epithelium cells were slight on electron microscopic examination, while those in the outer segment of the receptor cells were somewhat conspicuous (Fig. 11). The form of the synaptic bodies in the outer plexiform layer was comparatively normal, but there was a decrease in the number with the tendency for their diameter to become larger (Table 1).

stimulus intensity 80 joule

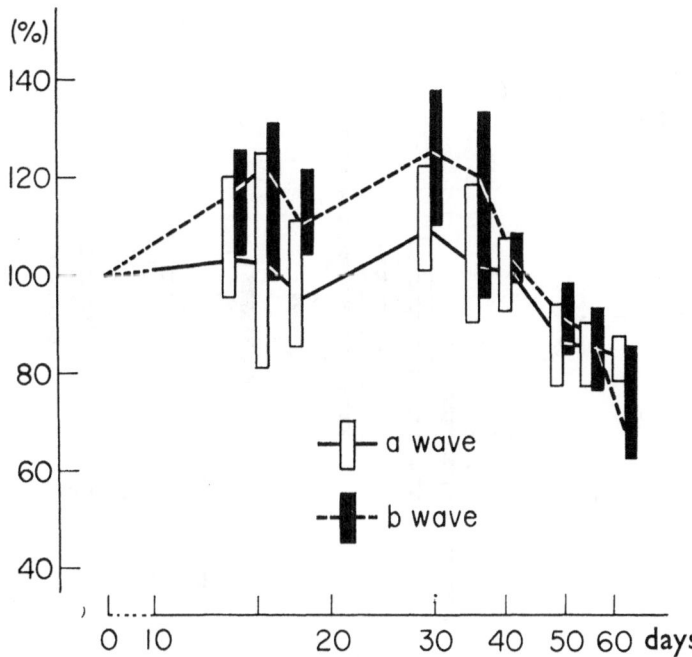

Fig. 7. The a- and b-wave amplitudes after injections of continuous small doses of sodium iodate.

4. *Glutamate continuous small dose group*

The daily changes of the a- and b-wave amplitudes showed a similar transitional pattern, with 2 peaks and 2 troughs. The time of appearance of the peaks, however, was entirely different from that of the iodate continuous small dose group (Fig. 8). The amplitudes of the a- and b-waves from the 40th day onward were higher than those recorded before the injection.

The light rise of the EOG for this group was similar to that of the iodate continuous small dose group in that both had 3 peaks. But the time of appearance of the peaks was later than in the case of the iodate group. No reversal in polarity of the transient phenomenon was observed (Fig. 10).

111

The electron microscopic examination did not reveal any conspicuous changes in Bruch's membrane, the pigment epithelium or the outer segment of the receptor cells, except for the changes in the myoid of the inner segment of the receptor cells (Fig. 12).

The number of the synaptic vesicles showed a daily decrease in their diameter tending toward becoming smaller (Table 1). On the other hand, in the inner

stimulus intensity 80 joule

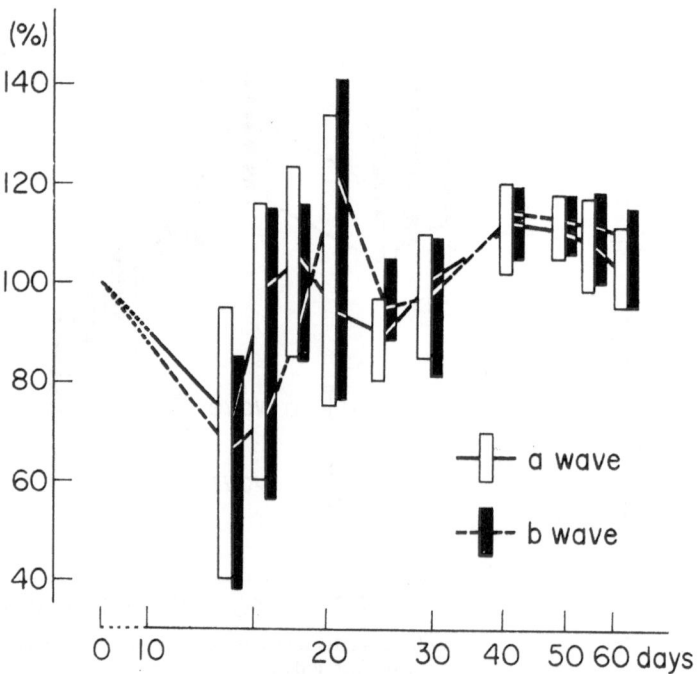

Fig. 8. The a- and b-wave amplitudes after injections of continuous small dose of sodium 1-glutamate.

nuclear cell layer, a decrease in the number of cells, and thinning of the layer was observed on light microscopic examination.

DISCUSSION

The light microscopic findings by HAMATSU (1969), YOSHIDA (1965) and IMAIZUMI (1969) showing that administration of a single large dose of sodium iodate triggered a change invading from the outer to inner layers of the retina were again confirmed in the present experiment by electron microscopic observations.

112

Corresponding to the histological changes, abnormality was first recognized in EOG prior to ERG.

On the other hand, in the glutamate single large dose group, the changes in the outer layer of the retina were slighter than those of the iodate group. The daily reduction in the a-wave amplitude and that of the light rise of EOG, however, were not so small in the glutamate group as compared to the iodate group. This difference in electrophysiological responses might be due to other effects, rather than the morphological changes.

The difference between the single large dose of iodate and glutamate administration was that in the former no recoveries in ERG or EOG were recognized, while in the latter the recovery was observed in ERG. The reversal in polarity of the transient phenomenon in EOG, which was observed in the iodate group,

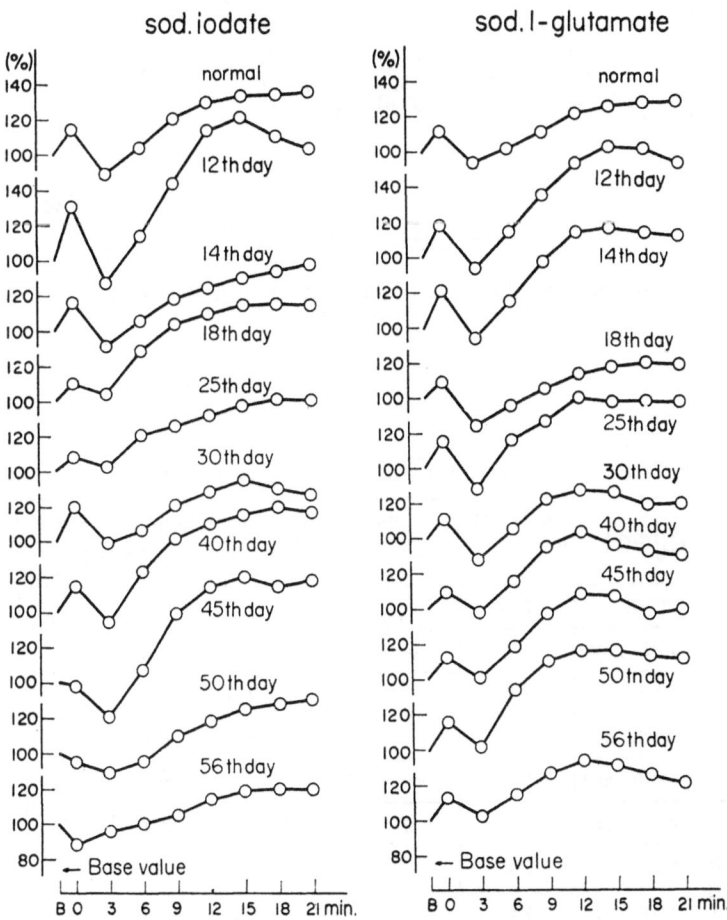

Fig. 9. The EOG time curves recorded at various stages after injections of sodium iodate or sodium 1-glutamate.

113

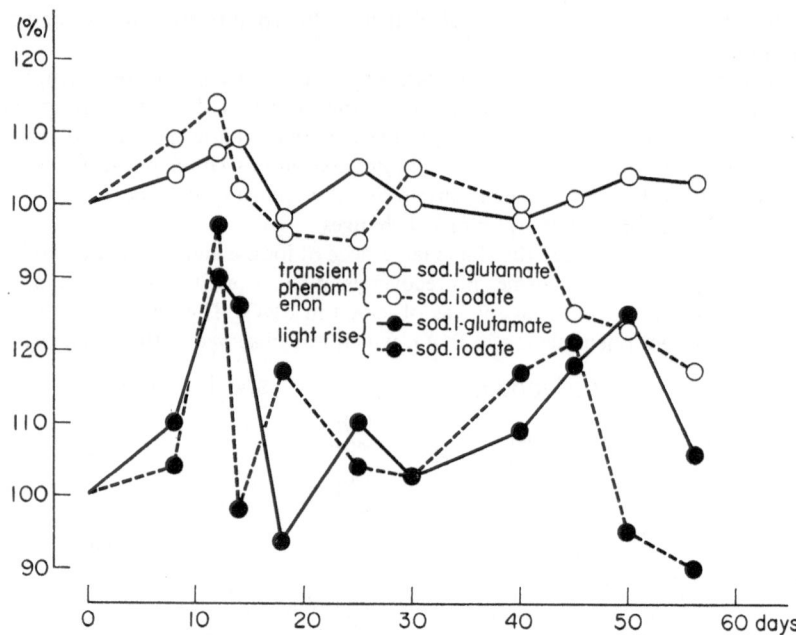

Fig. 10. Transitional changes of the transient phenomena and the light rises of EOGs.

Table 1. Distribution of the synaptic vesicles in the outer plexiform layer.

subject		number of the vesicles in 0.5μ	diameter and percentage of the vesicle					
			21-30 nm	31-40 nm	41-50 nm	51-60 nm	61-70 nm	71-80 nm
normal		29	—(%)	23(%)	72(%)	5(%)	—(%)	—(%)
Sod. iodate	2 th hour	34	—	16	71	13	—	—
	10th day	35	—	17	79	4	—	—
	30th day	28	—	—	37	43	19	1
	50th day	25	—	6	43	48	3	—
Sod. l-glutamate	4th day	16	2	6	52	37	3	—
	10th day	32	—	4	76	20	—	—
	30th day	25	—	34	52	14	—	—
	50th day	12	12	73	10	5	—	—

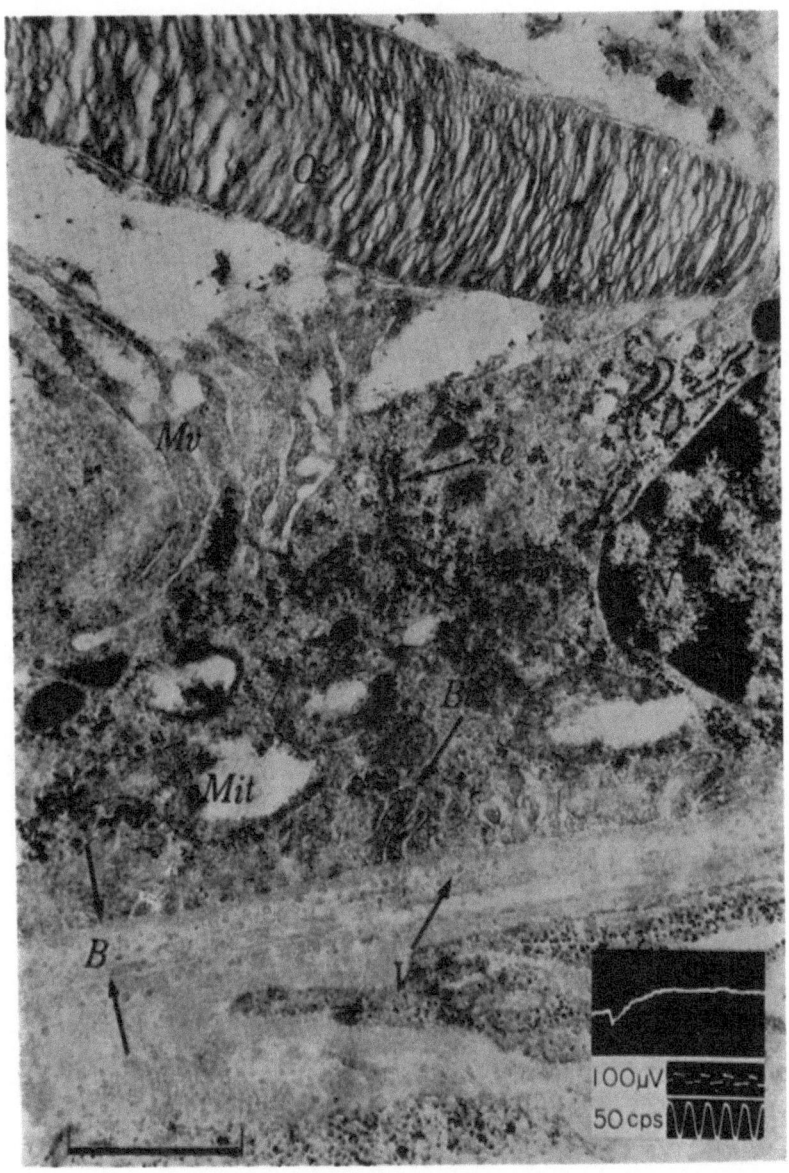

Fig. 11. An electron microscopic picture, injected with continuous small dose
of sodium iodate.

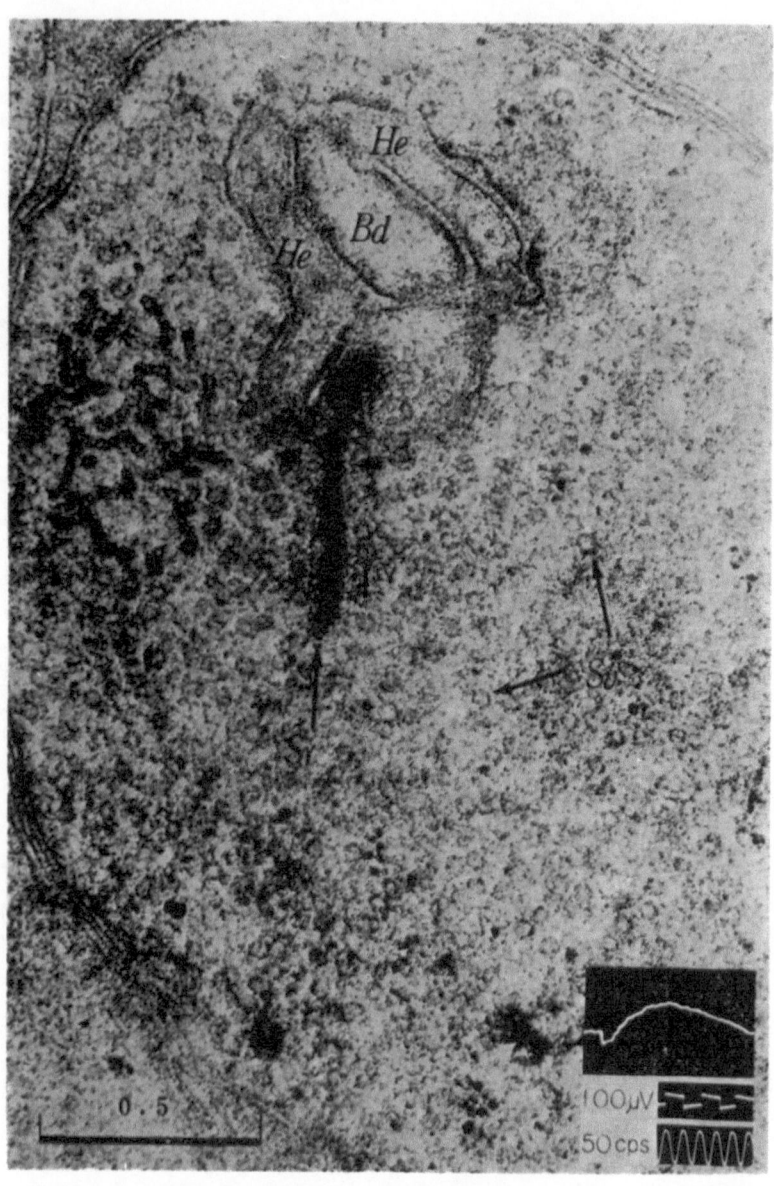

Fig. 12. An electron microscopic picture, injected with continuous small dose of sodium 1-glutamate.

was not seen in the glutamate group. Both groups were similar, however, in that both showed a greater inhibition of a-wave amplitudes than those of the b-wave, and that light rise of EOGs were markedly restrained. These findings on the large dose administration were identical to those of other reports, but the present authors have attempted to investigate further the different effects of the continuous small dose administration of these drugs on the ERG and EOG.

The histological changes of the retina treated with continuous small doses of sodium iodate or 1-glutamate were less than those recognized in the single large dose group with light (IMAIZUMI, 1970) or electron microscopic examination, but remarkable fluctuations were observed in ERG and EOG. The changes of the a- and b-wave amplitudes, the light rise and transient phenomenon in iodate groups were quite similar to the glutamate groups until the 40th day with little variations in the appearance time of the peaks. After the 41st day these groups took different courses. Careful examination of the histological findings did not allow us to obtain a simple correspondence between the histological changes and the complicated electrophysiological responses observed until the 40th day. It would also be difficult to account for the very similar electrophysiological findings in the first 40 days in terms of the distinct morphological difference induced by the 2 kinds of sodium. WALD (1961) states that sodium 1-glutamate has an affinity for the inner layer of the retina. FREEDMAN (1963) and POTTS (1965), on the other hand, studied the experimentally induced retinopathy in young animals and they claimed that this retinopathy was caused by the changes of activity of the enzymes involved in the metabolism of sodium 1-glutamate. We presumed that there were enzymatic changes going on in the retina of both groups during the first 40 days of the apparently similar transitional patterns of ERG and EOG, and that different electrophysiological findings after the 41st day were due to different effects of the two drugs on the retinal tissues. We interpreted in the same way the discrepancy between the electrophysiological responses and the histological changes induced by single large doses of sodium iodate or 1-glutamate. The interpretation seems to be possible in view of the systematic daily changes in the number and the diameter of the synaptic vesicles in the outer plexiform layer. Sodium iodate showed its distinct effect on the histology, after 40 days with a concomitant attenuation of ERG and EOG amplitude. This fact has also been stated by NOELL (1963). Sodium 1-glutamate showed milder effects on the histology of the retina than the iodate, as mentioned above, although synaptic bodies in the outer plexiform layer were more strongly affected by the glutamate than by sodium iodate.

After 40 days the attenuated amplitudes of the light rise of the EOG caused by the glutamate do not regain their original values. However, the a- and b-wave amplitudes of ERG, which fluctuated after the glutamate treatment, gradually showed recovery to the control values. This restoration might be effected by the recovery of the functions of the inner layer, as POTTS (1965) suggested that submaximal treatment with glutamate helped the damaged bipolar cell layer to recover.

With respect to the a-wave, a depressive effect was observed in the iodate group, while augmentation in the amplitude was seen in the glutamate group.

117

This phenomenon could be explained by a fact described by NOELL (1963) and WALD (1961), that sodium iodate affected the a-wave, and also by BUCKSER (1969) that the effects of sodium 1-glutamate on the a-wave was slight.

SUMMARY

The effects of sodium iodate and sodium 1-glutamate were studied by means of electrophysiological and electron microscopic examinations on adult albino rabbits treated with single large doses, or continuous small doses of each drug. The following results were obtained:

(1) The single large dose of sodium iodate rabbits showed the histological changes which began in the outer layers and then gradually moved into the inner layers. The amplitudes of the a- and b-wave of ERG, and the transient phenomenon and the light rise of EOG exhibited a gradual reduction.

The glutamate single large dose group had milder or lesser histological changes than the iodate group, and the degeneration began in the outer layers as in the cases of the iodate animals. However, the severity of the electrophysiological changes, especially in the EOG, was greater than that of the histological ones. The ERG showed a tendency to return to the original values.

Both in the glutamate and iodate groups, the EOG was affected earlier than ERG.

(2) In the groups of continuous small dose administration of iodate or glutamate, the histological changes appeared in the outer layer of the retina after 40 days. The changes brought about by glutamate injection were much less than those caused by iodate. The responses of ERG and EOG were similar during the first 40 days, but after that the 2 groups took different courses which could not be accounted for in terms of the changes in the histology.

(3) Sodium 1-glutamate was presumed to prevent the activity of certain enzymes in the retinal tissues.

(4) The changes in the number and diameter of the presynaptic vesicles of the outer plexiform layer were more marked in the glutamate group than the iodate animals.

REFERENCES

BUCKSER, S. *Jap. J. Physiol.* 19:547 (1969).
COHEN, A. I. *Amer. J. Anatomy* 120:319 (1968).
FREEDMAN, J. K. & POTTS, A. M. *Invest. Ophth.* 2:252 (1963).
HAMATSU, T. *Acta Soc. Ophth. Jap.* 68:1621 (1964).
IMAIZUMI, K., TAKAHASHI, R., KAMEI, M. & HAMATSU, T. *Acta Soc. Ophth. Jap.* 69:2150 (1965).
IMAIZUMI, K. TAKAHASHI, R. & HAMATSU, T. *Jap. J. Ophth.*, Suppl. 10:71 (1966).
IMAIZUMI, K., TAKAHASHI, R., TAKAHASHI, F., YOSHIDA, G., INOMATA, K. & OGAWA, K. *Acta Soc. Ophth. Jap.* 72:1512 (1968).
IMAIZUMI, K. *Acta Soc. Ophth. Jap.* 73:2347 (1969).
IMAIZUMI, S. *Acta Soc. Ophth. Jap.* 74:896 (1970).
KOBAYASHI, H. *Acta Soc. Ophth. Jap.* 74:902 (1970).
NOELL, W. K. *J. Ophth. Soc. Amer.* 53:36 (1963).
OGAWA, K. *Acta Soc. Ophth. Jap.* 71:1466 (1967).
POTTS, A. M. Biochemistry of the retina. 115, Academic Press, New York (1965).
WALD, F. & DE ROBERTIS, E. *Zeitsch. Zellforsch.* 55:649 (1961).
YOSHIDA, G. *Acta Soc. Ophth. Jap.* 69:1249 (1965).

EFFECT OF ALCOHOL-DEHYDROGENASE ACTIVATORS ON MOUSE ERG

K. K. GAURI, K. A. HELLNER, J. RICKERS & I. WATANABE*

Initially it was found that *in vitro* experiments N-alkyl substituted pyridones-2 (Fig. 1), depending upon the length of the carbon chain (n = 4 to 7), are capable of increasing the activity of the liver alcohol-dehydrogenase (ADH-L) (Gauri, 1971; Gauri & Kristahn, 1971).

In the retina this enzyme is associated with the rhodopsin synthesis (Fig. 2), in that it oxidizes retinol to retinal. The latter combines with opsin to yield rhodopsin (see Bliss, 1951).

Following a working hypothesis that an enhancement of the ADH activity in retina will lead to an increased synthesis of the rhodopsin, the effect of alcohol-dehydrogenase-L activators was studied on the mouse ERG. (Gauri et al., 1972). As is shown in Fig. 3, the compounds pentyl- and hexyl pyridones are capable of increasing b-wave amplitudes in the mouse ERG when compared to that of the control animals.

These experiments were conducted in the following way: Mice weighing 40 g were dark adapted overnight. Then ERG dark threshold was determined. This was followed by 5 min. of light adaptation with an intensity 6 log. units higher than that determined for the dark threshold. Growth of the b-wave amplitude was observed during 60 min. of dark adaptation.

Optimal activity is associated with the compound hexylpyridone. In *in vitro* experiments on the ADH-L maximum activity was shown. Pyridone-2 and its

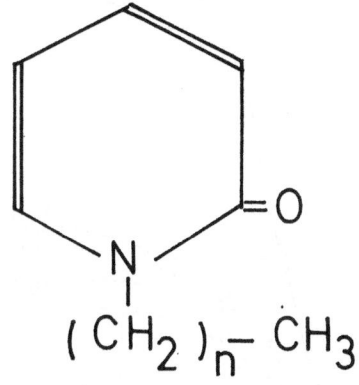

Alkyl pyridones -2

Fig. 1

---

* Institute of Pharmacology and Eye Hospital Hamburg University, Hamburg-20.

119

$$\underset{11-Cis}{Retinol \xrightarrow{\;ADH\;} Retinal} \quad +Opsin \underline{\quad\quad} Rhodopsin$$

Fig. 2

N-allyl, ethyl and propyl-derivatives were ineffective. They were also without effect on the ADH-L (GAURI, 1972).

These results lead to the conclusion that the activation of the ERG in mice should result from an activation of the ADH in the retina. An unexpected finding in further experiments was the observation that N-decylpyridone-2 (I, n = 9) [which in *in vitro* experiments has absolutely no effect on the ADH-L (GAURI, 1972)] activates the b-wave amplitude in mice ERG (Fig. 4). In comparison to hexylpyridone, it is much less active; but in each experiment this activity was present. Accordingly, the original hypothesis—activation of b-wave through increasing of ADH activity in retina—could not be supported anymore. Structural resemblance between retinine and the active alkyl-pyridones, specifically reflected in the length of the carbon chain, led us to postulate that in rhodopsin they might substitute for retinal (Fig. 5).

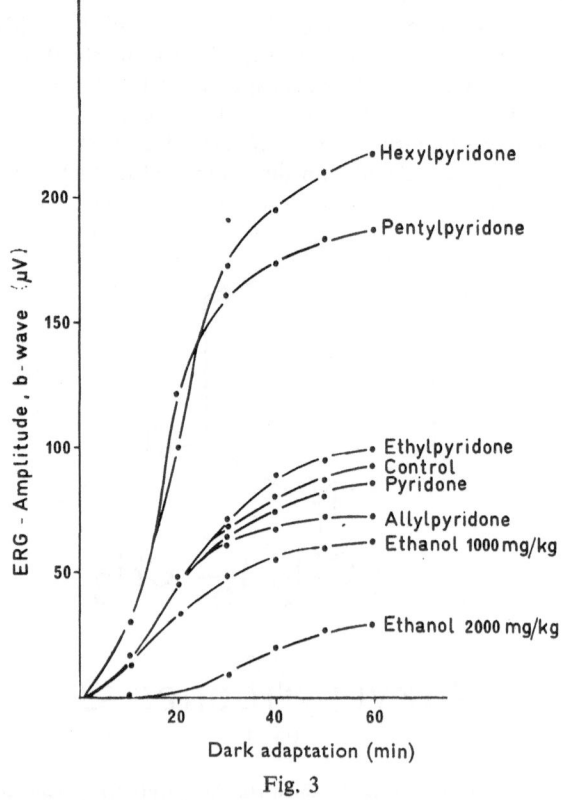

Fig. 3

120

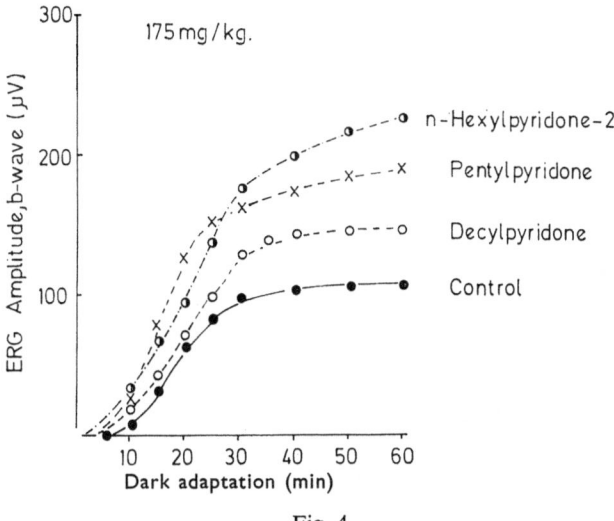

Fig. 4

In this case the *in vivo* active alkylpyridones-2 must primarily be converted into the corresponding ω-hydroxy derivatives to combine with opsin. Should this hypothesis be valid at all, then the ω-hydroxyalkylpyridones themselves constitute *in vivo* active compounds. Consequently ω-hydroxyhexylpyridone-2 was synthesized (GAURI, 1972). Results with this compound are shown in Fig. 6. In comparison to controls it activates the b-wave amplitude to about 200%, whereas the parent compound, hexylpyridone-2 activates to 100% only. These results indicate that the *in vivo* active alkylpyridones can act as analogues of retinine.

To varify this result—i.e. to see if the ω-hydroxyhexylpyridone-2 can actually substitute for retinol-one more experiment was conducted. 21 days old inbred WISTAR rats were maintained on standard laboratory diets (a) supplemented with synthetic vit. A, (b) vit. A-less and (c) vit. A-less + ω-hydroxyhexylpyridone-2 (GAURI & BARNASEK 1972). After 8 weeks ERG was recorded as described. Results show (Fig. 7) that in vit. A-less (i.e. deficient) animals the dark

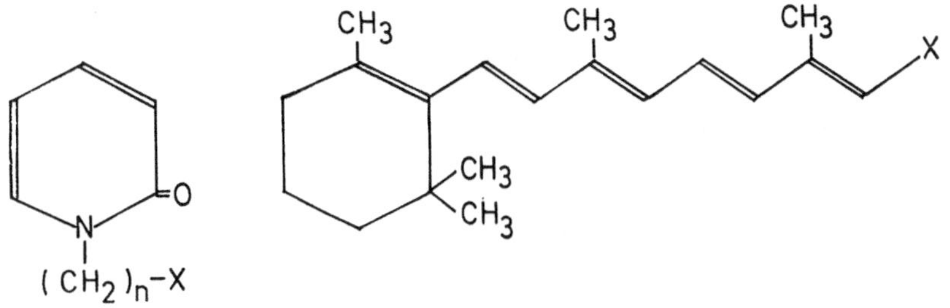

Fig. 5

121

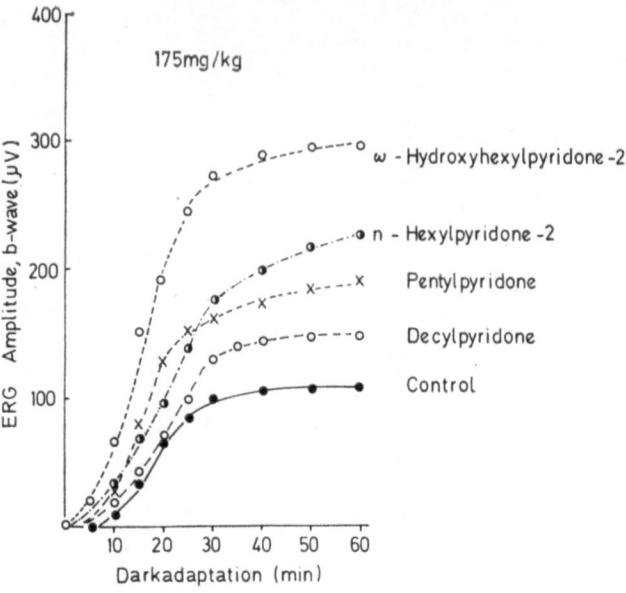

Fig. 6

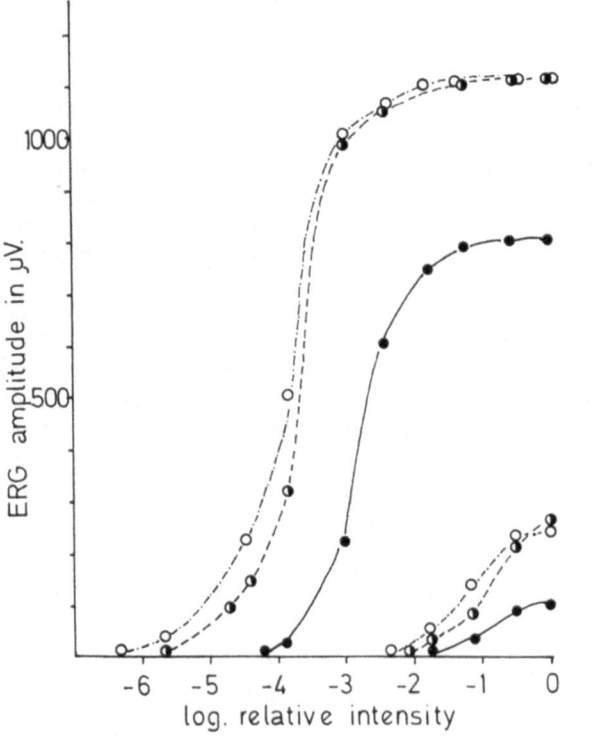

Fig. 7. ● Vit. A less
◑ Vit. A
○ Vit. A less + Analogue

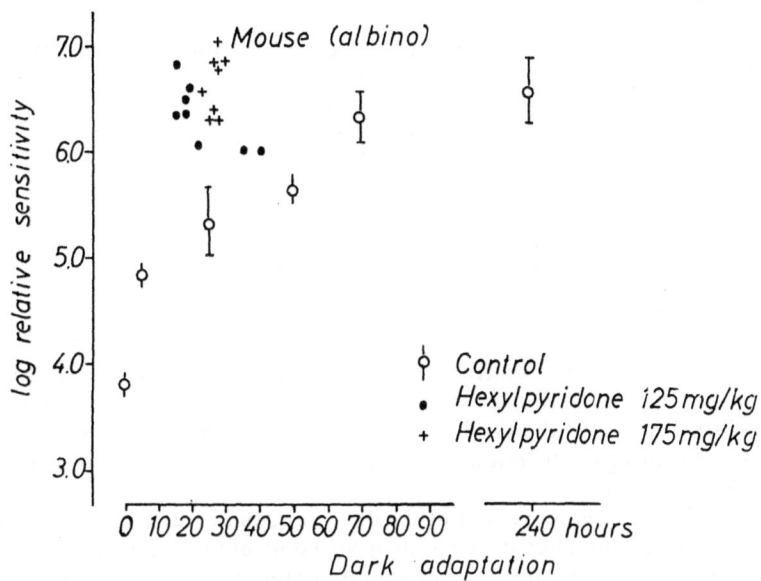

Fig. 8

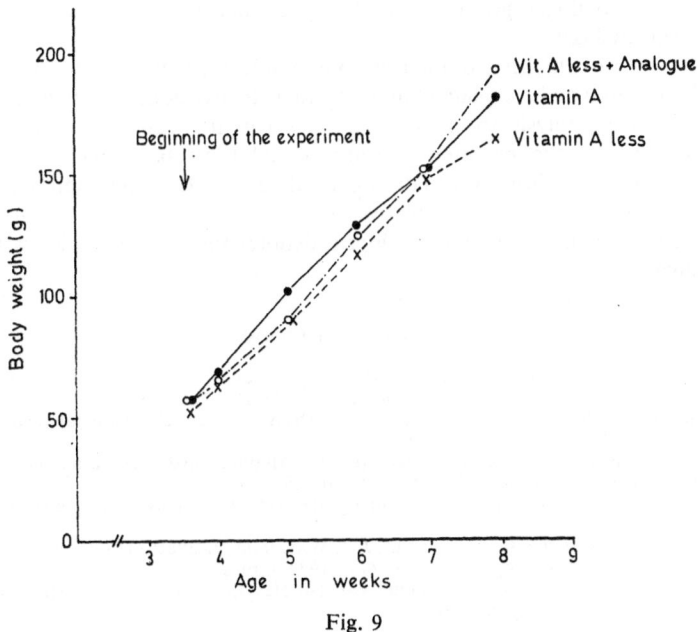

Fig. 9

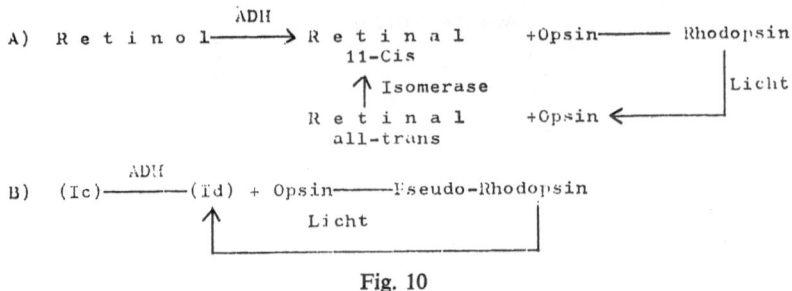

Fig. 10

threshold of b-wave is decreased by 2 log. units, as compared with the vit. A-supplemented ones. In these deficient animals the maximum b-wave amplitude is also reduced. In the third group of vit. A-deficient animals supplemented with the analogue, the threshold, as compared to that of the vit. A animals, is at least normal.

A still clearer improvement of the dark threshold is recorded in mice which were not fed, but injected with a single high dose of the analogue (Fig. 8). This activity is lost 70 h after the injection indicating that the analogue then gets replaced by vit. A.

In the previously mentioned dietary experiment with rats, the growth curve reveals that ω-hydroxyhexylpyridone-2 can also substitute for vit. A as growth factor (Fig. 9). According to the present status of this experiment, the growth rate in the analogue group is slightly higher than that observed in the vit. A supplemented one.

The superior efficiency of the new compounds in comparison to that of vit. A in rhodopsin may be explained in a way that the pyridone aldehyde derivatives after their photolysis from opsin-complex can immediately recombine with opsin, whereas the resulting all-trans retinal must be isomerised to 11-cis configuration first (Fig. 10). In this figure, the Ic and Id designations correspond to alcohol and aldehyde derivatives of the *in vivo* active N-alkylpyridones respectively, whereas pseudo-rhodopsin denotes the opsin complex with these aldehydes.

REFERENCES

BLISS, A. F. The equilibrium between vitamin A alcohol and aldehyde in the presence of alcohol dehydrogenase. *Arch. Biochem. Biophys.* 31:*197–204* (1951).

GAURI, K. K. N-alkylsubstituierte pyridon-2-Derivate. Deutsche Patentanmeldung M/11 435 (1971).

———. N-Alkyl-2-Pyridone als Aktivatoren der Alkoholdehydrogenase aus pferdeleber in vitro. Archiv d. Pharmazie; (submitted for publication)

———ω-Hydroxyalkylpyridone-2 als Analoga des Retinols. Archiv d. Pharmazie; (submitted for publication).

GAURI, K. K., HELLNER, K. A., RICKERS, J. & WATANABE, J. Effect of N-Hexylpyridone-2 on the Mouse Electroretinogram. *Ophth. Res.* (1972 in press).

GAURI, K. K. & KRISTAHN, M. Einfluß von 1-n-Hexylpyridon-2 auf die Alkoholdehydrogenase (ADH). (in preparation).

IS THE EOG INFLUENCED BY NICOTINE?
RELATIONS TO THE EEG*

P. HOCHGESAND, H. RIEGER & K. H. SCHICKETANZ**

(*Mainz*)

Cigarette smoking causes a number of effects in the human body, not the least of which may be attributed to nicotine. The problem under investigation is whether, by smoking retinal activity is influenced, and whether measureable changes are found by electrophysiological testing.

After smoking green American tobacco, spasms of retinal arteries with retinal bleeding was observed. In the first ten minutes after cigarette smoking HEIMBÖCK found a vasoconstriction of the fundus vessels. Strong smokers produced crystal clear degeneration spots of the posterior pole (HAGER), which are considered a consequence of circulation disturbance. According to HOLLWICH, nicotine in conjunction with the functional spasm found in hypertension, arteriosclerosis, and central vein occlusion plays a pathogenic role. Besides the nicotine effect on the nervous system, blood circulation, metabolism of the retina, and the intraocular circulation, it may also have a sclerosing influence. Aortic arteriosclerosis is more pronounced in smokers (WAHL & SCHLETTLER). However, a true relationship between smoking and arteriosclerosis is not yet proven.

It is known that cigarette smoking mainly causes b-wave changes in the ERG. As far as changes in the resting potential are concerned, there are only a few partially contradictory notes in literature: After smoking two filterless cigarettes, SCHMIDT found a statistically significant decrease in the first eight minutes of the dark-period of the EOG. She recorded two EOG's at ten minute intervals, the test subjects smoked during break. Furthermore, she noticed an increase of the ARDEN-ratio by 16.2 and related these changes to a nicotine effect.

On the other side, HAASE & MUELLER observed a marked decrease in the dark-period of the second EOG without nicotine and supposed a physiological regulatory process in the resting potential to be involved. They also recorded the EOG on different days with and without nicotine and determined that the dark-period had decreased after smoking. The latter was not considered statistically significant. In total, they could not prove a truly significant influence of cigarette smoking on the EOG. Therefore, another study was carried out to determine to what degree the mentioned changes were real effects related to smoking, or physiological effects in the oscillatory course of the EOG, and whether there would be parallel changes in the EEG.

* Supported by the Deutsche Forschungsgemeinschaft.
** From the Eye Clinic of the University of Mainz (Director: PROF. DR. A. NOVER), the Neuro-Psychiatric Clinic of the University of Mainz (Director: PROF. DR. U. H. PETERS) and the Institute for Medical Statistics and Documentation of the University of Mainz (Director: PROF. DR. S. KOLLER).

Ten male and seven female subjects were tested twice with each eye at ten minute intervals. The population ranged in age from 32 to 43 years. The test-subjects had no eye disease, except ametropias. Ten persons smoked during the break, seven didn't. Records were taken between 8 and 10 a.m. Beckman's skin electrodes were placed within 10 mm of each lateral and medial canthus. DC-amplification (Tönnies) was used. To avoid a baseline change through DC-drift at the electrodes, the baseline was kept at a constant value by automatic feed-back of the working point. Potentials were recorded on paper moving at a rate of 1 cm/min. The spikes of the EOG-trace were measured with an optical lens.

After placing the electrodes, the subject carried out eye-movement in the two dark-periods (12 min. each) and the light-periods (also 12 min. each) at a constant angle of 35°. These eye movements are controlled by two alternatingly energizing flashlight-bulbs, luminating in a ten second cycle (8 sec. right, 2 sec. left). Figure 1 shows the original records of a test-subject without smoking in the break, Fig. 2, the record of a smoking person.

Simultaneously, the EEG was recorded on both hemispheres with bipolar parieto-occipital leads on two channels and registered on magnetic tape.

Results

In the evaluation-process, the following parameters were considered (Fig. 3): Amplitude-height of the dark-period at the beginning of the test, expressed as a mean-value of the amplitude-height during the second minute; dark-trough and time to reach that point; amplitude-height at the beginning of the light-period (also calculated as mean-value of the amplitude-height during the second minute), light-peak and time to reach that point; and additionally the Arden-ratio. For the second EOG, the same parameters were used.

To reduce the effect of artifacts, a moving average was done with a width of three to five spikes. Empirically, a width of four spikes was most convenient.

Assuming an equal behaviour of both eyes in the EOG, the evaluation was based exclusively on the values of the right eye. When evaluating, the changes of the parameters in the first and second EOG, separated for the two groups, are considered: In comparison of the amplitude-height of the dark-begin in both periods, there is a potential-decrease in the non-smoking group in the second period, with an average 0.26 millivolt. The t-test for the paired observations confirmed this significant low begin (Fig. 4). In the smoking-group there is also a low begin to be observed, i.e. 0.06 millivolt. The related t-test for paired observations, however, was not significant. Between group-comparison in the t-test for unpaired observations there is also a statistically significant test-value, so that a systematic difference between smoking and non-smoking persons is supposed.

Comparing the amplitude-height of dark-trough I and II, non-smoking persons showed an average decrease of 0.06 millivolt, smoking ones an increase of 0.06 millivolt. These changes in the t-test cannot be valued significantly in both groups. There was also no significance in group-comparison regarding the

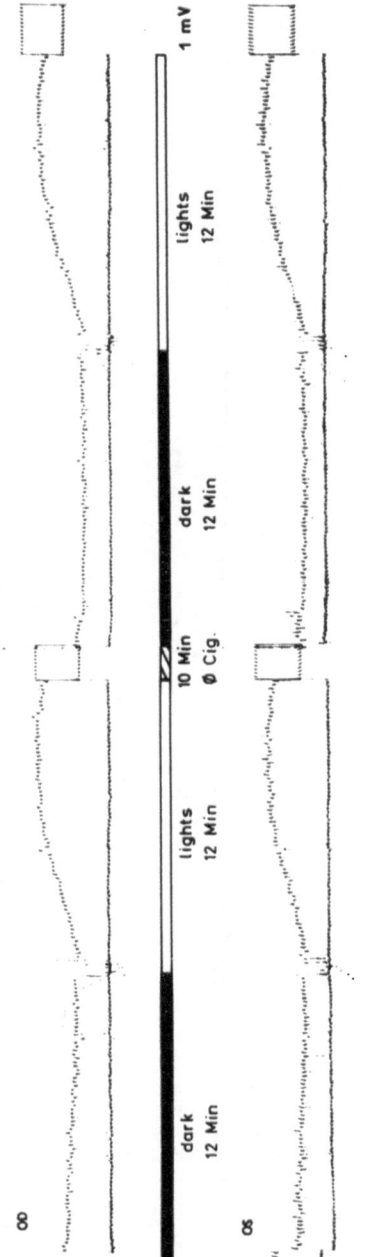

Fig. 1. Original-records of the right (above) and the left (below) eye of a test-subject that didn't smoke during the break. The potential decrease of the second EOG during the first minutes of the dark-period is obvious.

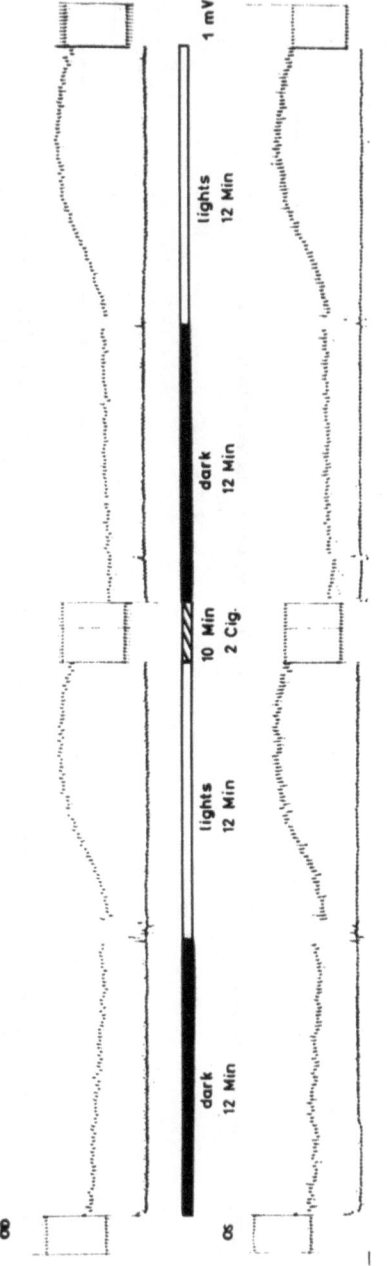

Fig. 2. Original-records of a test-subject, that had smoked during the break. The potential decrease in the dark-period of the second EOG is obvious, too.

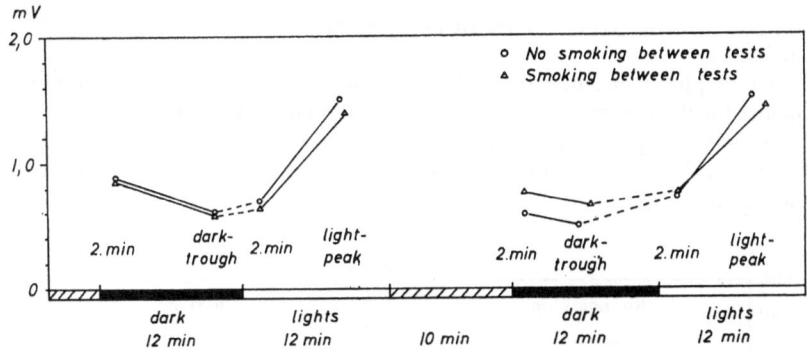

Fig. 3. Mean values of the parameters considered in the first and second EOG, smoking and non-smoking persons separated. In both groups potential-decrease during the second dark-period; non-smoking persons more, smoking persons less.

given differences. However, it should be mentioned that a decrease of the dark-trough in the non-smoking group can be observed against an increase of the same value in the smoking-group.

Looking at the time from test-beginning to dark-trough, we find that the latter was reached in the non-smoking group in the second period by an average of 281 seconds earlier than in the first period, and 185 seconds for the smoking group. In the t-test this time-difference was significant for the non-smoking, not

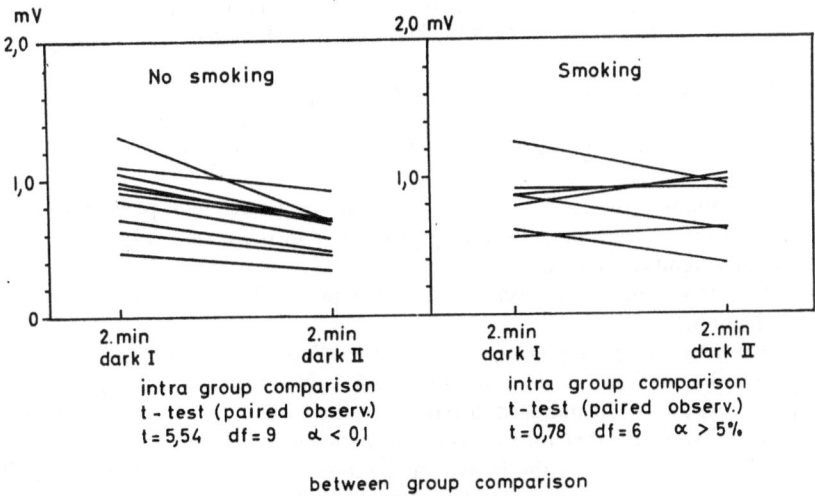

Fig. 4. Comparison of the dark-begin between first and second period and between smoking and non-smoking subjects.

129

for the smoking group. Between group-comparison there was no significant difference.

The amplitude-height at the beginning of the light-period II was 0.075 millivolts higher for the non-smoking subjects, and 0.08 millivolt for the smoking group, as against the light-period I. However, in the smoking group the increase in the t-test was significant. As expected, the t-test between group-comparison showed no significance.

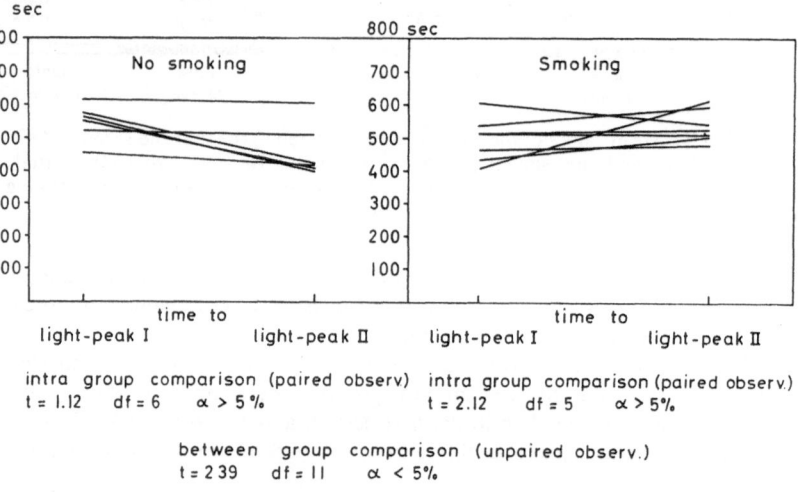

intra group comparison (paired observ) intra group comparison (paired observ.)
t = 1.12   df = 6   α > 5%   t = 2.12   df = 5   α > 5%

between group comparison (unpaired observ.)
t = 2.39   df = 11   α < 5%

Fig. 5. Comparison of the time to the light-peak between first and second period and between smoking and non-smoking subjects.

Regarding the non-smoking group, the light-peak II rose from the light-peak I at an average rate of 0.065, and regarding the smoking group 0.02, i.e. significant for the smoking group in the t-test. No significance between group-comparison.

In evaluating the time needed to reach the respective light-peak, the results showed that neither in the smoking group nor in the no-smoking group there was any significance (Fig. 5).

All t-tests carried out were based on a probability of error of <5% for evaluation.

For the non-smoking group in the first EOG the ARDEN-ratio was 262 ± 62 standard deviation, in the second EOG 298 ± 45; for the smoking group in the first EOG 238 ± 60 standard deviation, in the second 259 ± 72. No difference could be verified either for the groups *or between in number of cases*.

Above we compared the individual periods and groups; now we are going to study the results of correlation statistical investigations: In the smoking group we got a number of correlations differing statistically significant from zero, which can be mainly interpreted as curve-effects. Part of the correlation matrices, which were calculated separately for each group, and considered

130

particularly interesting, are shown in Fig. 6, and compared. It should be noted, that the correlation with a given variable, i.e. light-peak I and any other amplitude-parameters resulted in regularly high significantly positive significance in the non-smoking group; there is none in the smoking group, and, moreover, nearly all significances turn into negative correlations.

But it should be emphasized, that the correlation-coefficients in the smoking group with a view to the relatively low number of cases are no more differing

correlated variables		No smoking			Smoking		
		correlation coefficient	n	significant: + (α < 5%) not significant: -	correlation coefficient	n	significant: + (α < 5%) not significant: -
LP II with	DB I	0,96	6	+	- 0,62	7	-
	DT I	0,86	6	+	- 0,47	7	-
	DB II	0,99	6	+	0,05	7	-
	DT II	0,97	6	+	0,01	7	-
	LB I	0,84	6	+	-0,34	7	-
	LP I	0,99	6	+	- 0,11	7	-

Correlations coefficients between LP II (light-peak II) and other amplitude variables

DB I = dark begin I   DT I = dark - trough I
DB II = dark begin II   DT II = dark - trough II
LB I = light begin I   LP I = light - peak I

Fig. 6. Correlation coefficients between LP II (light-peak II) and other amplitude variables. DB I = dark-begin I, DT I = dark-trough I, DB II = dark-begin II, DT II = dark-trough II, LP I = light-begin I, LP I = light-peak I.

significantly from zero. Nevertheless, this relationship seems to document a systematic influence.

In evaluating the EEG, it is of interest, that the recording conditions with open eyes and rhythmic horizontal eye-movements differ very much from the usual EEG recording. However, there is a more or less distinct basic rhythm, mainly in the alpha-band. Even with the best recording technique, rhythmic ocular artifacts in the EEG cannot be completely avoided.

The visual EEG-evaluation showed no pathological changes in any test-subject, only the usual variability of the normal EEG. Due to the recording of eyes open, flat tracings were relatively frequent. In the test-course no systematically visible changes were found, in particular no pathological slowings or other anomalies in any case after cigarette smoking. That's why automatic methods were used for a more precise analyses of EEG; Amplitude-histograms as well as interval-histograms of the recorded EEG were done after AD-transformation.

The amplitude-histography divides the measured EEG-amplitudes into 1024 amplitude-classes. The result obtained with this method allows one to describe the amplitude-distribution of the EEG by one single number, i.e. the standard deviation. Fig. 7 shows such an amplitude-histogram with the cumulated

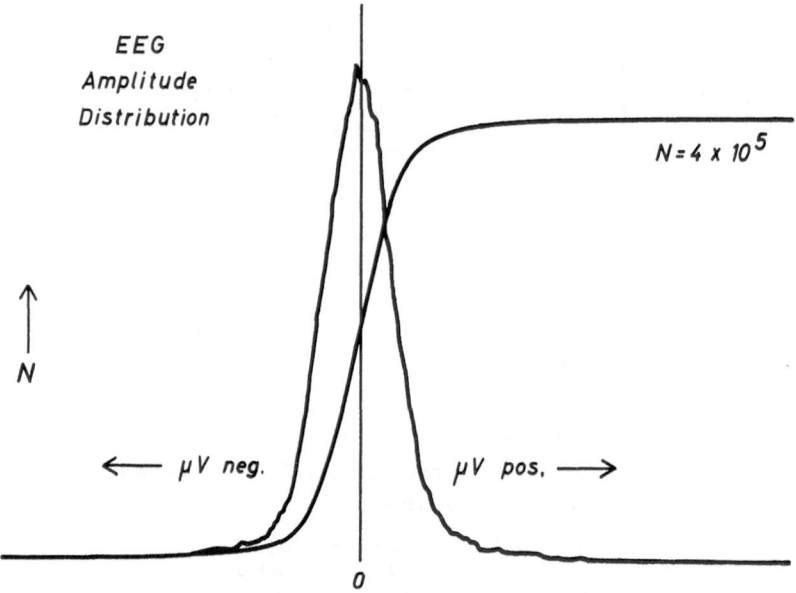

Fig. 7. Amplitude-histogram in the first light-period of the left hemisphere-EEG of a smoking subject. The distribution-function shows the number of the different amplitude-classes; high amplitudes lie at both extremities of the distribution. The mean-value in the EEG is always zero and corresponds to the maximum of the graph. The s-shaped curve shows the cumulated distribution. The time of analyses is always 160 sec.

distribution. This method of measurement reveals no significant inter- and intra-individual differences in the above described comparisons. Due to the large intra- and interindividual variability and the small number of test-subjects, no perceptible difference between smoking and non-smoking persons can be seen.

The interval-histography measures the frequency-composition of the EEG and can show relative acceleration or slowing of the waves. The time between two zero-line-crossings is measured and these intervals are distributed into 256 classes. The time-resolution is 2 msec. Fig. 8 gives an example of an interval-distribution. This distribution was transformed in the usual frequency-ranges and the number of waves in the beta-, alpha-, theta- and delta-band was calculated.

132

The test-course reveals an increase of the physiological alpha- and beta-activities during the second light-period in the non-smoking group. This increase is also perceptible after cigarette-smoking, however at a lower degree (Fig. 9). The increase from the first dark-period to the second light-period in this frequency-band is 23.2% in the non-smoking group, after smoking only 6.9%.

DISCUSSION

The resting potential originates mainly in the outer retinal layers and the pigment epithelium with part of the choroidal vessels. However, the origin and the light

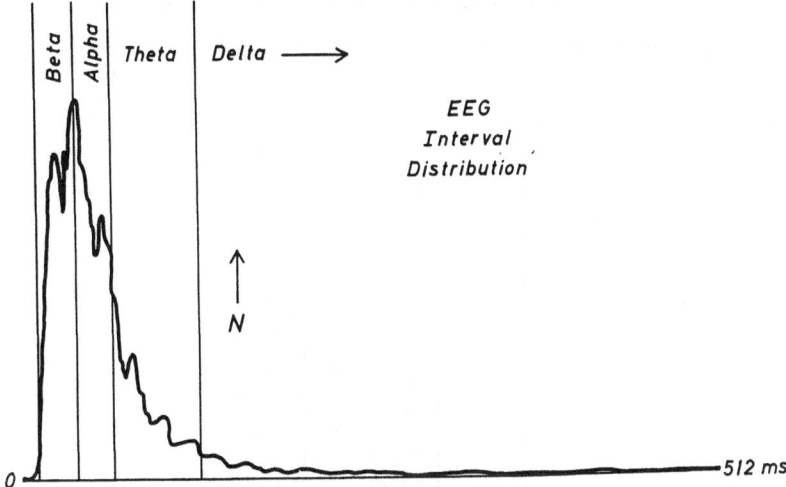

Fig. 8. The right hemisphere interval-histogram of a smoking subject in the second light-period. The curve shows the usual irregular distribution with maxima and minima within the physiological frequency-bands with a rather high amount of rapid rhythms in the beta-band, presumably due to open eyes.

dependent changes of the resting potential are not well understood. Since the studies of KOLDER we know that the resting potential underlies a physiological regulatory process in the form of a damped oscillation. Several attempts were made to express the potential-oscillations by mathematical or empirical equations (HOMER & KOLDER, KOLDER & HOCHGESAND).

Our study also shows such a regulatory process, i.e. the reciprocal influence of dark-period and light-period: that means, the correlation of a variable, for example, light-peak I to any amplitude-parameter show highly significant positive significances in the non-smoking group. On the other hand there are no significances in the smoking group, and nearly all turn out to be negative correlations.

Group comparison regarding the amplitude-height of dark-begin shows statistically significant test-value in both periods; therefore, a systematic difference between smoking and non-smoking persons may be assumed. It is supposed, that the oscillation-system of the resting potential is influenced by cigarette smoking.

Regarding the small number of test-persons it has to be emphasized, that the result of the statistical test is not sufficient to be the basis for a systematic interpretation. However, the mentioned differences, partly statistically significant, seem to prove, that there is a true influence of cigarette smoking on the EOG.

As expected, no visible or pathologic changes were observed in the EEG under the relatively low nicotine dosage. The automatic methods of analysis

α- and β-activity of the EEG.

Difference between test-end and test-begin.

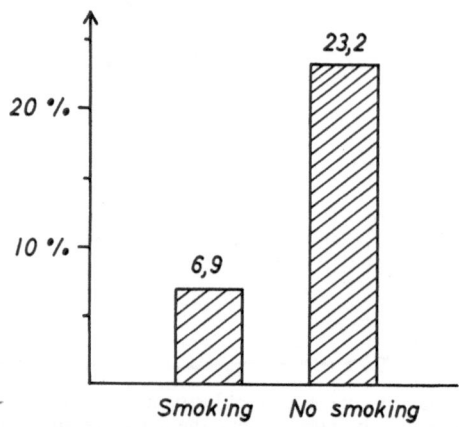

Fig. 9. Alpha- and beta-activity in the EEG. Difference between test-end and test-beginning non-smoking persons show a high increase. Average values of each group.

equally show only discrete systematic differences attributable to smoking. It is of interest, that the test-person has to adapt to the experimental conditions. The increase of physiological alpha- and beta-waves towards the end of the test suggests, that this adaptation is easier without smoking. This effect of relaxation seems to occur at a far lower degree in the smoking group.

This more psychological than pharmacological interpretation corresponds to the one of the BICKFORD-Group (HAUSER et al.), who observed a similar frequency-modification under the influence of smoking. Due to the different origins of EOG and EEG, and due to the completely different frequency-characteristics of these signals, it is impossible to establish direct correlations, which can be referred to the same basic process. Consequently, there was no result in cross-correlation-analyses, especially adapted to the rhythm of the EOG.

Smoking and non-smoking test-persons showed, however, a parallelism in the course of EEG and EOG during the second test-period.

134

SUMMARY

Two groups of volunteers having no eye disease were examined electro-oculographically twice at ten minute intervals. One group smoked in the break, one didn't.

In the non-smoking group there are a number of significant correlations between the tested parameters in the dark-period and in the light-period, which could not be found to the same degree in the smoking group. The fact that there were differences between the two groups—even though not interpretable systematically—suggests, that smoking influences physiological processes in the EOG.

In the second period of the test, a parallelism in the course of EOG and EEG was observed, the EEG-changes, however, are interpreted more psychologically than pharmacologically.

REFERENCES

HAASE, E. & MUELLER, W. Meßbare Beeinflussung des EOG durch Zigarettenrauchen? *Klin. Mbl. Augenhk.* Bd. 158:*677* (1971).

HAGER, H. Thrombangiitis obliterans und Auge. *Klin. Mbl. Augenhk.* Bd. 114:*238* (1949).

HAUSER, H., SCHWARZE, B. E., ROTH, G. & BICKFORD, R. G. Electroencephalographic changes related to smoking. *EEG clin. Neurophysiol.* Vol. 10:*576P* (1958).

HEIMBÖCK. *Wien. klin. Wschr. Bd.* 73:*529* (1961).

HOLLWICH, F., JÜNEMANN, G. & DAMASKE, E. Auge. In: Nikotin. Edited by Schievelbein. H. Georg Thieme Verlag, Stuttgart (1968).

HOMER, L. D. & KOLDER, H. Mathematical model of oscillations in human corneo-retinal potential. *Pflügers Arch. ges. Physiol.* 287:*197* (1966).

KOLDER H. Spontane und experimentelle Änderungen des Bestandpotentials des menschlichen Auges. *Pflügerrs Arch. ges. Physiol.* 268:*258* (1959).

KOLDER, H. E. & HOCHGESAND, P. Empirical Model of Electro-Oculogram. *Doc. Ophthal.* (1972) in press.

SCHMIDT, B. Einfluß des Zigarettenrauchens aud das EOG. *Klin. Mbl. Augenhk.* Bd. 156:*523* (1970).

WAHL, P. & SCHETTLER, G. Arteriosklerose und Fettstoffwechsel. In: Nikotin. Edited by Schievelbein. H. Georg Thieme Verlag, Stuttgart (1968).

135

LOCALIZATION STUDIES OF THE HUMAN VISUAL EVOKED RESPONSE*

WILLIAM R. BIERSDORF & ZENJU NAKAMURA**

Recent research has shown it possible to distinguish visual evoked responses from stimulation of the left and right half visual fields (REGAN & HERON, 1969; COBB & MORTON, 1970). The objectives of the present studies have been to identify components of the VER related to stimulation of the lateral halves of the visual field and to localize their brain origin. The approach has been by obtaining detailed spatial potential contour maps of the posterior scalp from multiple electrode placements. Previous reports have shown waveform differences over the two cerebral hemispheres from blank flash stimulation of the two lateral half-fields (BIERSDORF & NAKAMURA, 1971; NAKAMURA & BIERSDORF, 1971). The aim of the present study is to compare the VER's produced by patterned flash stimulation of the lateral half-fields.

The subject was maintained in a light-adapted condition with a 50 cm diameter hemisphere illuminated with white light at a level of 100 ft-L. The stimulus field was one-half of a 15° disc containing alternate opaque and clear checks each subtending 15 minutes at a fixation distance of 50 cm. The checkerboard was illuminated from behind through a red filter (Corning 2412) by a xenon flash lamp. The photic stimulator was enclosed in a sound-shielded box, and masking noise provided by a ventilating fan on the shielded recording enclosure made the clicks inaudible. The subject maintained fixation at the center of the vertical edge of the stimulus field or at other locations as specified.

Standard EEG electrodes (5 mm in diameter) of chlorided silver were attached to the scalp with electrode paste following the International 10-20 EEG system with interpolations. Monopolar recording was generally employed with the tip of the nose as the negative electrode, and a ground on the forehead at the midline. Ten channels were recorded simultaneously with a four channel signal averager (Fabri-Tek 1052) and an FM tape recorder. Responses were recorded on an X-Y plotter. For the potential contour mapping, ten electrode positions clustered around the occipital pole were recorded first. Then a second recording covered ten electrode positions on the periphery of the first, with certain positions repeated for reliability.

Stimulation consisted of the red checkerboard pattern flashing at the rate of 3.3 Hz for a summation of 256 flashes. Various flash intensities were investigated. Stimulation was monocular, with the other eye covered by an opaque black eye patch.

Representative evoked responses are presented in Fig. 1 from left and right half-field stimulation with subject fixation at the center of the vertical edge of

* This research was supported in part by USPHS Research Grant No. EY00454.
** From the Ohio State University and the Tokyo Medical & Dental University.

the stimulus. For right half-field stimulation over the left hemisphere (T_5, TO_5) a prominent positive deflection appeared at 84 msec which was replaced by a negative deflection recorded over the right hemisphere (TO_6, T_6). For left half-field stimulation the responses were inverted in polarity. Similar relations held for the next deflection of the VER occurring at 150 msec. These responses are consistent with the contralateral representation of the visual field at the visual cortex.

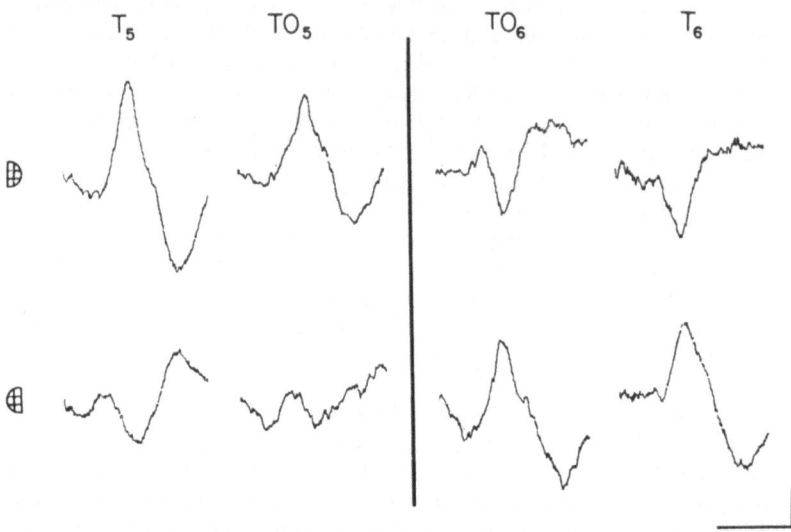

Fig. 1. Visual evoked responses from stimulation of right visual field (upper row) and left visual field (lower row) 15° half-disc. T_5 and TO_5 are electrodes over the left occipital scalp, with TO_6 and T_6 over the right scalp. Positive potentials are upward deflections. Calibration: 2 microvolts, 100 msec.

To obtain spatial potential maps of the VER, amplitudes of the components were measured peak-to-peak at constant latencies from all 17 electrode locations on the posterior scalp. The type of map obtained is represented in Fig. 2 for the full lateral-half field stimulus (one-half 15° disc). For the right half-field, a maximum positive potential occurred over the left hemisphere about half way between the occipital pole and the ear, with a negative maximum at a similar position over the right hemisphere. There is a zero crossing (represented by the dotted line) near the midline. For the left half-field, the map is reversed with the positive maximum potential now occurring over the right hemisphere. These maps were obtained for the 84 msec VER component. Similar maps were obtained for the following 150 msec component with accompanying polarity reversal. The mapping seems to be relatively independent of which eye is stimulated with similar distributions obtained for right and left eyes. Similar maps were also obtained with intensity settings of the photic stimulator from I-1 to I-16.

138

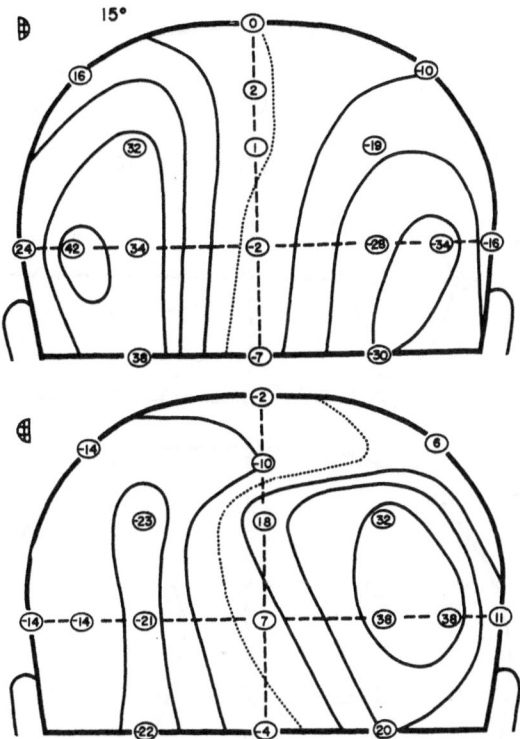

Fig. 2. Posterior scalp view of the potential distributions for the 84 msec peak. Subject C, right eye stimulation for right (upper plot) and left (lower plot half disc (15°). Electrode location at the bottom midline is the inion. Moving up are electrodes at 10% distance (O_z), 20%, 30% (P_z), and 50% (C_z). Moving left horizontally from O_z are electrodes at 15% distance (TO_5), 30% (T_z), and 50% (T_3). Also shown in the upper left quadrants are electrodes P_3 and C_3. Directly below the first electrode to the left of O_z is one on line horizontally with the inion. Similar positions are recorded on the right hemisphere (evennumbered). Potentials are microvolts × 10.

These potential distributions have been obtained with relatively large macular fields, but basically similar distributions are obtained for foveal sized fields (1° × 2° half-disc) as seen in Fig. 3. Again, we have a positive maximum for the 84 msec component over the left hemisphere for the right half-field, and the opposite result for the left half-field. The main difference for the smaller stimulus is the much smaller amplitude of the VER. There is also a tilt of the axis of the voltage distribution away from the nearly horizontal axis found with the larger stimulus. A tilt was also found for the blank field lateral half stimulation previously reported (BIERSDORF & NAKAMURA, 1971; NAKAMURA & BIERSDORF, 1971). The retinal area contributed to by these VER's apparently includes both the fovea and parafovea.

139

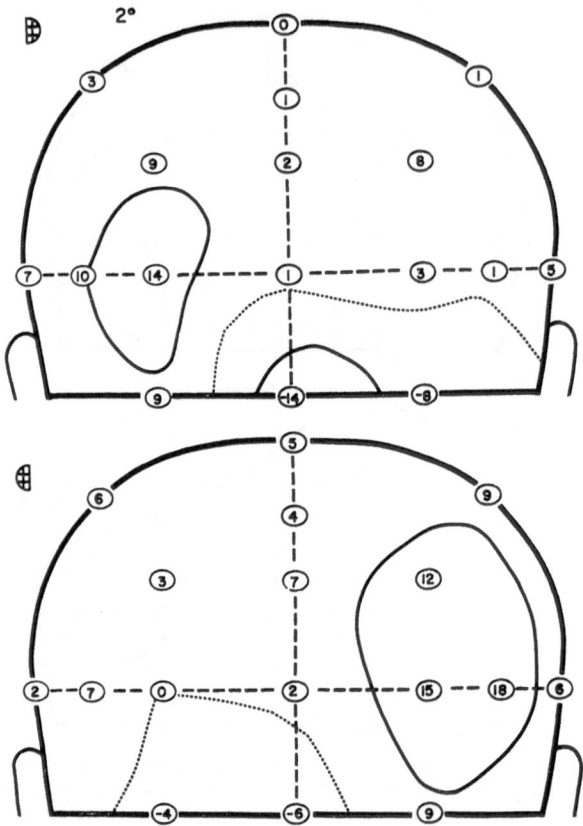

Fig. 3. Posterior scalp view of the potential distributions for the 84 msec peak, right and left half disc (2°). Other conditions, and electrode positions same as previous figure.

This question was further explored by using the large (15° diameter) half-disc and moving fixation away from the vertical edge of the stimulus. Fig. 4 shows the type of results obtained by moving fixation perpendicularly away from the edge of the left half-field. This graph is a cross-section of the previous potential contour map. Potentials shown are from a horizontal line of electrodes running through O_z, which is near the presumed location of the occipital pole. Large differences between the two sides of the head are obtained for fixation at the edge of the stimulus or 1°–2° off the edge, thereafter falling to low values for 5°–10°.

Fig. 5 illustrates the results obtained by moving fixation away from the edge of the right half-field. Differences between the two sides of the head drop rapidly with some difference still at 5° off the edge. These differences were absent at 10°. This type of result also indicates that the response comes from both fovea and parafoveal retina.

140

The question naturally arises as to where in the brain these visual evoked responses are generated. With the type of data represented here, we can start to answer this question. These voltage distributions can be related to the concept of a potential dipole which has been used to localize electrical sources in the heart and more recently in the brain. Two main types of potential distributions are those generated by a dipole source either tangential, or radial to the surface

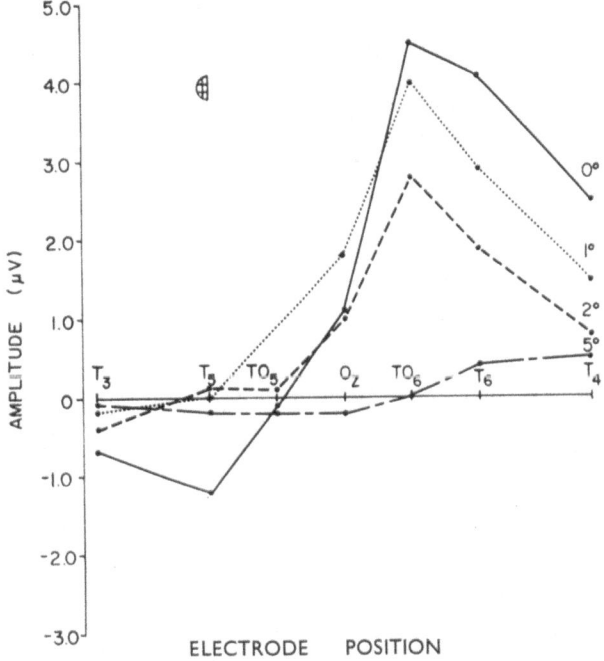

Fig. 4. Monopolar potentials for 84 msec peak at electrode positions along the horizontal line through O_z. Parameter: distance of fixation perpendicular to the center of the vertical edge of the left half-field (15°).

of a sphere, by which the head can be represented. A single dipole source radial to the surface produces a potential maximum at the surface over the source with potentials decreasing smoothly in all directions from this point. On the other hand, a single dipole tangential to the surface produces two potential maximum at the surface (one negative, and one positive) along a line parallel to the dipole axis. For example the voltage distribution at 0° in Fig. 5 can be represented by a single dipole with the positive end pointing left and the negative end pointing right. This dipole would be located somewhere near O_z and the occipital pole. All of the responses, maps, and graphs illustrated thus far have been obtained with monopolar recording. For precise EEG localization studies, bipolar recording has traditionally been used. In Fig. 6, bipolar recording has been made from the same horizontal row of electrodes. Both left and right

141

half-fields at 0° (stimulus edge) are presented. The shape of the expected voltage distributions is changed for bipolar recording, with a tangential dipole now producing a single maxima on the surface over the dipole. From this data, it is clear that the dipole is located in the correct (contralateral) hemisphere for each half-field. The right half-field dipole source is represented a short distance left of the occipital pole, while the left half-field source is located to the right of

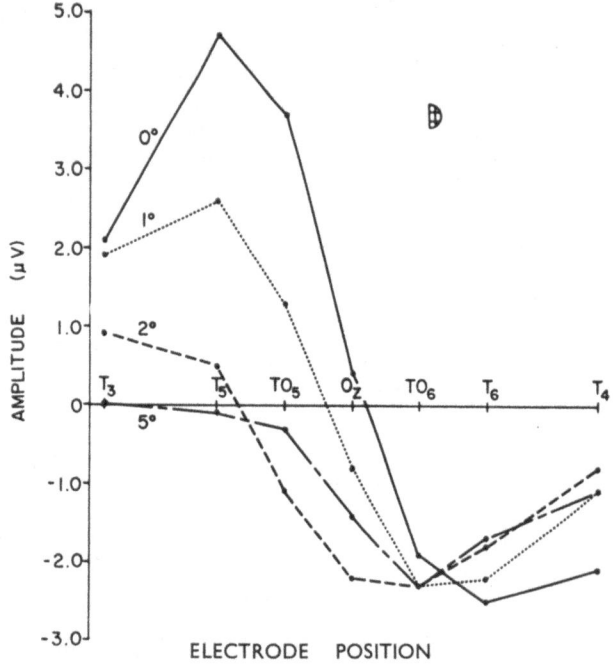

Fig. 5. Monopolar potentials for 84 msec peak at electrode positions along the horizontal line through O_z. Parameter: distance of fixation perpendicular to the centre of the vertical edge of the right half-field (15°).

the occipital pole. The distributions are not perfectly symmetrical, indicating that the dipoles are not completely tangential, but are tilted slightly toward the surface of the scalp.

The scalp potential distributions of these evoked responses to half-field stimulation suggest that these early components are generated in primary visual cortex. The single dipole is equivalent to a sheet of tiny dipoles all oriented in the same direction. These dipole sheets are probably located on the medial surfaces of the hemispheres normal to the surface in the median longitudinal fissure. Each visual half-field would be located on the medial surface of the contralateral hemisphere. It is expected that excitation on the upper and lower banks of the calcarine fissure would tend to cancel each other out at the scalp surface as each stimulus excites both upper and lower half visual fields. The

142

results from changing fixation indicate that excitation in the calcarine fissure probably does not contribute to these responses. Moving fixation away from the edge of the lateral half-field does not change the locus of the equivalent dipole as might be expected if calcarine excitation were contributory. This model has similarities to one proposed by Vaughan (1969) except that the model is here applied to foveal and parafoveal stimulation of retinal cones.

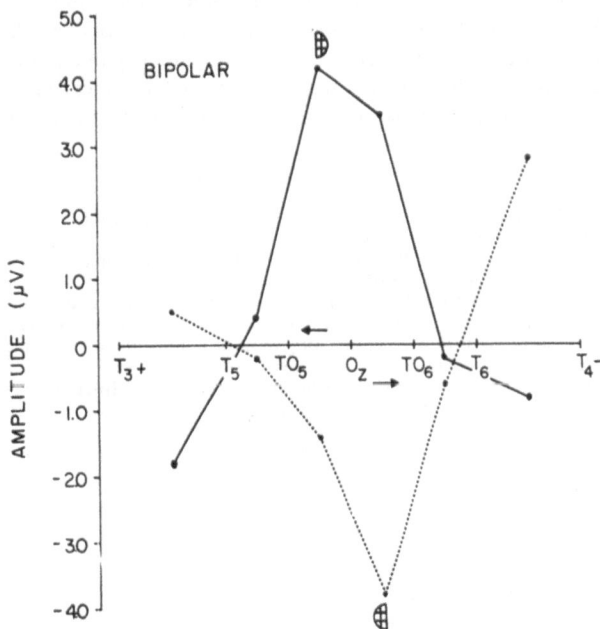

Fig. 6. Bipolar potentials for 84 msec peak at electrode positions along the horizontal line through O_z. For each electrode pair, the left one is positive. Right half-field is solid line, left half-field is dotted line. Arrows indicate approximate location laterally of postulated dipole sources. 15° half-discs.

These results compare quite well with results from blank half-field stimulation previously reported (BIERSDORF & NAKAMURA, 1971; NAKAMURA & BIERSDORF, 1971). The main difference is in the VER waveform. The blank response is quite complex. The check waveform is a simplified response with fewer peaks. The peak latencies are longer for the check VER with a latency to the first large peak of 84 msec compared to the blank VER peak latency of 74 msec under the same conditions. Scalp localization is correct for lateral half-field blank stimulation for peaks at 74 and 96 msec, but fails at 112 msec when either half produces a similar maximum near the occipital pole (NAKAMURA & BIERSDORF, 1971). Localization is correct for a longer time with the checkerboard VER including peaks at 84 and 150 msec.

The potential contour maps for both blank and check VER's are similar in showing tangential dipoles located over the correct (contralateral) hemispheres.

143

The large blank flash half-field dipole axes showed more tilt with the horizontal plane (NAKAMURA & BIERSDORF, 1971) than did the checkerboard half-fields for the present subject.

In summary, potential contour mapping of the posterior scalp has been utilized to study visual evoked responses to lateral half-field stimulation. The stimulus was a flashed checkerboard half-disc presented in a light-adapted surround of 100 ft-L. Both monopolar and bipolar recording have been used to show that each half-field is represented on the scalp over the contralateral hemisphere for early components of the VER. Intensity of stimulation, field size, and eye stimulated had no or minor effects on this localization. A model is presented postulating the sources of these early VER components in primary visual cortex.

REFERENCES

BIERSDORF, W. R. & NAKAMURA, Z. Electroencephalogram potentials evoked by hemi-retinal stimulation. *Experientia* 27:402 (1971).

COBB, W. A. & MORTON, H. B. Evoked potentials from the human scalp to visual half-field stimulation. *J. Physiol.* 208:39-P (1970).

NAKAMURA, Z. & BIERSDORF, W. R. Localization of the human visual evoked response. Early components specific to visual stimulation. *Amer. J. Ophth.* 72:988 (1971).

REGAN, D. & HERON, J. R. Clinical investigation of lesions of the visual pathway: a new objective technique. *J. Neurol. Neurosurg. Psychiat.* 32:479 (1969).

VAUGHAN, H. G., JR. Human brain potentials and vision. In: International Ophthalmology Clinics 9, No. 4, 1969 (Ed. S. J. Fricker) p. 899.

COMPUTER PROCESSING OF THE
VISUAL EVOKED RESPONSE*

KARL J. FRITZ, JOHN STEINHOFF, ATSUKO HIRATA,
DAVID BUFFUM, GILBERT NG & ALBERT M. POTTS**

(*Chicago*)

ABSTRACT

One of the chief problems in making the visual evoked response (VER) a usable tool in the clinic and laboratory is the complex nature of the response itself. Signal averaging removes much noise but the remaining complex waveform requires further processing. We have studied three processing techniques which analyze the shape of the waveform as a whole. These are: projection of the waveform onto a vector space spanned by orthogonal functions; least squares fitting with non-linear functions of the parameters; and integration of the product of the waveform and a template function. These studies were motivated by our need for computer methods to characterize waveforms during the course of experiments.

Projection of waveforms onto a vector space spanned by orthogonal functions has been valuable for both smoothing and characterization of the responses. Once an expansion in orthogonal functions has been obtained for a group of similar waveforms, additional computation is done to find another set of basis vectors which provides a more rapidly convergent expansion. It is possible to characterize a waveform with as few as six coefficients using this method.

Least squares fitting with non-linear functions of the parameters allows selection of descriptive parameters with a simple physical interpretation. It has proved difficult to find a simple non-linear function which faithfully represents a VER over the entire time range: however, portions of a VER are well fit.

Integration of the product of a waveform and a template function can be done very rapidly. A set of such integrals provides a convenient method of characterizing waveforms whenever a representation of the waveform itself is not necessary.

Our experience indicates that either projection of waveforms on a vector space of orthogonal functions or integration of products of waveforms and template functions will provide sufficient speed and accuracy to characterize a waveform during an experiment.

INTRODUCTION

The complex waveforms of visual evoked responses have been analyzed by a variety of methods. Many of these methods employ some means of locating critical points such as maxima, minima, zeroes and inflection points of the original waveforms (CIGANEK, 1961; KOOI & BAGCHI, 1964; RIETVELD, 1963). Smoothing using various digital filters is also frequently performed before an attempt to locate critical points is made (BENNETT et al., 1971). Whereas the

* Supported in part by USPHS Grant Number EY 00212, from the National Eye Institute, National Institutes of Health, Bethesda, Maryland, by the L. L. Sinton Trust Research Grant and the Fight for Sight Grant-in-Aid No. G-482, Fight For Sight, Inc., New York, New York.
** From the Department of Ophthalmology, The Eye Research Laboratories, University of Chicago, 950 East 59th Street, Chicago, Illinois 60637.

145

location of critical points is an intuitively attractive method and may be done without extensive computing equipment, it is sensitive to random noise and the location of the critical points is subject to ambiguity. The ambiguity in location of critical points becomes particularly troublesome when automatic processing is used. Our laboratory is developing an apparatus for fully automated experiments. Decisions regarding the sequence of experimental steps and the timing of those steps will be programmed for a digital computer. Frequently these decisions will depend on recognition of certain aspects of waveforms by the computer. It was for this reason we began studying techniques which could specify the structure of a waveform by an analysis of the shape of the curve as a whole. Our experience with three of these techniques is reported here. These are: projection of the waveforms onto a vector space of orthogonal functions, fitting the waveform with non-linear functions of the fitting parameters, and integrating the product of normalized waveforms and template functions.

The most familiar example of waveform analysis using a vector space of orthogonal functions is Fourier analysis. Sines and cosines provide the basis of this vector space. Other sets of orthogonal functions which we have used include Chebychev and Legendre polynomials. Chebychev polynomials provide an optimum fit over the entire range of a curve. Legendre polynomials are the most easily evaluated of the orthogonal functions we have used. The expansions for a selected set of waveforms may be used to compute a new set of orthogonal functions. This new set of functions allows an efficient representation of waveforms similar to those in the selected set. A reasonable approximation to a visually evoked response may be made with as few as six terms. The expansion coefficients provide a parameterization of the response.

Non-linear fitting of the waveforms allows choosing parameters to represent quantities with a simple physical interpretation such as amplitudes, frequency and phase of the response. Our computational algorithm permits the investigator to check the non-linear fit of the curve when he makes the initial estimates of the parameters. When the fitting function approximates the original data with reasonable accuracy, the computation of the parameters to produce a best fit becomes automatic.

The integral of the product of a waveform and a template function can be computed very rapidly. The integrals provide a quantitative measure of the similarity of the shape of the waveform and the template function.

DATA ACQUISITION

The VER waveforms are recorded from scalp electrodes and amplified through several stages. After amplification the signals are either recorded on magnetic tape using frequency modulation for subsequent digitizing and analysis or are transmitted directly to a PDP-15 digital computer. The conversion to digital form is done at the computer every millisecond for one-half second durations with twenty-five points converted before the stimulus and four-hundred and seventy-five converted after the stimulus. Summation of one-hundred and fifty responses is done digitally. Preliminary processing which includes scaling

146

of summed responses to represent the original voltage at the scalp electrodes is done at the end of each set of one-hundred and fifty responses. The scaled values are then stored in digital form on magnetic tape where they are accessible for further analysis.

Two broad classes of stimuli were used in assembling the data for these studies. Red and white flashes of one millisecond duration and a variety of intensities and target sizes were used. The flashes occurred one second apart and the subject was given rest periods between the groups of one-hundred and fifty flashes. The second class of stimuli consisted of checkerboard patterns of alternating light and dark squares which simultaneously changed from light to dark and dark to light once each second (POTTS & HIRATA, in preparation). The time of the change was taken to be the stimulus time. Normal subjects and patients with eye disease were studied.

ORTHOGONAL FUNCTIONS

A set of functions

$$S = \{\phi_1, \phi_2, \ldots, \phi_n, \ldots\} \tag{1}$$

is said to be orthogonal with respect to a weighting function ω and a range of integration L if:

$$\int_L \phi_m(t)\phi_n(t)\omega(t)\,dt = 0 \qquad m \neq n \tag{2}$$

The orthogonal functions are said to be orthonormal if in addition,

$$\int_L \phi_n(t)\phi_n(t)\omega(t)\,dt = 1 \text{ for all } \phi_n \in S \tag{3}$$

A set of orthogonal functions is complete if for any piecewise continuous function ψ there exists a set of numbers $a_1, a_2, \ldots$ such that

$$\int_L \left(\psi(t) - \sum_{\phi_n \in S} a_n\phi_n(t)\right)^2 dt = 0 \tag{4}$$

There are many complete sets of orthonormal functions which are suitable for representation of evoked response waveforms. The most commonly used is the set of sines and cosines:

$$\sin \omega t, \sin 2\omega t, \ldots, \cos \omega t, \cos 2\omega t, \ldots \tag{5}$$

This set is orthogonal over the range R to $R + (2\pi/\omega)$ where R is any real number. The sum

$$\bar{\psi}(t) = a_0 + \sum_{m=1}^{\infty} a_m \cos(m\omega t) + b_m \sin(m\omega t) \tag{6}$$

is called the Fourier series representing ψ if $\psi(t) = \bar{\psi}(t)$ for all values of t where ψ is continuous.

147

Two other sets of orthogonal functions we have used are Legendre polynomials, P, with the property

$$\int_{-1}^{1} P_m(t) P_n(t) \, dt = \begin{cases} 1 & m = n \\ 0 & m \neq n \end{cases} \tag{7}$$

and Chebychev polynomials, T, with the property

$$\frac{1}{\pi} \int_{-1}^{1} T_m(t) T_n(t) \, \frac{1}{\sqrt{1 - t^2}} \, dt = \begin{cases} 1 & \text{for} \quad m = n \neq 0 \\ \frac{1}{2} & \text{for} \quad m = n = 0 \\ 0 & \text{for} \quad m \neq n \end{cases} \tag{8}$$

It is easy to see from equation (2) and (4) that the expansion coefficients for an orthonormal set of functions are given by

$$a_m = \int_L \psi(t) \phi_m(t) \omega(t) \, dt \tag{9}$$

The interchange of summation and integration required for obtaining the result (9) is valid for all waveforms of biological interest. The operation illustrated in equation (9) is the projection of the function ψ on the function ϕ_m. Projection of ψ onto a member of an orthonormal set of functions yields the expansion coefficients, a_m, for the representation of the function ψ.

An approximation to the function ψ may be made by including only some members of a complete orthonormal set in the expansion (4). If

$$\bar{\psi}(t) = \sum_{m=1}^{N} a_m \phi_m(t)$$

then $\bar{\psi}$ is such an approximation to ψ. It is this type of sum we use to represent visual evoked responses. The order of the approximation (or representation) is the upper limit of the sum, N.

The approximation of an evoked response with either a Fourier, Legendre, or Chebychev sixth order series resembles the original data but does not give a very satisfactory representation. A thirtieth order approximation, however, provides an excellent representation for most regions of the original data. This is illustrated in Fig. 1 for a Legendre polynomial expansion. The parameterization using thirty numbers is too complex for practical use. Fortunately, the number of parameters can be reduced by exploiting the similarities in the shape of the evoked responses to construct still another set of orthonormal functions.

The procedure we have employed to select a new set of orthonormal functions is factor analysis of the expansion coefficients (HARMAN, 1969; JOHN et al., 1964; RUCHKIN et al., 1964). We begin with expansion of a typical set of waveforms to thirtieth order in Legendre polynomials. This gives a good representation of each waveform except at points of very high curvature (points with large absolute magnitude of the second derivative). The thirty coefficients of the Legendre polynomials representing each waveform characterize these waveforms. The jth expansion coefficient for each waveform is then modified by

148

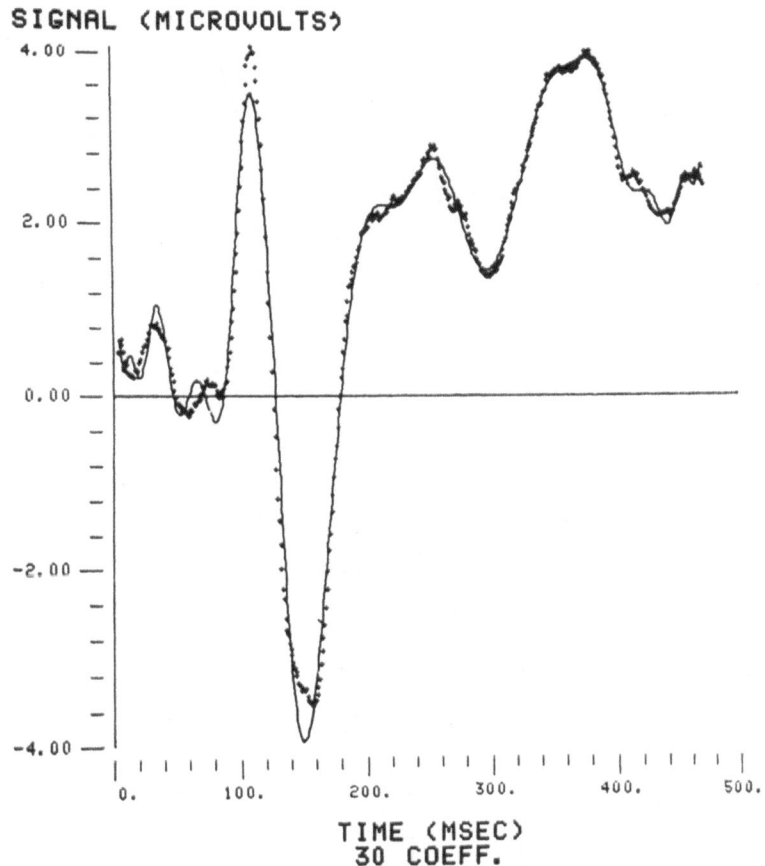

CH2 SIGNAL (MICROVOLTS)

TIME (MSEC)
30 COEFF.

Fig. 1. Thirtieth order Legendre polynomial representation of an evoked response. The original data are shown as discrete points and the approximation is a solid line.

subtracting the average of all the jth coefficients. These modified coefficients replace the representation of the waveform by a representation of its deviation from the average. A matrix is then formed from these new expansion coefficients by summing the product of the ith and jth coefficients over all the waveforms; for all i and j between 1 and 30. These sums, labeled by the indices i and j, form a symmetric matrix. The eigenvalues and eigenvectors of this matrix are then computed using an algorithm described by GARBOW (1969). The components of the eigenvectors are the Legendre expansion coefficients for the new orthonormal functions which, together with the mean, are used to expand the evoked responses. By making a slight abuse of the terminology, we sometimes call the new orthonormal functions eigenfunctions.

We have selected twenty-six responses from a checkerboard stimulus to use

149

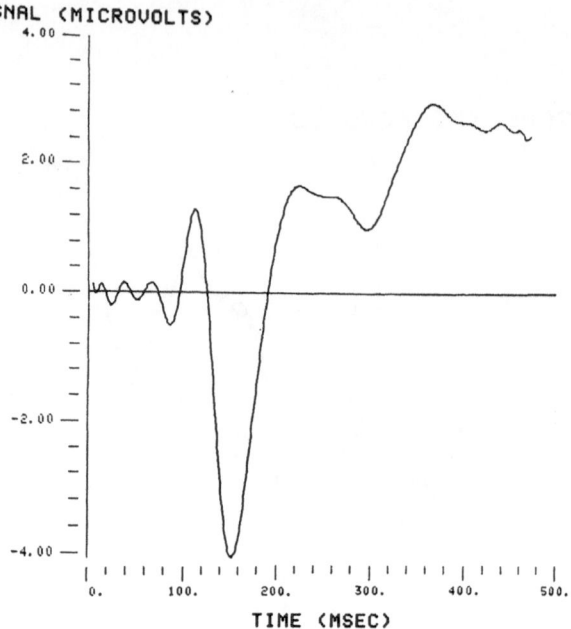

EIGENVALUE = 0.51467

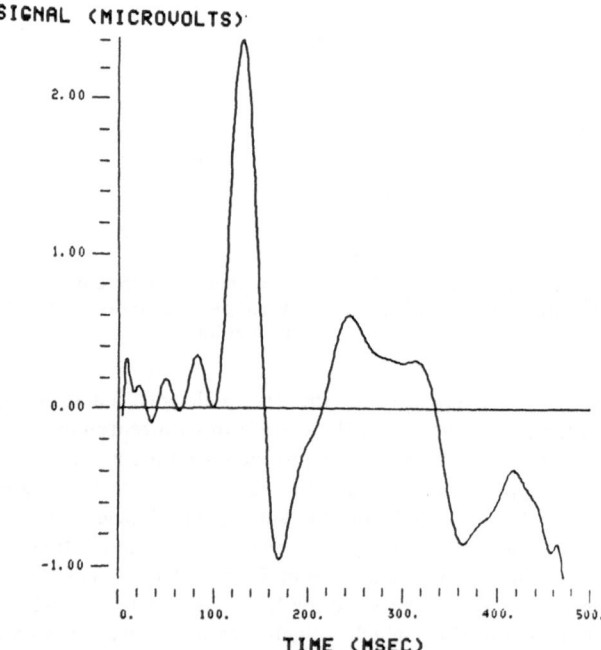

Fig. 2. The first six basis functions for expansion of evoked responses. The stimulus for the generating functions was a small checkerboard pattern illuminated with red light.

150

EIGENVALUE = 0.36925

SIGNAL (MICROVOLTS)

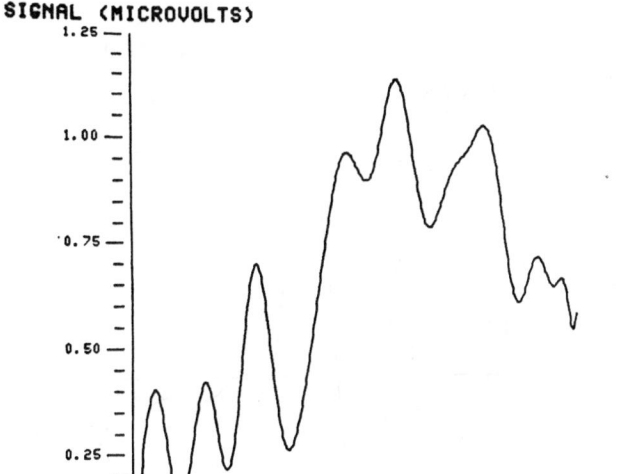

TIME (MSEC)

EIGENVALUE = 0.17222

SIGNAL (MICROVOLTS)

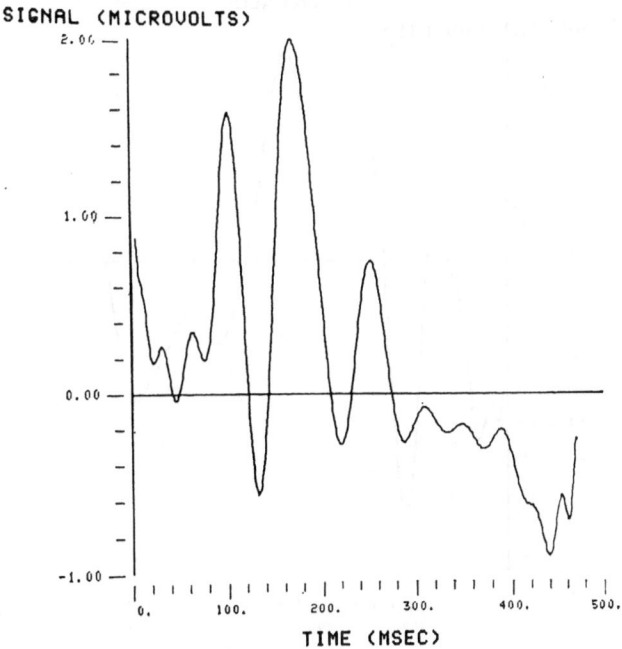

TIME (MSEC)

151

EIGENVALUE = 0.11675

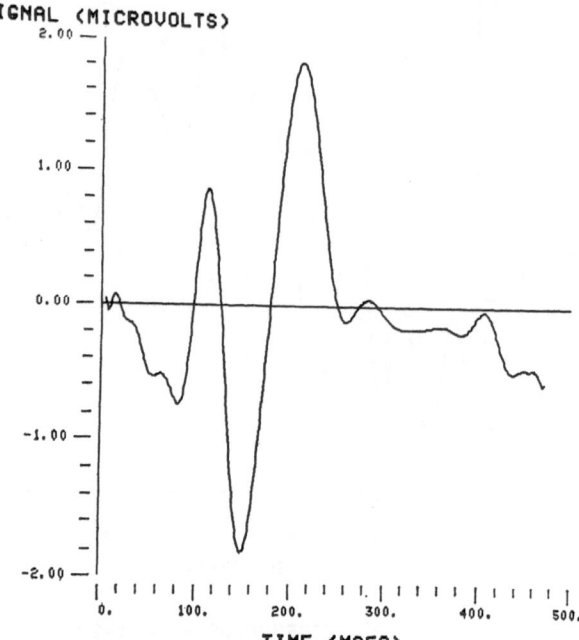

SIGNAL (MICROVOLTS)

TIME (MSEC)

EIGENVALUE = 0.06288

SIGNAL (MICROVOLTS)

TIME (MSEC)

152

as typical responses and have computed the new set of orthonormal functions based on these responses. We call the set of twenty-six responses the set of generating waveforms for the new orthonormal functions. The mean and the first five of the eigenfunctions are shown in Fig. 2. When a waveform is expanded by projection onto these new orthonormal functions, a reasonably good representation occurs in as few as six terms. Some examples of sixth order representation of waveforms is given in Fig. 3. The six expansion coefficients provide an efficient parameterization of the waveform. The square root of the sum of the squares for the coefficients not used in the expansion (RSS) provides a measure of the difference between the shape of the expanded waveform and the shape of the typical waveforms used to produce the orthonormal functions. This shape descriptor is tabulated for several responses. Table I shows that for waveforms which have been included in the generators of the eigenfunctions there is a

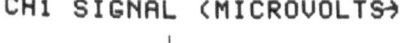

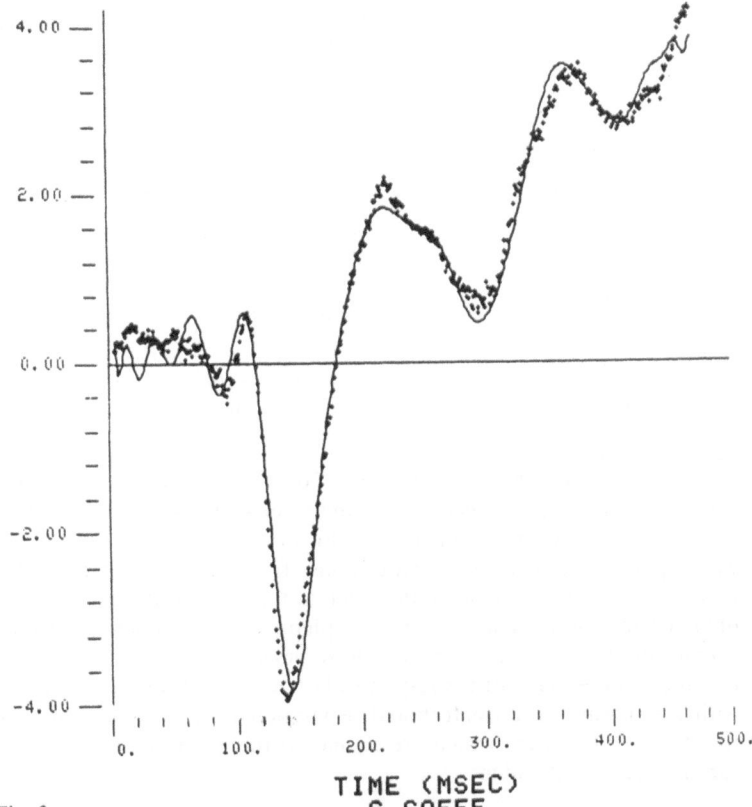

Fig. 3a

Fig. 3(a, b, c). Examples of sixth order representations of waveforms using an expansion in the functions shown in Fig. 2. The original data are shown as discrete points and the approximation is a solid line.

153

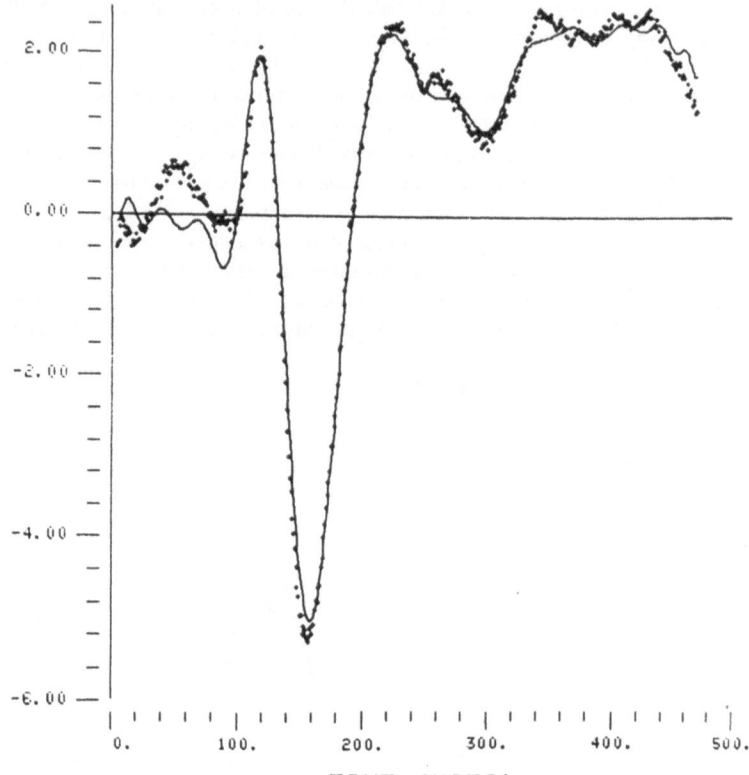

CH1 SIGNAL (MICROVOLTS)

Fig. 3b

TIME (MSEC)
6 COEFF.

value of about 0.3 to 0.4 for the RSS. For a subject whose evoked responses were not included in the generators, the value of the RSS is somewhat larger. The values of RSS for three patients with eye disease were also computed. It was impossible to select a typical response from these patients; therefore, it is necessary to show the range of the value of the RSS for these cases. The values obtained for the patients with retinal pigment degeneration are large on the average even though the responses were small. This indicates a considerable deviation in the shape of the responses because the RSS value changes linearly with overall waveform size. It should also be noted that the RSS value is sensitive to latency. Waveforms which are similar to the generators except for latency can have large RSS values.

Non-Linear Fitting

It is often convenient to express the approximating function describing a waveform as non-linear function of the descriptive parameters. In contrast to the

154

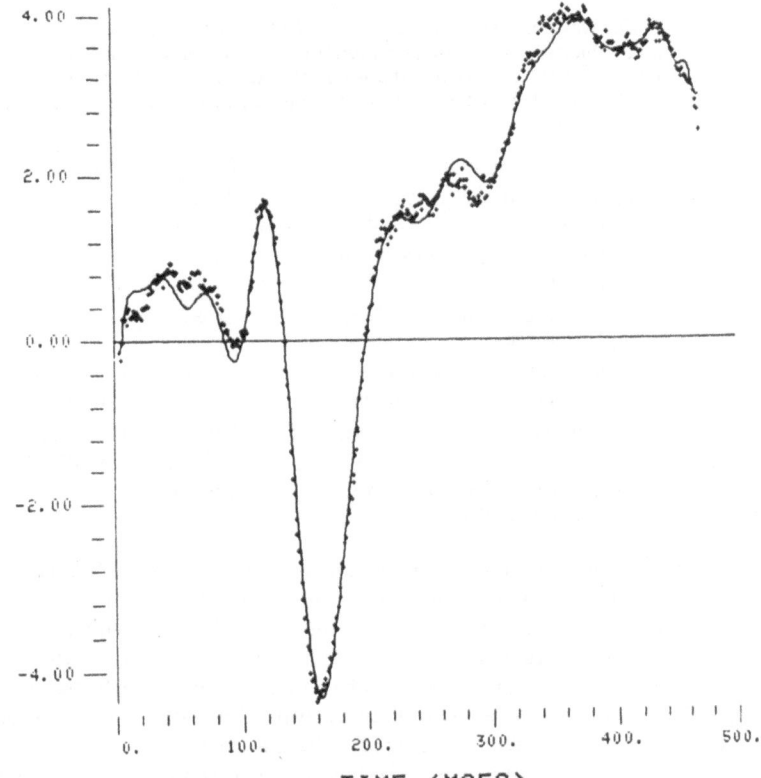

CH1 SIGNAL (MICROVOLTS)

Fig. 3c

TIME (MSEC)
6 COEFF.

orthogonal vector space expansions described in the previous section, the parameters in non-linear functions can frequently be given a simple physical interpretation. Quantities of interest describing responses include amplitudes of maxima and minima, mean frequency of response and phase of the response. An example of a non-linear fitting function which could be used to approximate a response is

$$\psi(t) = a + bt + ct^2 + d \cos(\omega t + \varphi)e^{-(t-t_0)^2/2\sigma^2} \qquad (10)$$

The coefficients a, b, c and d enter linearly but the frequency, ω, the phase, φ, the time of the maximum oscillation, t_0, and the width of the maximum oscillation, σ, enter non-linearly. It would be remarkable if the function (10) were to provide an accurate representation of any real response for the full time range. Nevertheless, the parameters, when adjusted for a best fit to a response, may provide consistent values for responses having specific shapes.

Adjustment of the parameters to make the best possible fit to a waveform is

11

155

Table I

The waveform shape descriptor (RSS) for VER's from normal subjects and subjects with eye disease are tabulated. A small checkerboard stimulus was used to produce the generators of the expansion functions. A small value of the RSS means that the tested waveform has a shape close to the generators.

Stimulus	RSS value	Comment
small checkerboard; normal subject waveform used in standard set	0.34	
small checkerboard; normal subject waveform used in standard set	0.38	
small checkerboard; normal subject waveform not used in standard set	0.69	
small checkerboard; patient with retinal pigment degeneration	0.9 to 1.6	low amplitude response
small checkerboard; patient with retinal pigment degeneration	0.7 to 1.2	low amplitude response
small checkerboard; patient with hysterical amblyopia	1.4 to 2.6	

done by minimizing the integrated square of the difference between the fitting function and the original data (BEVINGTON, 1969). The statistic used is chi-square, χ^2. Before an attempt to minimize χ^2 automatically is attempted, it is essential that the parameters be initialized to provide a fitting function which resembles the waveform to be approximated. This initialization is done by hand adjustment until a computer generated graph of the fitting function is similar in form to the evoked response. Then the automatic phase is started.

During the automatic phase, χ^2 is minimized by a combination of two methods. When the parameters are relatively far from their final values it is most efficient to compute the gradient of χ^2 with respect to the parameters. The parameters are then modified in the direction of the gradient. However, near the point of best fit, the parameters are adjusted more accurately by expanding χ^2 in a first order Taylor expansion of the fitting function. The minimum of χ^2 has an analytic expression relative to this linearized fitting function and can be easily computed. The criterion for a good fit is little change in successive values of χ^2. A check is made finally to ensure that the fitting function still resembles the original data.

The functional form shown in equation (10) was used to fit a set of waveforms from a normal subject viewing a small checkerboard stimulus illuminated with red light. The shape of the responses and several of the computed parameters are displayed in Table II. The first response was recorded when the subject had slightly too little positive correction to see the checkerboard clearly. The waveform has a wide and deep negative going portion which is represented in the parameters by the relatively large width of the maximum oscillation. The time of the maximum oscillation accurately represents the latency of this negative going portion. The second and third responses were obtained when the subject

Table II

	CHI-SQUARE	AMPLITUDE	TIME OF MAX. OSCILLATION	WIDTH OF MAX. OSCILLATION
1	0.146	2·113	200·117	59·867
2	0·308	5·005	142·639	29·815
3	0·290	4·980	147·939	26·016
4	0·015	0·260	203·488	71·105

(left column label: W A V E F O R M S)

was able to focus sharply on the stimulus. The responses are similar, both showing a narrowed negative going portion with an earlier latency relative to the first response. The parameters accurately reflect the similarities between the second and third as well as the differences from the first waveform. The fourth response was recorded when the subject had too much positive correction to see significant detail in the stimulus. This response has low amplitude (which is difficult to appreciate in the reproduction of the wave shape) and a form which differs drastically from that of the other waveforms. Most of the computed parameters are different for this final waveform.

TEMPLATE FUNCTIONS

A direct measure of the similarity in the shape of two functions, ψ and ϕ is given by the quotient

$$\rho = \frac{\int_L \phi(t)\psi(t)\, dt}{\sqrt{\left(\int_L \phi(t)\phi(t)\, dt\right)\left(\int_L \psi(t)\psi(t)\, dt\right)}}$$

where L is a time interval containing shape features of interest. This quotient is the correlation coefficient relating ψ to ϕ. It is easy to see by direct substitution

157

that if ϕ is a positive multiple of ψ (and therefore has the same shape), then ρ has the value 1 while if ϕ is a negative multiple of ψ, then ρ has the value -1. For functions of similar shapes, ρ will have a positive value less than 1 while for dissimilar shapes, ρ will have a negative value greater than -1.

Computation of the integrals can be done rapidly enough to allow the parameterization of a waveform during the course of an experiment. An example of the parameterization of a set of waveforms by template functions is shown in Table III. The shapes of the template waveforms and those waveforms tested against the templates are shown in the table. The first two of the template functions were selected from among the most typical of the responses to a small checkerboard stimulus illuminated with red light. The third template function is from stimulation by a white light flash of a millisecond duration and 0.06 degree angle while the fourth template function is the response to a red light flash of one millisecond duration and subtending 0.60 degree angle. The fifth template function is the response to a large checkerboard illuminated with incandescent white light. In all cases the subject had normal ocular and cerebral function and was able to form a sharp image of the stimulus on his retina. The waveforms tested against the templates came from a more varied selection of subjects. The stimulus was the same for all of the tested waveforms: the small checkerboard illuminated with red light was used. The first and second wave-

Table III

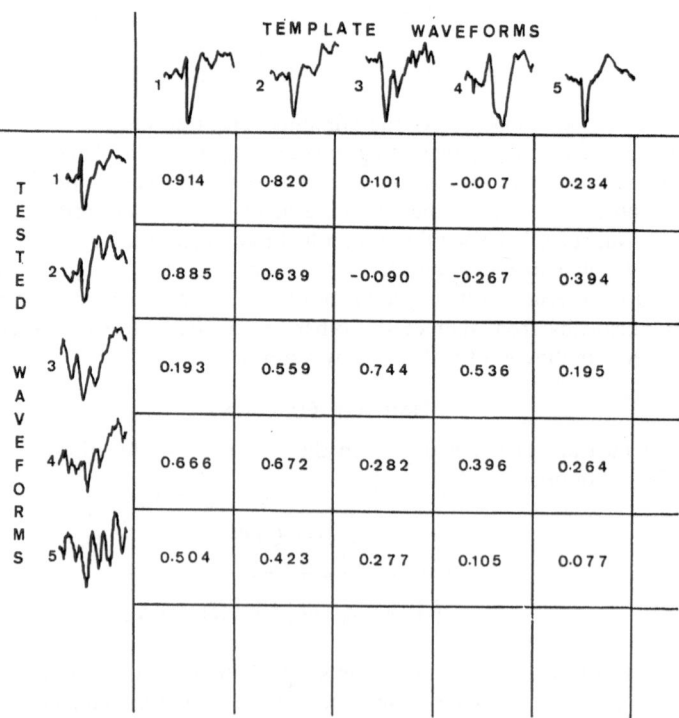

		1	2	3	4	5
T E S T E D	1	0.914	0.820	0.101	-0.007	0.234
	2	0.885	0.639	-0.090	-0.267	0.394
W A V E F O R M S	3	0.193	0.559	0.744	0.536	0.195
	4	0.666	0.672	0.282	0.396	0.264
	5	0.504	0.423	0.277	0.105	0.077

forms are from different normal subjects. The integrals show, as would be expected, a high correlation with the small checkerboard, a moderate correlation with the large checkerboard and poor correlation with the templates produced by light flashes. The third and fourth waveforms are from the same subject, a patient with retinal pigment degeneration. The two responses were obtained two days apart. The considerable variation in the shape of the waveforms is reflected in the differences in the values of the integrals. The final tested response is from a patient with hysterical amblyopia. This response correlated fairly well with the small checkerboard templates but poorly with the large checkerboard template. There is a slight correlation with the template functions from the red and white light flashes.

Discussion

This study was undertaken to find methods for parameterizing waveforms which would be useful in digital computer control of experiments. The methods considered all produced results which reflected the shape of the waveform as a whole. All three methods are suitable for certain applications although the second method discussed, non-linear parameterization, will probably not be useful for control of experiments.

Orthogonal functions provide the most accurate representation of the waveforms. They provide a parameterization of the waveform and in addition smooth noisy data so that other processing such as location of critical points can be more accurately done. The accuracy of the representation is sufficient in the high order expansion to allow storing the information contained in the waveform by recording the expansion coefficients. This, for our experimental procedure, means a saving of a factor of seven times in storage. To represent the waveform with reasonable fidelity with a sixth order expansion it is necessary to use a special set of orthonormal functions generated by a functions similar to the represented curve. These low order expansions provide a very concise parameterization of the waveform although the parameters have little to do with any quantities of physical meaning. At this point our experience is insufficient to state whether we will find a means of attaching significance to specific changes in the expansion coefficients. We expect to use the expansion coefficients to classify the differences between the responses from normal subjects, as well as the more pronounced differences that occur with ocular and cerebral disease. Should it be possible to classify changes, the low order expansions will provide excellent criteria for computer control of experiments. The time required for us to make a high (thirtieth) order expansion for a five-hundred point waveform is about 40 seconds. However, our computer at present does not have floating point hardware. For a computer endowed with floating point hardware, a high order expansion should take about one second.

Non-linear fitting of waveforms seems to be useful only where an estimate of the functional form of the curve to be approximated is quite well known or where parameters with physical meaning are required. Unfortunately, there seem to be no models at present which represent, with a function of known form, the myriad of waveforms found for visually evoked responses. If such a model is ever created, it will probably not be linear. Therefore, a non-linear

159

technique will have to be used. The computation of the best non-linear fit to waveforms is only conditionally stable when done by the methods we have used. It proved absolutely essential to begin the computation with the parameters adjusted close to their final values. Finding these initial values for the parameters was not particularly time consuming because the interactive display system of our computer allowed seeing the result of a parameter change within a few seconds. Without an interactive display system the task of selecting appropriate initial values would be formidable. Once the initial values have been selected the actual computation is quite time consuming. On our computer the time required for one alteration of the parameters is about four minutes. Approximately ten such alterations are usually required before chi-square becomes stable. Floating point hardware would reduce the time required to make a complete non-linear fit to about one minute.

The template function integrals we have used were restricted to real waveforms with integration carried out over the full experimental waveform duration. There is no theoretical reason why the template functions should be waveforms or even closely resemble waveforms. Upon gaining further experience we anticipate that we will be able to construct artificial template functions which will differentiate quite sharply between normal individuals and those who have eye disease which changes the evoked responses in a characteristic way. It is more difficult to predict whether template functions will provide a way to differentiate between the responses from normal individuals.

In the immediate future we plan no further study of non-linear fitting methods. Our experience has demonstrated that these methods are cumbersome and excessive amounts of computing time are required to produce a few parameters. Furthermore, the instability encountered during the search for parameters of best fit is intolerable during completely automatic digital computer control of an experiment. Development of template functions capable of sharp discrimination between classes of waveforms is underway. We are currently examining the use of artificial template functions made from square and triangular waves.

Projection of waveforms onto orthogonal functions will be the method under most intensive study by our laboratory in the near future. Much larger sets of generators will be used to produce expansion eigenfunctions. The maximum allowable size of the cluster of waveforms (as defined by the RSS or some similar measure) will be studied and the dependence of the convergence of expansions on the cluster size will be determined. Finally, the correlation between expansion coefficients and changes in experimental conditions or the ocular status of the subject will be determined. These correlations will allow using the expansion coefficients as numerical indicators of certain eye diseases as well as providing the parameters necessary to automatically control experiments.

REFERENCES

BENNETT, J. R., McDONALD, J. S., DRANCE, S. M. & UENOYAMA, K. Some statistical properties of the visual evoked potential in man and their application as a criterion of normality, I.E.E.E. *Trans. Bio-Med. Eng.* 18:23 (1971).

160

BEVINGTON, P. R. Data Reduction and Error Analysis for The Physical Sciences, New York, McGraw-Hill Book Co. 1969.

CIGANEK, L. The EEG response (evoked potential) to light stimulus in man. *Electroencephalogr. Clin. Neurophys.* 13:*165* (1961).

GARBOW, B. S. ANL FZOZS-1, Eigenvalues and Eigenvectors of a Real Symmetric Matrix, Argonne National Laboratory System/360 Library Subroutine, Revision, December 1969.

HARMAN, H. A. Modern Factor Analysis, Chicago, University of Chicago Press (1969).

JOHN, E. R., RUCHKIN, D. S. & VILLEGAS, J. Experimental background: signal analysis and behaviorial correlates of evoked potential configurations in cats, *Ann. N. Y. Acad. Sci.*112: *362* (1964).

KOOI, K. A. & BAGCHI, B. K. Visual evoked responses in man: normative data. *Ann. N. Y. Adad. N. Y. Sci.* 112:*254* (1964).

POTTS, A. M. & HIRATA, A. The objective measurement of foveal function by means of the VER and structured stimuli; manuscript in preparation.

RIETVELD, W. J. The occipitocortical response to lightflashes in man. *Acta. Physiol. Pharm. Neerl.* 12:*373* (1963).

RUCHKIN, D. S., VILLEGAS, J. & JOHN, E. R. An analysis of average evoked potentials making use of least mean square techniques, *Ann. N. Y. Acad. Sci.* 115:*799* (1964).

161

PSYCHOPHYSICS AND ELECTRO-PHYSIOLOGY OF A ROD-ACHROMAT

L. H. VAN DER TWEEL* & H. SPEKREIJSE*

(*Amsterdam*)

INTRODUCTION

Since HERING (1891) there has been a continuous interest in the phenomenon and especially the psychophysical aspects of rod-achromatism. Rod-achromats are suitable subjects for a study of scotopic vision, since the scotopic sensitivity curve holds even at luminance levels where normals exhibit a photopic component. On the other hand a fast branch is reported in the dark adaptation curve of most "monochromatic" subjects (SLOAN, 1958).

Some authors assume the existence of rod-like cones; an assumption supported by anatomical data (LARSEN, 1921) and the presence of a Stiles-Crawford effect (ALPERN, FALLS & LEE, 1960). These findings should be kept in mind whenever the term rod-achromatism is used.

In rod-achromats increment thresholds were studied extensively by ALPERN et al. (1960), BLAKEMORE & RUSHTON (1965) and by MEULENBRUGGE & ROUFS (1970). Apart from rod-saturation, these thresholds obey Weber's law over a large range of retinal illuminations (4 log units), and sensitivity increases with stimulus field. The latter applies also for flicker (MEULENBRUGGE & ROUFS, 1970). The flickerfusion curves (Modulation Transfer Function, MTF plots) show an overall decrease in sensitivity; at 30 tld the flickerfusion frequency (100% modulation depth) is on the average at 20 Hz, a value about 14 Hz below that of normals. (BREUKINK, 1962).

The literature about VEP's in rod achromats is scarce and there only are a few reports on ERG's (GOODMAN & BORNSCHEIN, 1957; DODT, VAN LITH & SCHMIDT, 1967).

To fill this gap we performed a study whose aim was to compare electro-physiology and psychophysics in rod-achromatism both for luminance and spatial contrast stimulation. To estimate the defects one normal subject went also through the entire series of experiments.

METHODS

Subjects

The present study is based on a rather large number of psychophysical and electro-physiological experiments on the same subject who was studied by MEULENBRUGGE & ROUFS (1970).

This subject is a male student of 25 years old with congenital binocular rod-achromatism. Also his brothers and two of his sisters are reported to have the

---

* Laboratory of Medical Physics, University of Amsterdam.

same aberration. His visual acuity for the C test object is reported to be as high as 1/3. Some stereopsis is present. The subject is photophobic and both pupils are fixed at approximately 3 mm. His dark adaptation curve does not show a typical cone or fast branch (Fig. 1). Increment thresholds for various combinations of wavelength indicate that no functional photopic mechanism is present. No electro-physiological data were available for this subject.

Experimental set up

The light stimulator has been described before (SPEKREIJSE 1966, VAN DER TWEEL & SPEKREIJSE, 1968). It consists of two independent, well-controlled

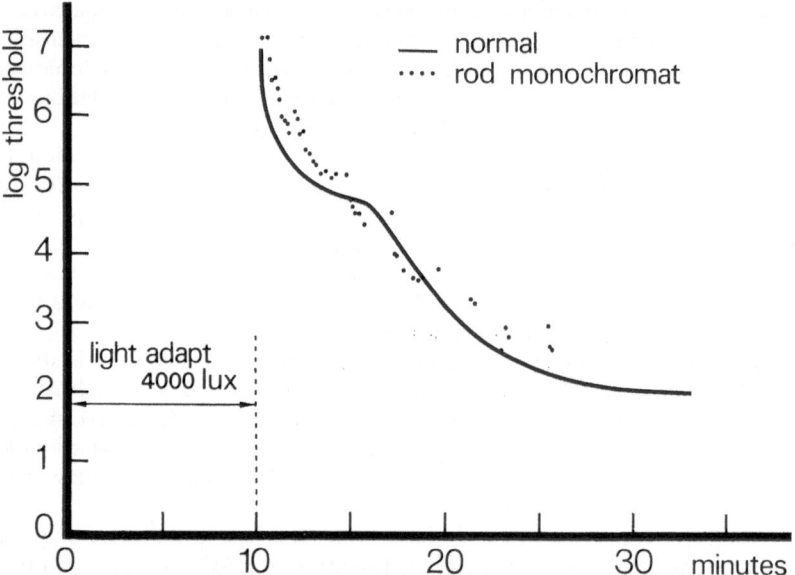

Fig. 1. Dark adaptation curves of a normal subject (drawn line) and of our rod monochromat (dashed line). The curves were determined with the Goldmann adaptometer.

(within 0.1 %) fluorescent tube light sources which are viewed through a checkerboard patterned mirror. The luminances of the two modulated light sources can be set in such a way that an appearing-disappearing checkerboard or a pattern reversal can be produced at constant average luminance. We used sinusoidal modulation for all psychophysical experiments and for the electrophysiological experiments on homogeneous fields. We used square-wave counterphase modulation of the light sources in our electro-physiological study of spatial contrast responses. Checkerboard and bar patterns were used. Relative contrast is defined as $\dfrac{L_{\max} - L_{\min}}{L_{\max} + L_{\min}} \times 100\%$. Note that this is the equivalence of modulation depth and half the conventional measure for steady contrast. Thresholds were

164

determined first to increasing and then to decreasing modulation depth and the average was taken. No artificial pupil was used in the achromatic subject. All experiments were done monocularly and usually with the left eye, which enabled some fixation. The field size used was generally 8° with checks ranging from 20′ to 200′. In most experiments the luminance was roughly 12 tld, a level at which a normal still has color vision. Our monochromat did not experience this light level too uncomfortably.

Recording-data analysis

The responses were recorded either from inion to vertex or monopolarly with the right ear as a reference. Averaging was performed by a CAT-computer. The power spectrum of the spontaneous activity was determined by fast Fourier transform. The harmonic content of the average responses to luminance stimulation was determined on the PDP-9 computer.

RESULTS

Theoretical and experimental problems of flickering spatial patterns, especially bars, have been treated in a number of recent publications and reviews. KELLY (1969, 1971) compared flicker sensitivity to counterphase modulated bars and to sinewave modulated homogeneous fields, and presented a theoretical model based on his material.

In our opinion checkerboard patterns are preferable as a research tool for the following reasons: considering the symmetry of retinal receptive or integrative fields, checkerboards* are the best fit. Bar patterns will only behave as a contrast stimulus in one direction; they are subject to integration along their length. However, they provide a simpler tool if concepts of spatial Fourier analysis are employed. A practical reason for the use of checkerboards in our experiments is that they provide much larger responses than bar patterns.

Psychophysics

Fig. 2 shows the fusion (MTF) curves of a normal subject to homogeneous field flicker, and to counterphase stimulation of bar and checkerboard patterns. The behaviour of these three curves—obtained at a luminance of 12 tld—differs distinctly at the low and high frequency end.

At *high frequencies* psychophysical sensitivity to counterphase stimulation is lower than to homogeneous field stimulation, but the slope of the two curves are similar. Psychophysical sensitivity to bars is higher than to a comparable checkerboard pattern, although still lower than to homogeneous field stimulation.

At *low frequencies* the difference between the homogeneous field and counterphase curves is more striking. The counterphase curves become practically horizontal whereas the homogeneous field curve (without surround) shows a

---

* Although polygons of a higher order are of course more disklike, every polygon would have more than four neighbours so that they are not feasible for counterphase experiments.

continuous drop in sensitivity as frequency is progressively reduced. This low frequency attenuation becomes stronger at higher luminances and/or field sizes. The flat low frequency tail of the counterphase curves is not surprising, since finally the steady contrast level will be reached.

Fig. 3 shows a similar set of de Lange curves (MTF plots) measured for our achromatic subject. These data differ markedly from those of Fig. 2. Whereas the sensitivity for homogeneous fields is still about half of that of the normal subject, the sensitivity for counterphase modulation has dropped distinctly. For checks of 50′ it is about 1/5th of that of the normal, although the shape of the curves resemble those of the normal subject. For 25′ checks the sensitivity

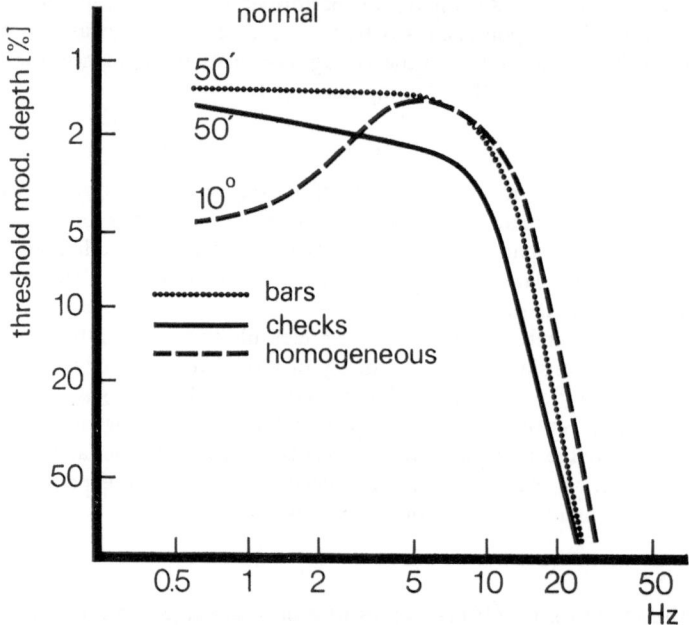

Fig. 2. Fusion curves (MTF plots) of a normal subject to a sine wave modulated homogeneous field and to pattern reversal.

becomes so low that at higher frequencies the achromate could apply two criteria: one for detecting reversal of contrast, the other for flicker perception. The sensitivity of the latter is slightly higher than for the reversal of contrast. Bars of 25′ show a much higher sensitivity than checks of the same size, although still below that of a normal. A reduced sensitivity, compared to a normal, is also present at 0.12 tld level both for homogeneous field and checkerboard stimulation.

Fig. 4 gives the dependency on field size for homogeneous fields and checker-boards. We were able to confirm the results of ROUFFS & MEULENBRUGGE for homogeneous fields as that up to 10° there was an overall gain in sensitivity. The same occurs also for sinusoidally counterphase modulated checkerboards.

166

1. *Homogeneous fields*

The evoked responses to sine wave modulated fields of about 90° subtense were similar to those recorded for normal subjects (at generally higher luminances). A quantitative judgement of possible differences is difficult due to interindividual variation (VAN DER TWEEL & VERDUYN LUNEL, 1965, KAMPHUISEN,

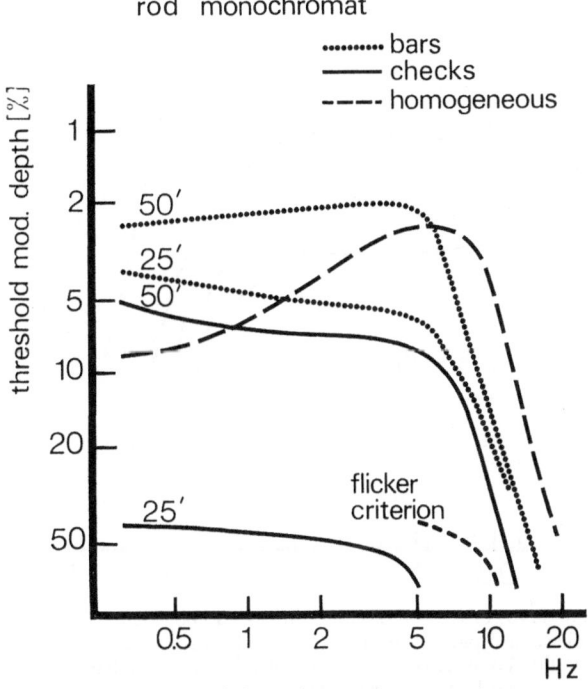

Fig. 3. Fusion curves of the rod monochromat to homogeneous field flicker and to counterphase stimulation of bar and checkerboard patterns. For dashed line, labeled flicker criterion, see text.

1969). In any case sine wave stimulation with frequencies from 4–7 Hz gave rise to a strong second harmonic component, whereas stimulation with frequencies from 10–13 Hz evoked a response, in which the fundamental component dominates. The peak sensitivity for the second harmonic is at a stimulus frequency of 5.5 Hz, the strongest fundamental is found at 11 Hz. This peak frequency coincides with the peak in the spectrum of the spontaneous α-activity (Fig. 5).

High frequency responses were also recorded. Second harmonics were strong at about 19 Hz, whereas fundamental components were dominant for stimulus frequencies above 30 Hz. The latency of the high frequency response, as calculated from the phase characteristic of the fundamental component, amounts to 100 msec. Within the restricted accuracy of such measurements, this value is of the same order as found for the normal subject.

It is noteworthy that even with the scotopic function of an achromat high frequency cortical responses are found above the fusion frequencies, especially since the high frequency responses in the ERG are reported to be largely depressed (GOODMAN & BORNSCHEIN, 1957 and DODT et al., 1967).

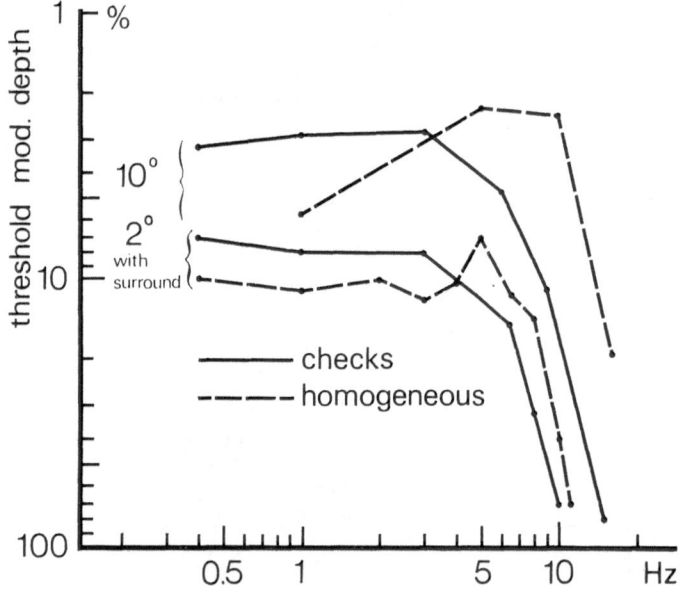

Fig. 4. Fusion curves of the rod monochromat to homogeneous field stimulation and checkerboard pattern reversal (50′ checks) as a function of fieldsize. For both stimulus conditions an increase of stimulus field from 2° to 10° results in an overall gain in sensitivity.

2. *Appearance and disappearance of checkerboards*

The responses to this type of stimulus are also comparable to those of normals. Because of the concentration required of the subject not all sessions were successful. However, the appearance response which we obtained, exhibited many of the features found in normals. Fig. 6 gives an appearance response for a monochromat and a normal subject. The two waveforms seem identical but the "latency" of the response of the monochromat is about 40 msec longer. There is another difference: whereas in a normal subject checks of approx. 25′ give the largest response, the achromat needs larger checks (>50′) to give optimal responses (Fig. 7).

The depressing effect of a trellis, which occurs in normals (SPEKREIJSE, 1966), was also present. Outlining with contrasty 6′ lines suppresses the response

168

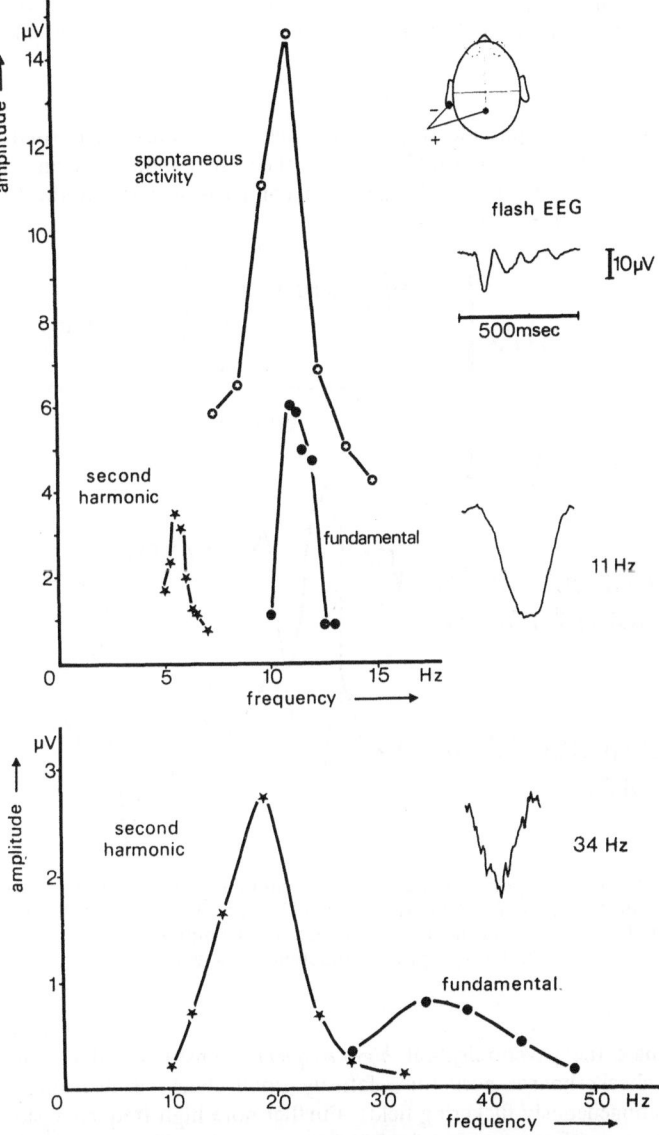

Fig. 5. Amplitude characteristics of fundamental and second harmonic for low frequency (top half figure) and high frequency (bottom half figure) sine wave modulated light. For stimulus frequencies around 11 Hz the fundamental component in the occipital response dominates. The peak frequency coincides with the peak in the spectrum of the spontaneous activity. At the right the VEP to flash stimulation with a 10° field. Flash "energy" is 25 asb. sec. Also the average responses to a 30° field sinusoidally modulated at 11 Hz and 34 Hz respectively are shown.

169

completely (Fig. 7). The lines are broader than needed to obtain the same reduction for a normal subject, but still narrow compared to the checksizes involved.

Firstly we will recapitulate some of the results obtained in normals, next compare them with the data obtained under the same conditions from the rod-achromat, and finally discuss the latter in comparison with another case of reduced visual acuity: amblyopia.

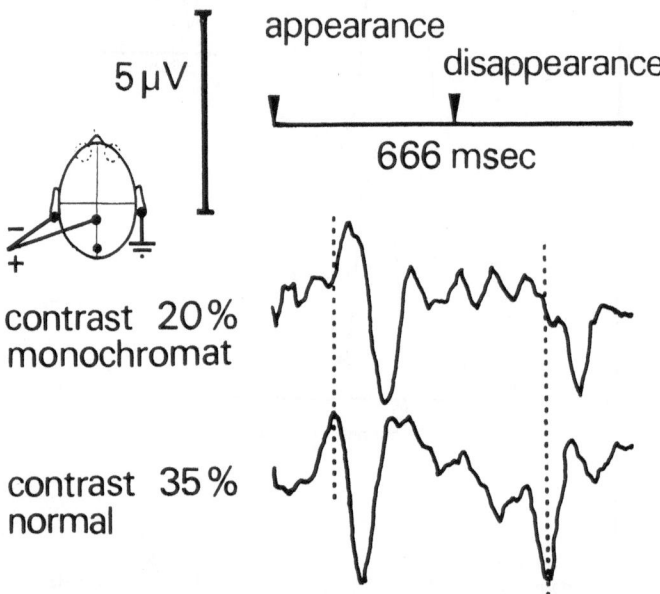

Fig. 6. Occipital responses to the appearance and disappearance of a checker-board with 50′ checks for the normal, and 200′ checks for the monochromatic subject. The responses of the normal subject and the monochromat are rather similar, except for a difference in latency.

Normal subjects

In normals the psychophysical *high frequency* sensitivity to counterphase flickering checkerboards even for relatively small checks is not much below that to homogeneously flickering fields. Furthermore high frequency slopes for counterphase and homogeneous field flicker are similar. This suggests that also for counterphase stimulation (pattern reversal) luminance flicker is the deter-mining factor at high frequencies; in other words contrast components do not contribute to threshold at these frequencies. The lower sensitivity for counter-phase flicker is due to partial cancellation of the luminance variations within any individual integrative field. For very small checks the sensitivity is also reduced by geometrical optical defects. Our data point to relatively small integrative

170

fields, since even for small checks the sensitivity is not much reduced. However, the real picture is certainly more complicated because sensitivity increases with total field size up to several degrees.

The *low frequency* tails of the homogeneous field and counterphase curves show a large difference both in sensitivity and slope. For homogeneous field stimulation sensitivity drops as frequency is reduced. For counterphase stimulation the

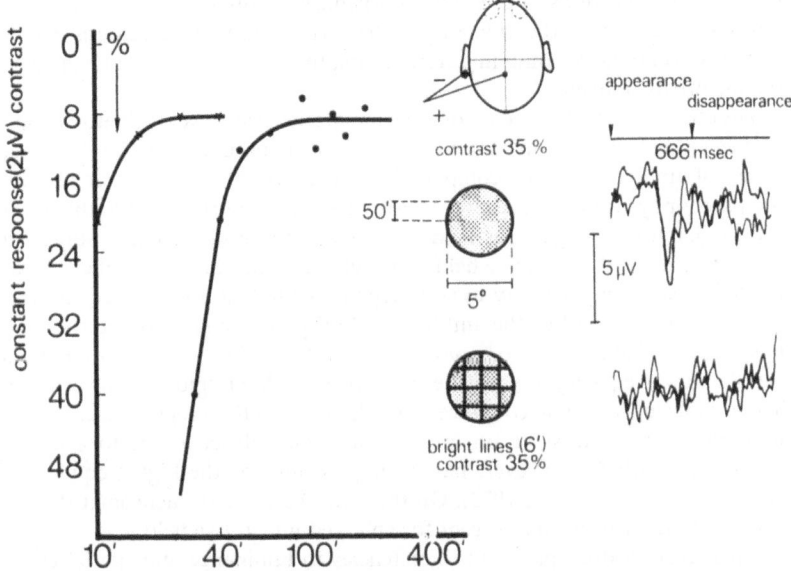

Fig. 7. Amplitude of the appearance response as a function of checksize for a normal subject and a monochromat. The normal subject gives optimal responses for half the checksize, needed for the monochromat. The right side responses show that outlining of the checkerboard pattern with bright 6′ lines (for printing reasons black in the figure) suppresses the occipital response of the monochromat.

thresholds are practically independent of frequency; they approach the static contrast threshold. Integration along the lengths of bars can explain the higher sensitivity at all frequencies to a bar pattern than to a comparable checkerboard.

Monochromatic subject

The results from our achromatic subject fit in with the existence of large integrative fields in the rod system. The integrative fields should be of the order of 1°, because even for checks of 50′ the reduction in sensitivity is considerable at all frequencies. In all other respects the flicker curves to homogeneous field and counterphase stimulation are similar for our achromatic and normal subject. There remains an interesting problem about the relation between integrative fields and visual acuity: the large integrative fields (about 1°)

171

do not seem to be in accordance with the subjects visual acuity; our subject could resolve details of 3-7'.

Because of the overall lower sensitivity and the larger integrative fields the situation seems simpler in the achromat than in the normal:

a. Psychophysical experiments are not contaminated by possible optical defects because they are much smaller than the actual sizes of the spatial elements used.

b. Since the sensitivity of normals exceeds that of the achromat, the influence of quantal noise can also be neglected. Therefore experiments on achromats can give clearer indications of their visual organization than similar experiments on normal subjects. That the difference at the various stimulus conditions (e.g. bars and checks) are larger than in a normal, might also be attributed to the lack of the factors mentioned.

The above assumed existence of large integrative fields over the entire temporal frequency scale is not compulsory for cases of reduced acuity. For example, in a case of amblyopia with a comparably reduced visual acuity as our achromat, the psychophysical *high frequency* sensitivities of the normal and amblyopic eye are similar for homogeneous field and counterphase (20' checks) stimulation, suggesting normal integrative fields for high frequency luminance flicker. Solely the low frequency sensitivity to counterphase stimulation is reduced. Moreover the low frequency tail of the amblyopic MTF plot to counterphase stimulation has the same shape as that to homogeneous field stimulation. This is in contrast to the flat low frequency tail of the counterphase MTF plot of the achromat. These data suggest, in accordance with the electrophysiological data, that the impairment of contrast vision in the amblyopic subject is due to a defect in organization which, however, has no implication for the high frequency sensitivity (SPEKREIJSE et al., 1972). On the other hand, in the achromat the visual organization seems normal except for enlarged integrative fields.

Apart from a discrepancy in the latencies to luminance and spatial contrast stimulation, our electro-physiological data also agree with such concept. All features of normals, such as second harmonic formation, frequency selectivity, presence of high frequency responses and contrast responses are found. The spatial coarseness as expressed in the spatial contrast EP's is, however, greater for the achromat (Fig. 7). This could indicate that once the ganglion cells are excited, all subsequent processes are similar in normal and achromat. Hence impaired visual acuity as such seems not necessarily to cause a deviating organization of the visual system. The difference in acuity of the two eyes of the anisometropic amblyopic subject studied by us (SPEKREIJSE et al., 1972) and the indeed deviating organization reflected in i.a. the spatial contrast evoked responses, seems therefore to be significantly related.

AKCNOWLEDGEMENTS

We are grateful to Mr. C. M. J. MOONS for his continuous and most pleasant co-operation during the experiments and to Mrs. L. H. DE VRIES and Mr. O. ESTÉVEZ for technical assistance. We are indebted to Drs. H. J. MEULEBRUGGE and J. A. J. ROUFS for introducing the subject and for allowing the use of all their

172

data. This research was supported by the Organisation for Health Research TNO, The Hague.

REFERENCES

ALPERN, M., FALLS, H. F. & LEE, G. B. The enigma of typical total monochromacy. *Am. J. Ophthal.* 50: *996–1011* or *326–341* (1960).

BLAKEMORE, C. B. & RUSHTON, W. A. H. Dark adaptation and increment threshold in a rod monochromat, *J. Physiol.* 181: *612–628;* The rod increment threshold during dark adaptation in normal and rod monochromat. *J. Physiol.* 181: *629–640* (1965).

BREUKINK, E. W. De frekwentiekarakteristiek van het menselijk oog onder normale en pathologische omstandigheden. Thesis, R. U. te Utrecht, Publ.: Elinkwijk, Utrecht (1962).

DODT, E., LITH, G. H. M. VAN & SCHMIDT, B. Electroretinographic evaluation of the photopic malfunction in a totally colour blind. *Vision Res.* 7: *231–241* (1967).

GOODMAN, G. & BORNSCHEIN, H. Comparative Electroretinographic Studies in Congenital Night Blindness and Total Color Blindness. *Archs. Ophthal. N.Y.* 58: *174–182* (1957).

HERING, E. Untersuchung eines total Farbenblinden. *Pflüg. Arch. ges. Physiol.* 49: *563–608* (1891).

KAMPHUISEN, H. A. C. Average EEG response to sinusoidally modulated light in normal subjects and patients. Thesis Univ. of Utrecht. Publ.: Fa. L. G. Strubbe, Zeist (1969).

KELLY, D. H. Flickering Patterns and Lateral Inhibition. *J. Opt. Soc. Amer.* 59: *1361–1370* (1969).

KELLY, D. H. Theory of Flicker and Transient Responses, I. Uniform Fields, *J. Opt. Soc. Amer.* 61: *537–546*, II. Counterphase Gratings, *J. Opt. Soc. Amer.* 61: *632–640* (1971).

LARSEN, H. Demonstration mikroskopischer Preparate von einem monochromatischen Auge. *Klin. Monatsbl. f. Augenh.* 67: *301–302* (1921).

MEULENBRUGGE, H. J. & ROUFS, J. A. J. Thresholds of flashes and flickering light in relation to stimulus diameter for a rod achromat. I. P.O. *Ann. Progr. Rep.* 5: *137–144* (1970).

SLOAN, L. L. The photopic retinal receptors of the typical achromat. *Am. J. Ophthal.* 46: *81–86* (1958).

SPEKREIJSE, H. Analysis of EEG responses in man evoked by sine wave modulated light. Thesis Univ. of Amsterdam, Publ.: Dr. W. Junk, The Hague (1966).

SPEKREIJSE, H., KHOE, L. H. & TWEEL, L. H. VAN DER, A case of amblyopia: Electrophysiology and psychophysics of luminance and contrast. In: The Visual System ed. G. B. Arden: 141–156 (1972).

SPEKREIJSE, H., TWEEL, L. H. VAN DER & ZUIDEMA, T. Contrast evoked responses in man. *Vision Res.* (1973 in press).

TWEEL, L. H. VAN DER & SPEKREIJSE, H. Visual Evoked Responses. ISCERG Symp. Ghent 1966. The Clinical Value of Electroretinography. Basel/New York, Karger, 83–94 (1968).

TWEEL, L. H. VAN DER & VERDUYN LUNEL, H. F. E. Human visual responses to sinusoidally modulated light. *Electroenceph. Clin. Neurophysiol.* 18: *587–598* (1965).

173

GENERAL CONE DYSFUNCTION WITHOUT ACHROMATOPSIA

G. H. M. VAN LITH*

(*Rotterdam*)

INTRODUCTION

Cone dysfunctions generally have a colour vision defect. Of these defects, also called dyschromatisms, several types are known (SPIVEY, 1964). They may be classified into dichromatisms (protan, deutan, tritan), monochromatism (cone monochromate) and achromatism (rod achromat). Sometimes the term monochromatism is used instead of achromatism. This may be confusing.

The typical symptoms of the rod achromat are a total lack of cone function, i.e. total colour blindness, low visual acuity (about 0.1), nystagmus, photophobia, absent Purkinje shift, low flicker fusion frequency and absent photopic ERG. ALPERN et al. (1960) demonstrated, however, that even in rod achromatism signs of cone function are present. They found a two-receptor-system, one of which works at high luminances and shows directional sensitivity. Histological examination proved the existence of cones, too (FALLS et al., 1965). Nevertheless, when all the symptoms mentioned above are completely present the syndrome is called a complete, total or typical achromatism.

A group that is not well understood is the incomplete, partial or atypical achromatism. This group does not show all the symptoms of the rod achromatism. The cone monochromatism originally belonged to this group, before it was recognized as a separate entity (WEALE, 1953, 1959; BLACKWELL & BLACKWELL, 1961; GIBSON, 1962; SPIVEY, 1965; ALPERN, LEE & SPIVEY, 1965; IKEDA & RIPPS, 1966; POKORNY et al., 1970). FRANCOIS & VERRIEST (1959) divided the group of the incomplete achromatisms into eight classes, supposing these classes to be intermediate stages between the real achromatism and the dichromatism.

In our electro-ophthalmological department we saw a patient who seemed to have an incomplete achromatism, but he did not show the symptoms of one of the eight types mentioned by FRANCOIS & VERRIEST. The diagnosis was difficult for us and for those ophthalmologists, who saw the patient before we did. As the disturbance was congenital, showed no fundus abnormalities and remained stable until now, it is surely not a cone dystrophy, but a cone dysfunction. In this paper we will therefore not delve into the problems of the cone dystrophies. A thorough and recent review of the latter is given by KRILL & DEUTMAN (1972, 1973).

CASE HISTORY

The patient is a healthy boy, born in 1960. He was examined several times over a period of eight years. Shortly after birth the parents noticed a nystagmus.

---

* Eye Clinic, Medical Faculty, Rotterdam, The Netherlands.

175

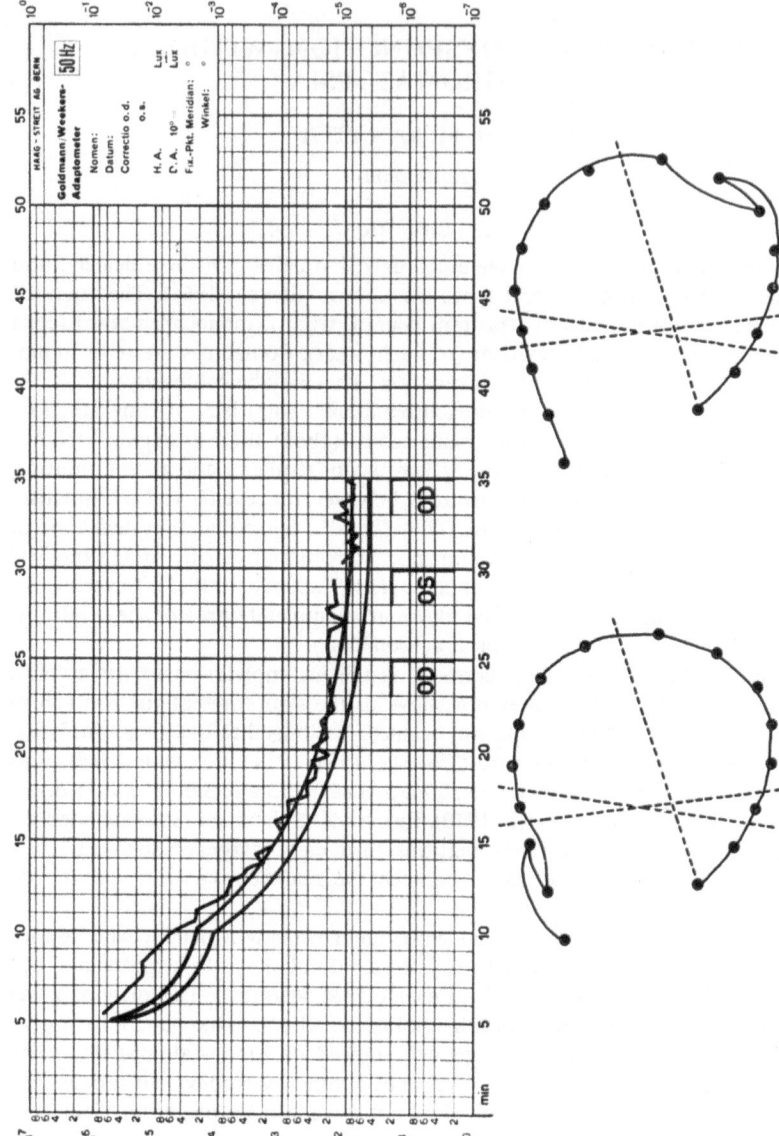

Fig. 1. Upper: The dark adaptation curve, made with the Goldmann-Weekers adaptometer, using full-field stimulation. Lower: The results of the Panel D-15 test.

Later on low vision appeared to exist, too. The ophthalmologist, consulted at that time, did not find any retinal abnormalities ophthalmoscopically. Parturition was normal. There are no visual abnormalities in the family, and there is no consanguinity between the parents. His three year older sister shows no visual abnormalities.

In 1965–66 the boy was examined more thoroughly. The nystagmus is horizontal and undulatory with a frequency of more than 5 per second. The visual acuity is about 0.1. Since the boy has flaxen hair, attention was primarily drawn to an ocular albinism. The absence of photophobia and the absence of diaphanous irides both in the boy himself and his relations make this diagnosis very improbable. Simple colour tests were done fairly well, so that an achromatism was not likely to exist either, although the electroretinogram, made under general anaesthesia, showed an almost absent photopic response.

In 1967 and 1970 the examination was repeated and extended. The visual field showed a slight reduction of the central sensitivity and the dark adaptation only a heightened cone branch (Fig. 1). The flicker fusion frequency (FFF) was lower than 15, psychophysically as well as in the electroretinogram. The Hardy-Rand-Rittler test, the anomaloscope and 100-Hue test revealed a slight deuteranomaly, while the Panel D-15 and colour naming tests were carried out with only small errors.

The electro-oculogram was normal as well as the electroretinogram of the rod system (scotopic ERG). The electroretinogram of the cone system (photopic ERG) was much reduced. In Fig. 2 the electric responses of the rod and cone system of the patient are compared with those of a normal subject and those of a typical achromat. The achromat has no photopic response at all; our patient a small response of about 20 μV with a lengthened latency time. The foveal electroretinogram (F-ERG) and visually evoked responses (VER) were absent.

During these years the symptoms remained stationary, so that a dysfunction instead of a dystrophy had to be assumed.

DISCUSSION

The patient, reported here, has symptoms of a defect in the function of the cone system, viz. the low visual acuity, the low Flicker Fusion Frequency and low photopic ERG. As the latter is not totally absent and colour vision is only slightly defective, he surely does not have a rod achromatism. A macular aplasia or macular dysfunction, in which only macular cones would be absent or would function abnormal, could not exist either in our patient, as a disease, restricted to the macular area does not show such a lowered photopic ERG (JACOBSON, 1961).

The diagnosis, therefore, was incomplete achromatism. However, we were not very happy with this diagnosis. It covers a multitude of sins, although less than the initial diagnosis bilateral amblyopia does. Our patient, moreover, did not fit any of the categories of the incomplete achromatism as described by FRANCOIS & VERRIEST (1959). The first six types all have normal visual acuity; the last two types a marked dyschromatopsia.

177

In the literature we found similar cases described by FRANCOIS & VERRIEST in 1960, by GOODMAN et al. in 1963 and by KRILL in 1968. FRANCOIS & VERRIEST presented three patients of which two were cousins, while the other was a solitary case like our patient. The two cousins had a deutan defect, the third patient showed only slight alterations in colour vision, but also of the deutan type. GOODMAN et al. described three unusual cases in their paper on cone

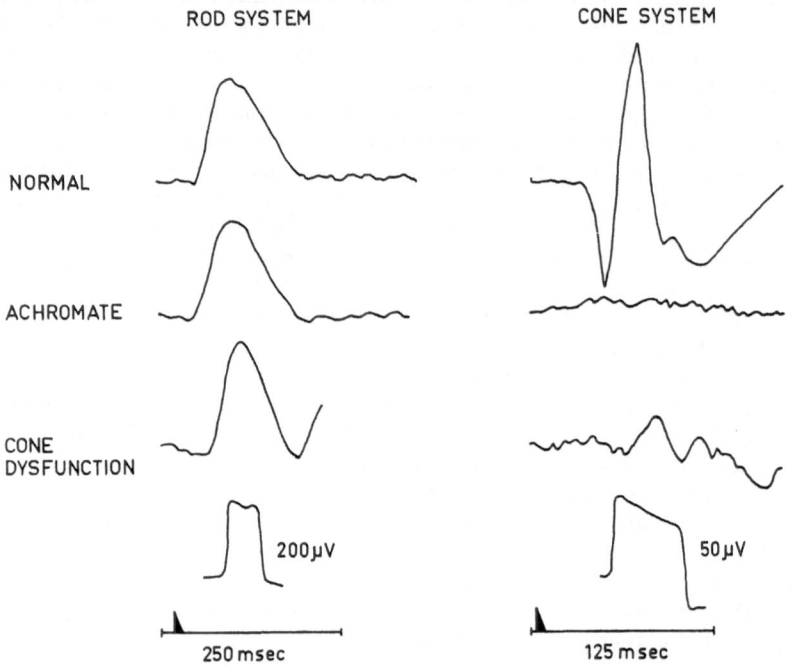

Fig. 2. ERGs of the rod system (left) and those of the cone system (right) of a normal subject, of a rod achromat and of the patient described. The ERGs of the rod system have been made in the dark adapted state with blue flashes in a frequency of 1 per second (9 responses averaged); the ERGs of the cone system in the light adapted state (blue background) with white flashes in a frequency of 4 per second (90 responses averaged).

dysfunctions. The second of the three showed the same symptoms as our patient. The authors supposed this patient to be suffering from a cone dystrophy. KRILL saw four siblings with also the same symptoms as our patient. The siblings, two males and two females, were children of related parents. KRILL supposed that they had mainly a central cone disturbance.

Now that we knew the type of dysfunction, we spotted three more patients last year: one is a solitary case, the other two are siblings. All three are children too young to be thoroughly examined, but they all have a lowered visual acuity, an extremely lowered photopic ERG and a good colour recognition.

178

We do not think that these cases are intermediate stages between the typical achromatism and the dichromatism, as FRANCOIS & VERRIEST (1959) supposed for the other categories of the incomplete achromatism. The patient described here and probably our other three patients as well, have a trichromatism in which the total number of functioning cones is diminished. ALPERN et al. (1960) found two kinds of receptors in the typical achromatism, one for low luminance vision, the other for high luminance vision. The high-luminance-receptors seemed to be cones, but not chromatic cones. The number of these cones was variable. BLACKWELL & BLACKWELL (1961) came to the same conclusion in blue cone monochromatism, in which only one cone system, the blue one, functions. Also in this disturbance the number of cones was variable. From our patient it appeared, that the same may happen in trichromatism.

It is known that in the typical achromatism the photopic ERG is extremely lowered or absent (KRILL 1968). In our set-up a bright blue adaptation light, suppressing all rods, and a Flicker Frequency of 4 flashes per second is used (VAN LITH & HENKES, 1968). This may be the reason that we do not find recordable photopic ERGs in the rod achromat, as in the latter CARR & SIEGEL (1964) and DODT et al. (1967) found a present photopic single flash ERG together with an absent Flicker ERG. In the blue cone monochromatism IKEDA & RIPPS (1966) found photopic activity in the electroretinogram. Blue sensitivity was normal, red sensitivity depressed as in protanopia. They did not furnish data concerning the degree of reduction. In general, the photopic ERGs from the incomplete achromatisms will be lowered to a lesser degree than those of the complete achromatism (KRILL, 1968).

In the photopic ERG of our patient both a- and b-wave are disturbed. The b-wave probably derives from the Müller cells (DOWLING, 1970). If this is true the b-wave does not inform us directly about the receptor system, but only indirectly after signal processing in the retina. The photopic a-wave, being a receptor potential (DOWLING, 1970), is surely a better indicator for the function of the cone receptors. The presence of both a- and b-wave in our patient indicates at least that there are functioning cones. As the value of the photopic ERG is only 15–20%, the number of functioning cones is very low.

The almost normal photopic visual field may mean that these cones are spread over the whole retina. The visual acuity, on the other hand, is probably determined by that part of the retina in or near the fovea, where cone density is highest. This place is very small in the boy examined as he can read small print more easily than large print. Large print has to be scanned before it can be recognized.

As colour vision is almost undisturbed in these patients, we do not think it right to use the term incomplete, atypical or partial 'achromatism'. It would be better to use the term 'general cone dysfunction with trichromatism' or to use the terminology of BLACKWELL & BLACKWELL (1961). In the latter case the name should be 'oligocone trichromacy'. From our patients and those of FRANCOIS & VERRIEST (1960) and KRILL (1968) it may be deduced, that the inheritance of this abnormality is autosomal recessive.

179

SUMMARY

This report deals with a patient, who has many symptoms of an achromatism, but he has good colour vison and a small (15-20%) photopic ERG. Probably three more of these patients have been observed in our department. In the literature, too, some of these cases have been described. We suppose, that in this disturbance some cones of each of the three colour systems function. Therefore this syndrome may be called 'oligocone trichromacy'. The inheritance is autosomal recessive.

REFERENCES

ALPERN, M., FALLS, H. F. & LEE, G. B. The enigma of typical total monochromacy. *Amer. J. Ophthal.* 50:*326* (1960).
ALPERN, M., LEE, G. B. & SPIVEY, B. E. Cone monochromatism. *Arch Ophthal.* 74:*334* (1965).
BLACKWELL, H. R. & BLACKWELL, O. M. Rod and cone receptor mechanisms in typical and atypical congenital achromatopsia. *Vision Res.* 1:*62* (1961).
CARR, R. E. & SIEGEL, I. M. Electrophysiological aspects of several retinal diseases. *Amer. J. Ophthal.* 58:*95* (1964).
DODT, E., LITH, G. H. M. VAN. & SCHMIDT, B. Electroretinographic evaluation of the photopic malfunction in a totally colour blind. *Vision Res.* 7:*231* (1967).
DOWLING, J. E. Organization of vertebrate retinas. *Invest. Ophthal.* 9:*655* (1970).
FALLS, H. F., WOLTER, R. & ALPERN, M. Typical total monochromacy. A histological and psychophysical study. *Arch. Ophthal.* 74:*610* (1965).
FRANCOIS, J. & VERRIEST, G. Contribution à l'étude des dyschromatopsies congénitales à symptomes intermédiaires entre ceux des systèmes dichromatiques classique et ceux de l'achromatopsie typique. *Ann. Oculist.* 192:*81* (1959).
FRANCOIS, J. & VERRIEST, G. Trois nouvelles observations d'achromatopsie congénitale atypique. *Ann. Oculist.* 193:*123* (1960).
GIBSON, I. M. Visual mechanisms in a cone-monochromat. *J. Physiol.* 161:*10* (1962).
GOODMAN, G., RIPPS, H. & SIEGEL, I. M. Cone dysfunction syndromes. *Arch. Ophthal.* 70:*214* (1963).
IKEDA, H. & RIPPS, H. The electroretinogram of a cone-monochromat. *Arch. Ophthal.* 75:*513* (1966).
JACOBSON, J. H. Clinical electroretinography; Proceedings 3rd ISCERG Symposium. Springfield, Thomas (1966).
KRILL, A. E. The electroretinogram in congenital color vision defects. In: The clinical value of electroretinography; Proc. 5th ISCERG Symposium Ghent 1966; ed. by J. Francois, p. 205. Basel, Karger (1968).
KRILL, A. E. & DEUTMAN, A. F. Dominant macular degenerations: the cone dystrophies. *Amer. J. Ophthal.* 73:*352* (1972).
KRILL, A. E. & DEUTMAN, A. F. The cone degenerations. *Doc. Ophthal.* 35, 1:*1–80* (1973).
LITH, G. H. M. VAN. & HENKES, H. E. The local electric response of the central retinal area. In: Advances in electrophysiology and -pathology of the visual system; Proc. 6th ISCERG Symposium Erfurt 1967; ed. by E. Schmöger. p. 163. Leipzig, Thieme (1968).
POKORNY, J., SMITH, V. C. & SWARTLEY, R. Threshold measurements of spectral sensitivity in a blue monocone monochromat. *Invest. Ophthal.* 9:*807* (1970).
SPIVEY, B. E. The office diagnosis of congenital achromatopsia (total color blindness). *J. Pediat. Ophthal.* 1:*30* (1964).
SPIVEY, B. E. The X-linked recessive inheritance of atypical monochromatism. *Arch. Ophthal.* 74:*327* (1965).
WEALE, R. A. Cone monochromatism. *J. Physiol.* 121:*548* (1953).
WEALE, R. A. Photosensitive reactions in foveae of normal and cone monochromatic observers. *Opt. Acta* 6:*158* (1959).

BOOLEAN NOTATION FOR OCULAR ELECTRO-PHYSIOLOGY (ERG AND VER) AND DIOPTRIC FACTORS

R. ALFIERI, P. SOLÉ & P. RENAUD*

(*Clermont-Ferrand*)

ABSTRACT

It often proves impossible to make an optical examination of the retina (funduscopy) when the transparent eye components are damaged, particularly in the case of lens opaqueness. In such cases the electric investigation (electroretinogram or ERG and visual evoked responses or VER) assumes its full value, since it then becomes the only objective means available to evaluate the sensorial function. However, when confronted with a change in the electric tracings, we have to be able to distinguish an actual retinal lesion from a 'pseudo-lesion' corresponding to a quantitative modification (energetic density) and a qualitative modification (spectral distribution) of the luminous flux reaching the retina. In order to emphasize the role of these dioptric factors, we have, (1), carried out a coupled electrophysiological exploration (ERG and VER) of the subjects before and after removal of the lens with a cataract; and (2), we have adopted a two-valued (all or nothing) Boolean notation to depict the result of each test: 1 if the test is normal, 0 if the test is altered.

I. PRINCIPLE

A. *Electroretinography*

We have only used static electroretinographic examinations, i.e. adapted to a high mesopic level. In white light, the ERG is usually purely photopic with a negative a-wave of medium amplitude, a positive b_1 wave of medium amplitude, and e-waves, or oscillatory potentials, which are located on the ascending slope of b_1. In orange light (Kodak Wratten filter), the ERG is composite: we find the previously mentioned photopic waves followed by a positive scotopic b_2-wave which is generally of smaller amplitude than the b_1-wave.

B. *Visual evoked responses*

We consider the VER in white light as a mere sign of the permeability of the optic pathways. In red monochromatic light (Schott interferential filter) the VER explores the conduction of the macular bundle of the optic nerve and allows an electric translation of the activity of the central cones since the cortical projection of the macula is preponderant.

C. *Coupled ERG and VER*

Assuming that the optic pathways are unimpaired between the multipolar cells and the occipital areas, the coupled survey of the ERG and VER allows a

---

* From the Faculty of Medicine, Clermont-Ferrand, France

global exploration of the retinal photoreceptors (ALFIERI et al., 1971): i.e. the rods (wave b_2 of the orange Wratten ERG), the peripheral cones (waves a, e and b_1 of the orange Wratten ERG) and the central cones (red interferential VER); the latter are not numerous enough to allow an electrical translation on the ERG under the usual recording conditions (ALFIERI et al., 1970).

D. *Boolean notation*

The result of a test, whether ERG or VER, is noted 1 if the test is normal, 0 if it is not. The findings of the electrophysiological exploration of a subject suffering from a cataract will thus be coded by a four-bit binary number where the first digit (extreme left) designates the pre-operative ERG; the second digit, the preoperative VER; the third digit, the post-operative ERG; and the fourth digit, (extreme right) the post-operative VER. Hence, the number 0011 will indicate a postoperative recovery of the ERG and VER tracings previously altered. Such a binary notation is valuable as it ensures an exhaustive enumeration of all possible cases (here $2^4 = 16$); it also ensures a thoroughly simple pattern, sparing us the out-of-date descriptions of purely morphological nosologies.

II. PROCEDURE

A. *Equipment*

Photostimulation with a xenon flash tube and recording of the potentials on a computer (ART 1000, SAIP), the curves being photographed on a polaroid film.

B. *Subject*

Adapted to a high mesopic level after dilation of the pupil with mydriatic solution. For the ERG: active corneal electrode (contact lens) and indifferent temporal electrode. For the VER, we use an active occipital electrode (2 cm from the median line and 2 cm above the external occipital bump) and an indifferent electrode fastened to the lobule of the ipsilateral ear. In addition, a grounded electrode is placed on the forehead and the distance between the subject and the luminant is 10 centimeters. We also allow a period of at least two months to elapse between the operation and the postoperative electric examination.

C. *Physical parameters*

(1) The ERG: Photostimulation: 4 Hz, first in white light, then in orange light (Kodak Wratten filter no. 26). Amplification: a time constant of 0.2 sec., band pass: between 0.8 and 250 Hz, with a 100 gain. Summation: analysis duration 200 ms, number of sweeps: 50.
(2) The VER: Photostimulation: 1 Hz, first in white light, then in red monochromatic light (Schott interferential filter 658 nm with a band pass of 14 nm). Amplification: time constant of 1 sec., band pass: 0.2 to 400 Hz, gain: 1000. Summation: analysis duration 500 ms, number of sweeps: 100.

182

III. Results

The global possible results may a priori be sorted into four groups, according to the electrophysiological results obtained before the operation, as follows:

11 xy: normal ERG and VER before the operation;
10 xy: normal ERG, but altered VER before the operation;
01 xy: altered ERG, but normal VER before the operation;
00 xy: altered preoperative ERG and VER;

Each group may then be divided into 4 sub-groups according to the electrophysiological results obtained after removal of the lens with a cataract, i.e. according to the values (0 and 1) assumed by x and y, which are:

- -11: normal (or improved) ERG and VER after the operation;
- -10: normal (or improved) ERG, but altered VER after the operation;
- -01: altered ERG, but normal (or improved) VER after the operation;
- -00: altered ERG and VER after the operation.

We shall now comment upon our observations (RENAUD, 1972) with such a classification:

A. *First group: 11 xy*—The preoperative results are normal: this corresponds to a comparatively minor opaqueness of the lens. After the operation, the electrophysiological results usually remain normal (Fig. 1: 1111, also noted ERG − VER → ERG − VER): it is the most common case. Infrequently, the post-operative results show a global "aggravation" (or 1100 which we also note as ERG − VER → $\overline{\text{ERG}}$ − $\overline{\text{VER}}$, the bar drawn above indicating the anomaly): we have for instance seen a diabetic retinopathy become rapidly progressive after ablation of the lens with a cataract. We have never come upon the following possible cases: 1110 (independent damage of the macula occurring between two electrophysiological explorations) and 1101 (postoperative detachment of the retina without any macular damage).

B. *Second group: 10 xy*—The VER alone is altered before the operation: this represents a slight opaqueness of the lens associated with a major or minor lesion of the macula. After the operation the results may show an improvement (Fig. 2: 1011, or ERG − $\overline{\text{VER}}$ → ERG − VER): the macula is only slightly affected and the gain in retinal illumination is significant enough to bring the VER back to normal. In exceptional cases, the postoperative results remain unchanged (1010, or ERG − $\overline{\text{VER}}$ → ERG − $\overline{\text{VER}}$): the macular damage is more serious. We have never come upon the possible cases 1001 (slight macular damage with intercurrent peripheral retinopathy) and 1000 (progressive macular retinopathy with peripheral extension).

C. *Third group 01 xy*—The ERG alone is altered before the operation. This means a moderate opaqueness of the lens (scotopic-type ERG) possibly associated with a retinopathy. After the operation, the results may show an improvement (Fig. 3: 0111 or $\overline{\text{ERG}}$ − VER → ERG − VER). If there is no coexisting

183

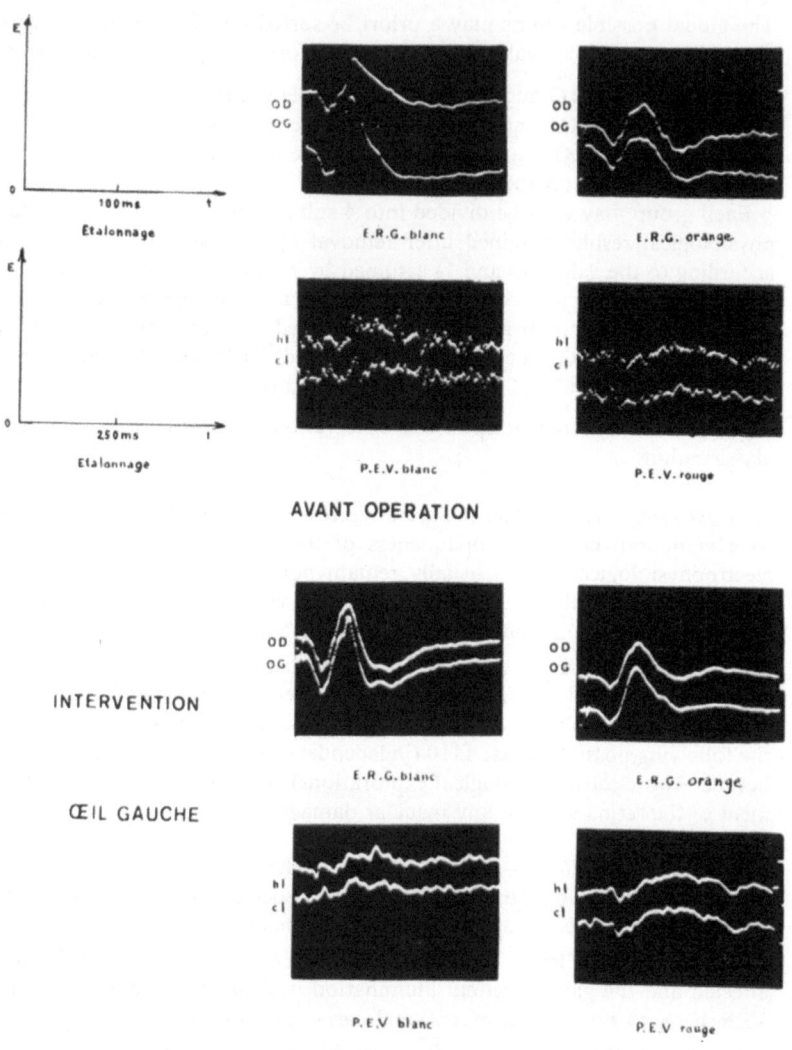

E.R.G.-P.E.V. ⟶ E.R.G.-P.E.V.

AVANT OPERATION

INTERVENTION

ŒIL GAUCHE

APRES OPERATION
Fig. 1.

Figs. 1, 2, 3 and 4.
Etalonnage: time scale
ERG blanc: white ERG
ERG orange: orange ERG   OD: RE = Right eye
PEV blanc: white VER   OG: LE = Left eye
PEV rouge: red VER   hl: homolateral
Avant operation: before operation   cl: controlateral
Après opération: after operation

184

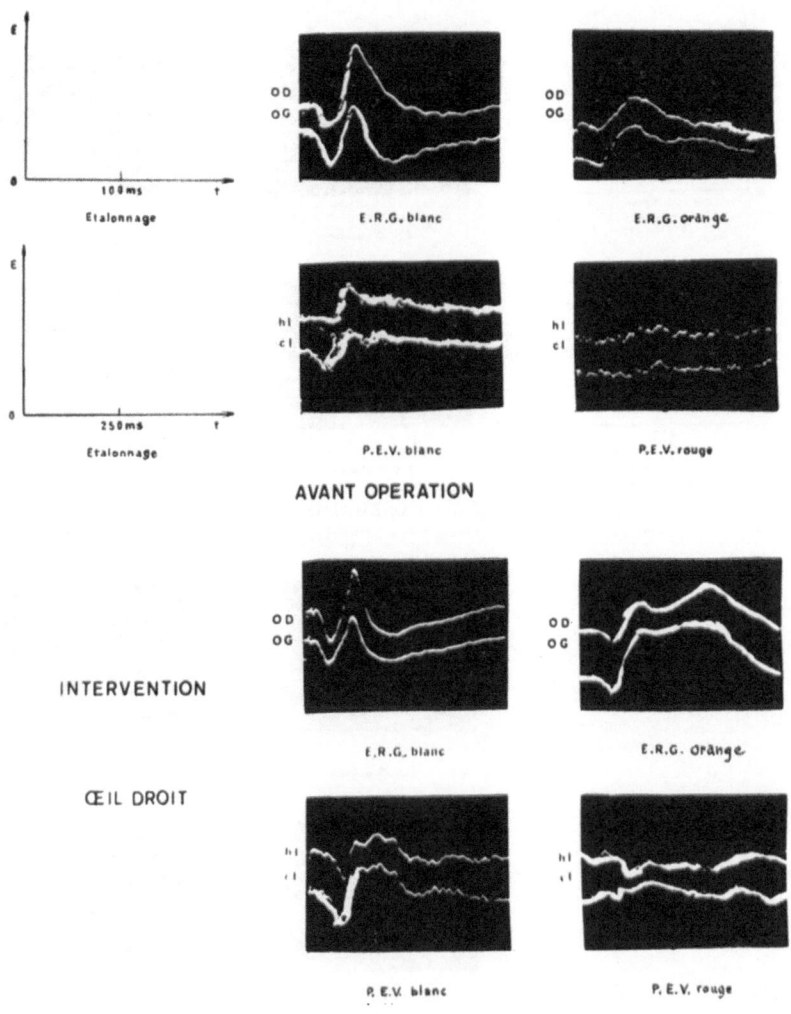

E.R.G. – $\overline{P.E.V.}$ ——→ E.R.G.–P.E.V.

Fig. 2.

retinopathy, the gain in retinal illumination allows a normalization of the $\overline{ERG}$. Sometimes the postoperative results remain unchanged (0101, or $\overline{ERG}$ – VER → $\overline{ERG}$ – VER): damage of the peripheral cones can be expected. Finally, the postoperative results may show a deterioration (0100 or $\overline{ERG}$ – VER → $\overline{ERG}$ – $\overline{VER}$): this reveals a progressive macular damage. We have

185

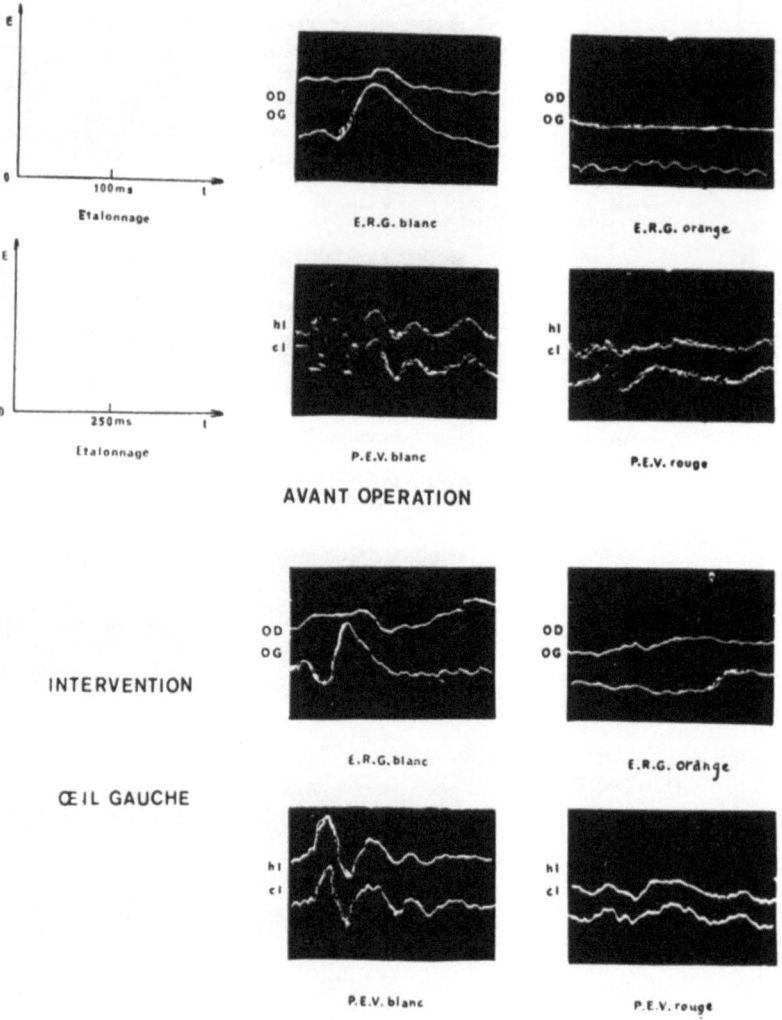

E.R.G. – P.E.V. ⟶ E.R.G. – P.E.V.

AVANT OPERATION

INTERVENTION

ŒIL GAUCHE

APRES OPERATION
Fig. 3.

never come upon the possible case 0110 (improvement of the ERG resulting from a gain in retinal illumination but weakening of the VER owing to an evolutive macular damage).

D. *Fourth group 00 xy*—Both preoperative ERG and VER results are abnormal: this means an important opaqueness of the lens if we exclude the possibility of a

186

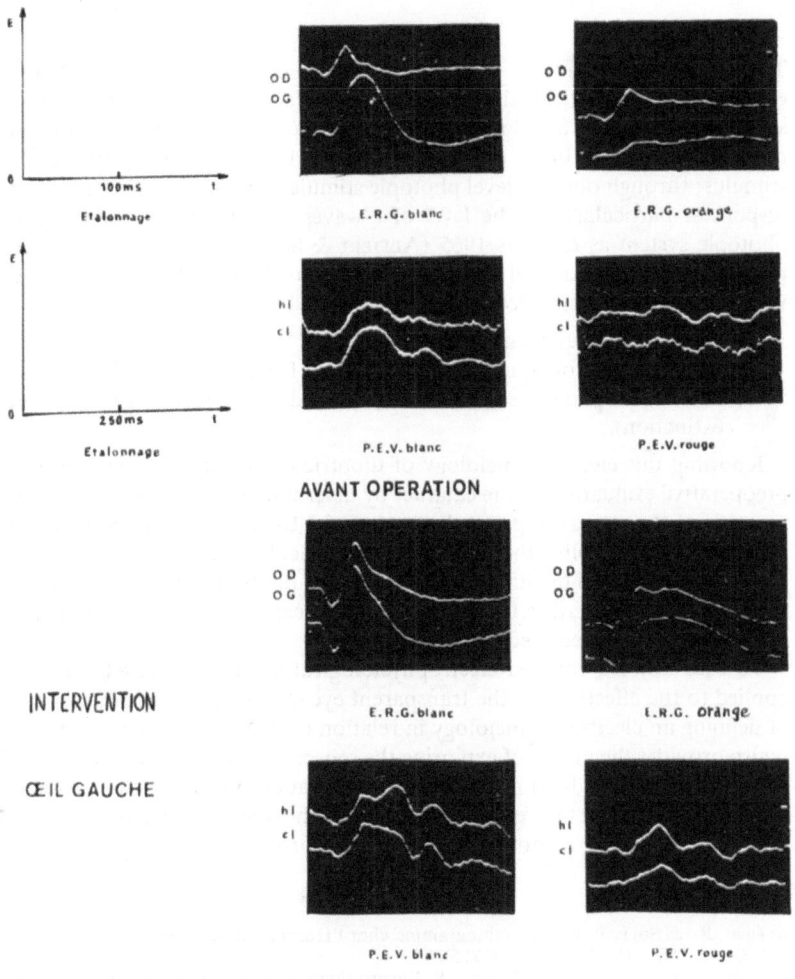

AVANT OPERATION

APRES OPERATION
Fig. 4.

concomitant retinopathy. After the operation, the results may become normal (Fig. 4: 0011, or $\overline{\text{ERG}} - \overline{\text{VER}} \rightarrow \text{ERG} - \text{VER}$): the electric anomaly was provoked by the dioptric factors alone. In some cases, the postoperative results show an improvement of the ERG only (0010 or $\overline{\text{ERG}} - \overline{\text{VER}} \rightarrow \text{ERG} - \overline{\text{VER}}$): this is macular retinopathy. In other cases, the postoperative results show an improvement of the VER alone (0001, or $\overline{\text{ERG}} - \overline{\text{VER}} \rightarrow \overline{\text{ERG}} -$

13

VER): peripheral retinopathy. Finally, the postoperative results may remain unchanged (0000, or $\overline{ERG} - \overline{VER} \rightarrow \overline{ERG} - \overline{VER}$): global retinopathy.

IV. DISCUSSION

The influence of a change in the transparency of the eye components on the electric responses of the retina is not equally recognized by the various authors; some will even deny any such influence (RENAUD, 1972). We think that these differences can most likely be explained by too high a luminance of the photo-stimulus; through our low-level photopic stimulations, we sensitize the electrical responses, particularly at the level of e-waves, which we associated with the photopic system as early as 1965 (ALFIERI & SOLÉ). Accordingly, the electro-physiological translation of an independent perturbation of the dioptric factors will be summarized as follows:

(1) For slight opaqueness, normal ERG and VER results;
(2) For moderate opaqueness, scotopic-type ERG and normal VER results;
(3) For high opaqueness, altered ERG and VER results (even down to extinction).

Knowing this electric semeiology of dioptric origin, it is possible to make a preoperative evaluation of the cataract by determining the value of the sensorial function of the retina; in particular a normal VER in red monochromatic light will practically establish the integrity of the macula at the date of examination (whether the ERG is disturbed or not). Finally, the Boolean notation will prove particularly convenient if the electrophysiological data are to be entered on a subject's computerized medical record.

To sum up, the coupled electrophysiological exploration (ERG and VER) applied to the affections of the transparent eye components provides the means of defining an electrical semeiology in relation to the degree of opaqueness, and it also provides the means of exploring the sensorial function of the retina during the preoperative evaluation of a cataract. In addition, this Boolean notation of the results ensures an exhaustive electropathogenic classification and facilitates their entry in a computerized medical record.

REFERENCES

ALFIERI, R. & SOLÉ, P. Electrorétinogramme chez l'Homme: ondes *e* et vision des couleurs. *C.R. Soc. Biol.* 159:*2362–2367* (1965).

ALFIERI, R., RIGAL, DANIELLE & SOLÉ, P. Electrophysiological nosology (ERG and VER) of retinopathies. In: Symposium on electroretinography; Proc. 8th ISCERG Symp., Pisa 7–12 Sept. 1970., p. 305. Pisa, Pacini (1972).

ALFIERI, R., SOLÉ, P. et ROUHER, F. Exploration électrophysiologique de la fonction visuelle en photostimulations monochromatiques. *Sciences médicales* 2:*157–166* (1971).

RENAUD, P. Etude comparative pré- et post-opératoire de l'électrorétinographie et des potentiels évoqués visuels dans la cataracte. (Thèse de médecine, Clermont-Ferrand, 1972). (90 references are mentioned in this paper).

ON THE SPECTRAL SENSITIVITY OF
OSCILLATORY POTENTIALS*

I. WATANABE, J. RICKERS & K. A. HELLNER**

(Hamburg)

Previously it was believed that in human beings the oscillatory potentials were photopic in nature (HECK & REMDAHL, 1957; REMDAHL, 1958). Later on it was pointed out that these potentials were either composed of photopic and scotopic elements, or they originated by interaction of both of these components (JACOBSON & MASUDA, 1963; NAGATA, 1964; AUERBACH, 1967; ALGVERE, 1969; ALGVERE & WESTBECK, 1972).

In animals, similar potentials were recorded both from predominant cone retinae as well as in predominant rod retinae (HECK & REMDAHL, 1957; REMDAHL, 1958; JACOBSON & MASUDA, 1963; NAGATA, 1964; AUERBACH, 1967; ALGVERE, 1969; ALGVERE & WESTBECK, 1972; NOELL, 1951, 1953; ARMINGTON, 1954; GRANDA, 1962; CRESCITELLI, 1961). To see whether the assumption of the dual photopic and scotopic nature of the oscillatory potentials is true, we measured the spectral sensitivity curves in a number of animal species.

The results of these investigations in mice, rats, guinea pigs and rabbits are reported.

MATERIAL AND METHODS

Whereas mice, rats and guinea pigs were examined under the general anesthesia with urethane, the experiments with rabbits were conducted under local anesthesia. Rabbits were dark adapted for 2 h and the other animals for 12 h. A halogen lamp (26 Volt, 25 Watts) built in a normal slide projector was used as a light source. Our optical system was almost the same as previously reported by HELLNER (1966). To get monochromatic light, Schott's interference filters were used. A second beam of this optical system was employed to achieve the selective colour adaptation.

The interference filters were equalized energetically, using a neutral light absorbing thermoelement in combination with a galvanometer. At the wavelengths used, the neutral filters were measured spectrophotometrically and their density was corrected, if necessary.

All the experiment were done both with pigmented and albinotic animals.

The spectral sensitivity curves were obtained from the diagrams showing the relationship of amplitude to light intensity (the amplitude versus intensity). As a threshold criterion an amplitude of 20 μV was chosen in all experiments.

RESULTS

As shown in Fig. 1 and 2, all animals showed distinctly 3 or more oscillatory potentials. The absolute b-wave threshold was calculated according to LE GRAND

* This study was supported by the Deutsche Forschungsgemeinschaft.

** From the University Eye Clinic, Hamburg, Germany.

189

(1957) and amounted in our experiments for mouse 1.7×10^{-10} lm/mm², for rat 1.1×10^{-10} lm/mm², for guinea pig 3.0×10^{-8} lm/mm² and for rabbit 8.3×10^{-9} lm/mm². The threshold of the a-wave was about 3.0 to 3.5 log units higher than that of the b-wave. Threshold for O_1 was essentially equal to that of the a-wave, whereas that of O_2 and O_3 lies about 1 log unit lower (Fig. 3 and 4).

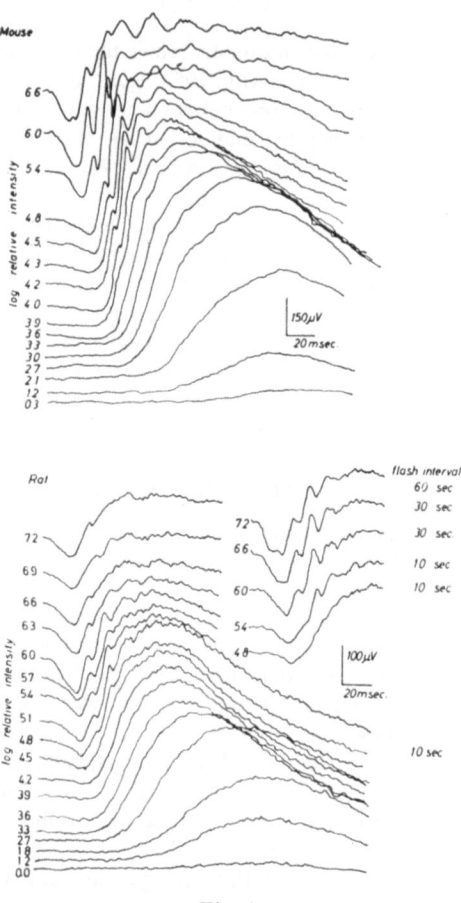

Fig. 1.

In all the animals the maximum of the spectral sensitivity curve was found at 500 nm. All types of albinotic animals showed a subpeak at ca. 600 nm. In the pigmented ones this subpeak was not constant. It was observed distinctly in rats and guinea pigs, missed in mice and rabbits. The spectral sensitivity curve of the oscillatory potentials coincided fairly well with the absorption curve of rhodopsin (CRESCITELLI & DARTNALL, 1953; DARTNALL, 1953; LEWIS, 1957). The spectral sensitivity curve of mice was broader than that of rhodopsin absorption spectrum.

190

In order to investigate the origin and nature of the subpeak, the following experiments were performed:

1. The effect of selective colour adaptation was studied.

  a: in mice;

    Here, the spectral sensitivity curve lost its subpeak at 600 nm while using 590 nm background illumination. This illumination amounted to 3.0 log

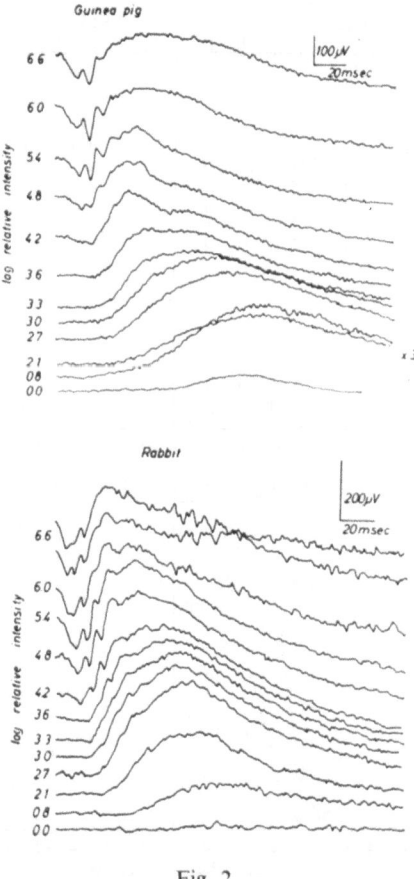

Fig. 2.

units higher that that determined for the b-wave threshold. However, under background illumination of 500 nm the subpeak at ca. 600 nm rose in comparison to those in experiments without background illumination.

  b: in rats and in guinea pigs

    The small hump at 600 nm was lost under the background illumination of 590 nm light. With 500 nm background illumination the increment of the subpeak was not as remarkable as in mice.

c: in rabbits

The subpeak at 600 nm could not be abolished with background illumination of 590 nm light. The change in intensity of the background illumination did not vary this result. The effect of 500 nm background illumination was not investigated.

2. Effect of an intravenous injection of Patent blue:

This experiment was performed as we could not abolish the subpeak in

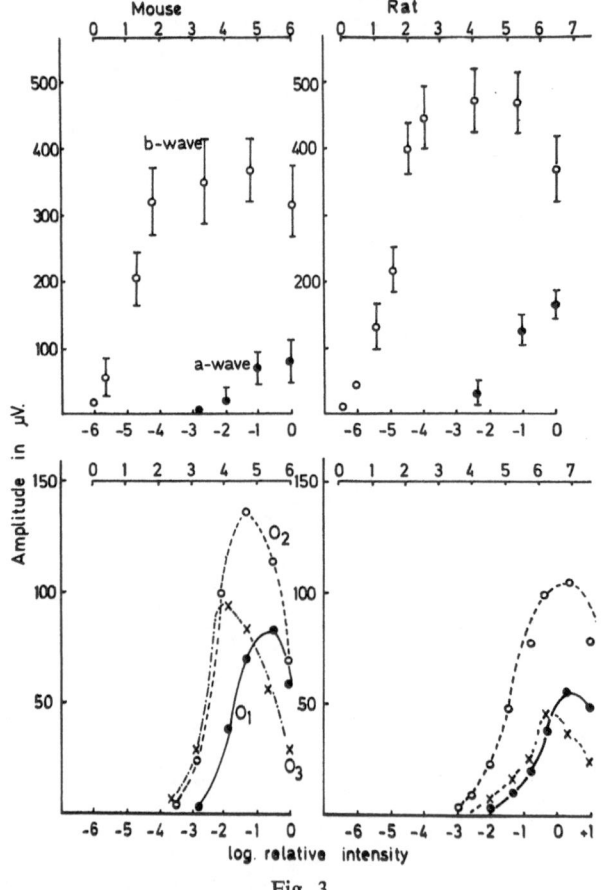

Fig. 3.

rabbits through background illumination. Patent blue was selected to eliminate the effect of blood reflection on the spectral sensitivity.

a: in rabbits (Fig. 8)

At first, the spectral sensitivity curve of the oscillatory potentials showed a remarkable subpeak at 600 nm. Thirty minutes after intravenous injection of Patent blue (0.2 g/kg), the subpeak was still present, but the sensitivity curve became slender at the shorter wave lengths. Then, a still higher dose of Patent blue (0.6 g/kg) was injected. Now, a monophasic curve with maximum at 500 nm without the subpeak at 600 nm was observed. Three hours later a reappearance of subpeak at 600 nm was found. An examination 20 h later yielded a curve resembling the one recorded before the Patent blue injection.

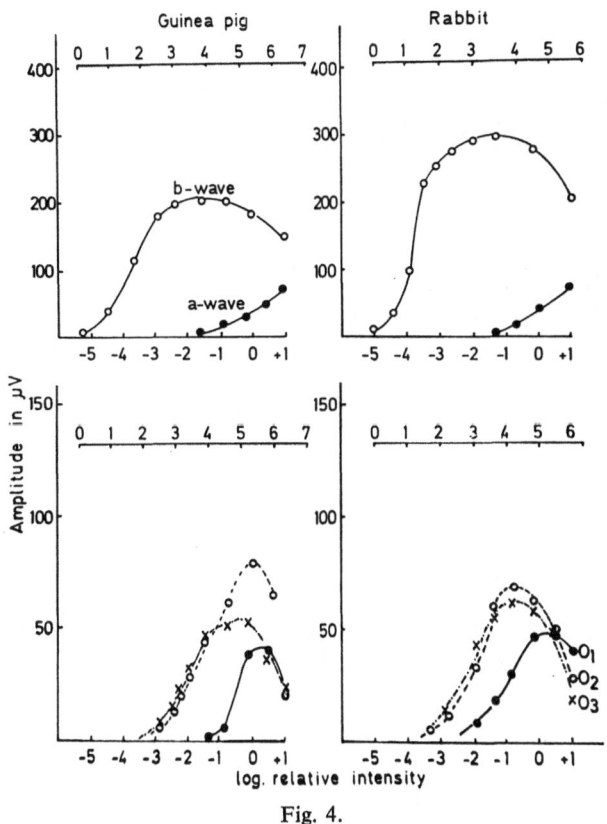

Fig. 4.

b: in rats (Fig. 9)

In this experiment the curve after the injection of Patent blue (1.0 k/kg) showed a hump at 600 nm and the whole curve corresponded well with the one without dye, within the range of experimental error.

DISCUSSION

The animals used here are believed to possess mixed retinae. However, mice and rats have so few a number of cones that sometimes they are regarded as rod animals (NOELL, 1951; CONE, 1963). GRANIT (1942) showed in the rat the existence of two modulators at 500 and 600 nm. Whereas, in the guinea pig, he found three narrow modulators at 450, 500 and 530 nm and a subpeak at

193

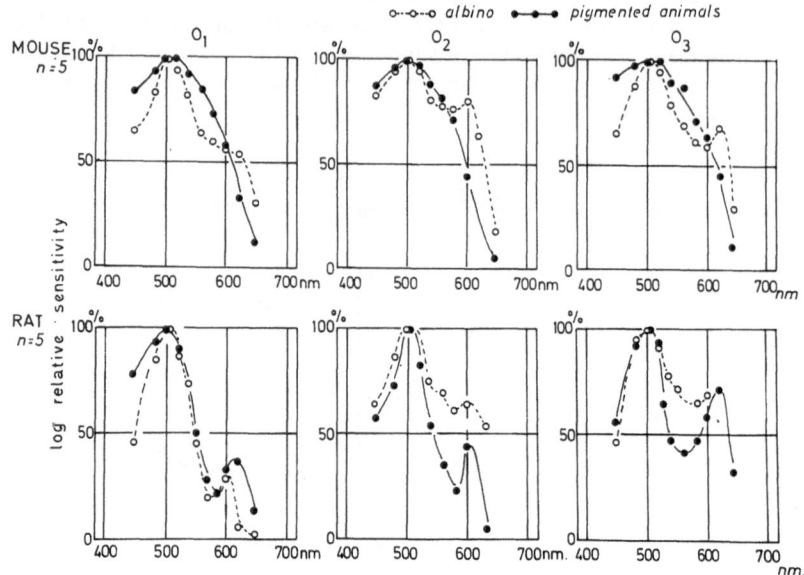

Fig. 5.

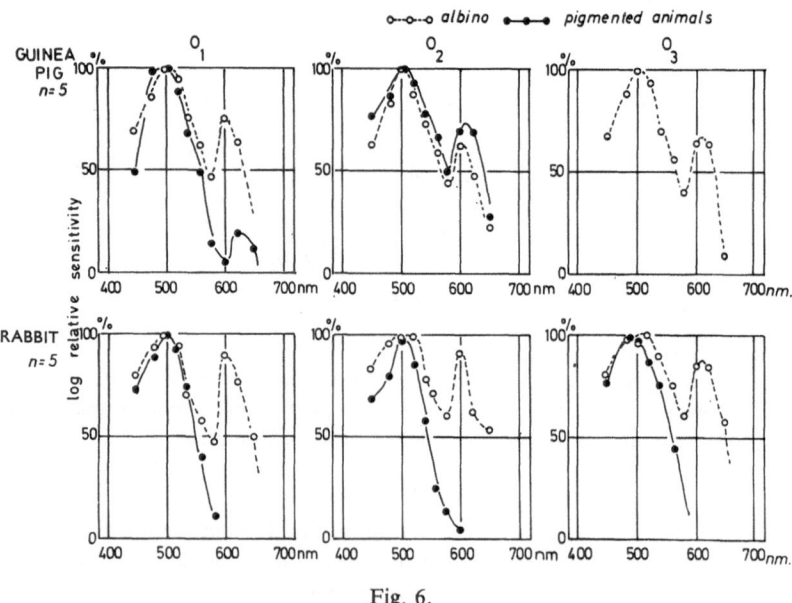

Fig. 6.

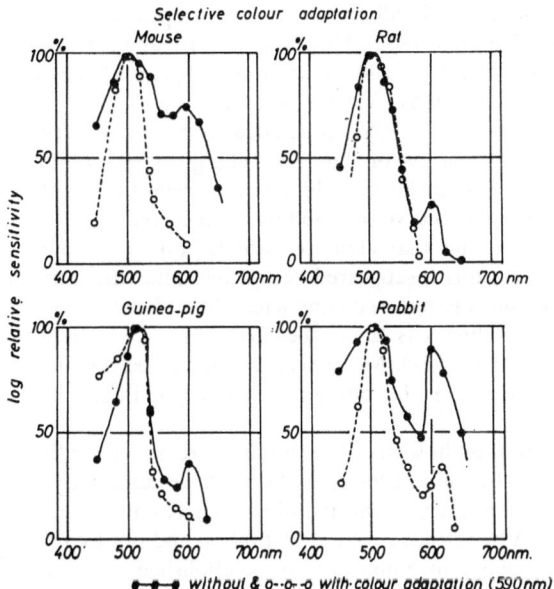

Fig. 7.

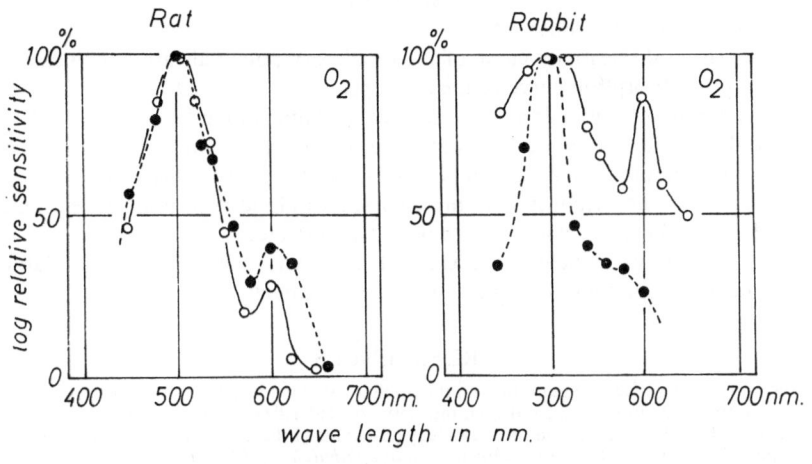

Fig. 8 and 9.

195

ca. 600 nm (1942). Also in albinotic rabbits a subpeak at ca. 600 nm was found (WIRTH, 1953; ELENIUS, 1958). However, in mice and rats, only a monophasic curve with a maximum at 500 nm without subpeak at the red end has been demonstrated (NOELL, 1951; VATTER, 1965).

DODT & WALTER (1959, 1958) concluded from their experiments concerning the spectral sensitivity curve of albinotic and pigmented rabbits that the subpeak at ca. 600 nm is due to a choroidal blood vessel reflection. In these experiments, the spectral absorption curve of blood was considered.

We have now found that albinotic rabbits show a distinct subpeak at ca. 600 nm. However, this disappeared completely after the intravenous injection of Patent blue and was restored completely 20 h after the injection. Therefore, in the rabbit this subpeak is due to the effect of choroidal light reflex as proved by DODT & WALTER (1958). Moreover, the pigmented rabbit did not show any subpeak at this region. So far our results are in good agreement with DODT & WALTER (1958).

Our present results show that these findings are not generally applicable to all types of animals. Because in the case of the rat we can clearly demonstrate that the subpeak does not arise from the blood reflection: In the rat the subpeak can be abolished by selective colour adaptation and not by Patent blue. On the contrary, the subpeak in rabbit can not be abolished by selective colour adaptation, but with Patent blue. This finding indicates the existence of a further retinal mechanism for the origin of the subpeak at ca. 600 nm.

SUMMARY

To summarize our results:
1. The spectral sensitivity curve of the oscillatory potentials are in coincidence with the absorption curve of the rhodopsin.
2. In all albinotic animals a subpeak at ca. 600 nm is found.
3. In the pigmented mouse and rabbit the subpeak is absent.
4. In the albinotic rabbit this subpeak is due to the blood reflection.
5. In the rat the origin is not only confined to blood reflection. An existence of a retinal component is accordingly demonstrated.
6. In general, we conclude the spectral sensitivity curves of the oscillatory potentials represent photopic and scotopic elements.

REFERENCES

ALGVERE, P. The effect of adaptation on the oscillatory potentials of the human electroretinogram to stimulation by flash of high intensity. 7th ISCERG Symposium. (1969).

ALGVERE, P. Clinical studies on the oscillatory potentials of the human electroretinogram with special reference to the scotopic b-wave. *Acta ophthal.* 46:993 (1969).

ALGVERE, P. & WESTBECK, S. Human ERG in response to double flashes of light during the course of dark adaptation: A Fourier analysis of the oscillatory potentials. *Vision res.* 12: *195–214* (1972).

ARMINGTON, J. C. Spectral sensititivy of the turtle, Pseudemys *J. Comp. Physiol. Psychol.* 47: *1–6* (1954).

AUERBACH, E. The human electroretinogram in the light and during dark adaptation. *Documenta ophthal.* 22:*1–7* (1967).

CONE, R. A. Quantum relations of the rat electroretiongram. *J. gen. physiol.* 46:*1267–1963* (1963).

196

CRESCITELLI, F. The Electroretinogram of the antelope ground squirrel. *Vision Res.* 1:*139–153.* (1961).

CRESCITELLI, F. & DARTNALL, H. J. A. Human Visual Purple. *Nature (London)* 172:*195–196* (1953).

DARTNALL, H. J. A. The interpretation of spectral sensitivity curves. *Brit. Med. Bull.* 9:*24–30* (1953).

DETWILER, S. R. Studies on the retina observation on the rods of nocturnal mammals. *J. comp. Neurol.* 37:*481–489* (1924).

DODT, E. & WALTHER, J. B. Elektroretinographische Messung der Spektralsensitivität von Albinoaugen bei direkter und diaskleraler Belichtung. *Pflügers Archiv.* 268:*435–443* (1959).

DODT, E. & WALTHER, J. B. Spektrale Sensitivität und Blutreflexion. Vergleichende Untersuchungen an pigmentierten und albinotischen Netzhäuten. *Pflügers Arch. ges. Physiol.* 266:*187* (1958).

ELENIUS, V. Recovery in the dark of the rabbit's electroretinogram in relation to intensity, duration and colour of light-adaptation. *Acta physiol. scand. suppl.* 150 (1958).

GRANDA, A. M. Electrical response of the light and dark adapted turtle eye. *Vision Res.* 2: *343–346* (1962).

GRANIT, R. Isolation of colour sensitive elements in a mammalian retina. *Acta physiol. scand.* 2:*93–109* (1942).

GRANIT, R. Spectral properties of the visual receptor elements of the guinea pig. *Acta physiol. scand.* 3:*318–328* (1942).

HECK, J. & REMDAHL, I. Component of the human electroretinogram. *Acta physiol. scand.* 39:*167–175* (1957).

HELLNER, K. A. Das adaptive Verhalten der Mäusenetzhaut. *Albrecht v. Graefes Arch. klin. exp. Ophthal.* 169:*166–175* (1966).

JACOBSON, J. & MASUDA, Y. Oscillatory potentials of the cat b-wave. III ISCERG Symposium. (1963).

LE GRAND, Y. Light, Colour and Vision. Chapman and Hall, London. (1957).

LEWIS, D. M. Retinal photopigment in the albino rat. *J. Physiol.* 136:*615–623* (1957).

NAGATA, M. Photopic flicker ERG in cases of congenital night blindness. *Documenta ophthal.* 18:*352–366* (1964).

NOELL, W. K. The effect of iodate on the vertebrate Retina. *J. cell. comp. Physiol.* 37:*283–307* (1951).

NOELL, W. K. Studies on the electrophysiology and the metabolism of the retina. USAF School of Aviation Medicine. Project No. 21-1201-0004. Report Nr. 1 Randolph Field, Texas. (1953).

RENDAHL, I. Component of the human electroretinogam. *Acta physiol. scan.* 44:*189–202* (1958).

VATTER, O. Das Elektroretinogramm der weißen Maus. *Naturwissenschaften* 52:*85–86* (1965).

WIRTH, A. Electroretinographic evaluation of the scotopic visibility function in cats and albino rabbits. *Acta physiol. scand.* 29:*22–30* (1953).

HUMAN SCOTOPIC FAST RETINAL POTENTIALS (FRP'S)

RICHARD STODTMEISTER*

(*Frankfurt*)

Introduction

Power spectral analysis of ERG responses reveals different frequency bands as shown by Jones et al. (1969) and by Kozak (1971) in animals, and by Algvere & Westbeck (1972) in humans. When the 150–200 Hz frequency band is selected (Dawson & Stewart, 1968) the so-called fast retinal potentials are recorded. Adams & Dawson (1971) showed luminosity functions obtained from averaged FRP's in humans and concluded that the FRP's obtained by means of active electronic filtering are primarily of photopic origin. In the present study FRP's were elicited from the dark adapted human eye by single stimuli. Relative spectral sensitivity values were obtained by the method of constant responses.

Methods

An 18 year old female and a 30 year old male, both in good health, were subjects. Their eyes showed no abnormalities. The subjects lay on a couch with the head held by a rubber band. Mydriaticum ROCHE and Neosynephrine 10% were used for maximal dilatation of the pupil and Chibro-Kerakain for topical anaesthesia of the cornea. After 20 minutes of dark adaptation the contact lens was inserted under dim red light. Then the dark adaptation was continued for an additional 10 minutes. The light stimulator was a two-beam adaptometer consisting of two series of optical relay systems (Scheibner, 1970). The light source was a 150 W short-arc xenon bulb. Rectangular stimuli were produced by an electromagnetic shutter driven by a square wave impulse generator. The stimulus duration was 100 msec, the rise time 1.0 msec. The stimulus interval was 90 sec. The test beam evenly illuminated a neutrally absorbing and diffusing disk positioned just in front of the contact lens, thus providing Ganzfeld illumination. The maximal luminance was 9000 cd/m². Monochromatic stimuli were obtained with the aid of interference bandfilters of known spectral peak transmittance (type AL, Schott & Gen., Mainz). In spectral energy measurements a thermopile with neutral characteristics was used in conjunction with a galvanometer. The electroretinogram was picked up by a Henkes low-vacuum contact lens electrode and differentially amplified by an AC coupled amplifier system (bandwidth 0.16–1300 Hz). The responses were both photographed from the oscilloscope screen and stored on a tape recorder (Bell & Howell VR 3200).

* Arbeitsgemeinschaft Universitäts-Augenklinik Frankfurt/Main (Direktor: Prof. Dr. W. Doden) und II. Physiologische Abteilung des W. G. Kerckhoff-Instituts der Max-Planck-Gesellschaft, Bad Nauheim (Direktor: Prof. Dr. E. Dodt).

For the display of the FRP's an active electronic variable filter was used in highpass mode (−3dB point: 87 Hz; −72dB/octave attenuation slope; type EF 2—Barr and Stroud, Glasgow).

With a 472 nm light ca. 2.5 log units above the first appearance of the FRP's, 5 FRP's were clearly seen. They were labelled 1–5 reading the records from left to right. The amplitudes of FRP's evoked by stimuli of 575 and 601 nm were compared with those of FRP's evoked by 472 nm light. FRP's of the same amplitude and latency were assigned the same numbers. The amplitudes were measured vertically from the FRP peak to the preceding depression.

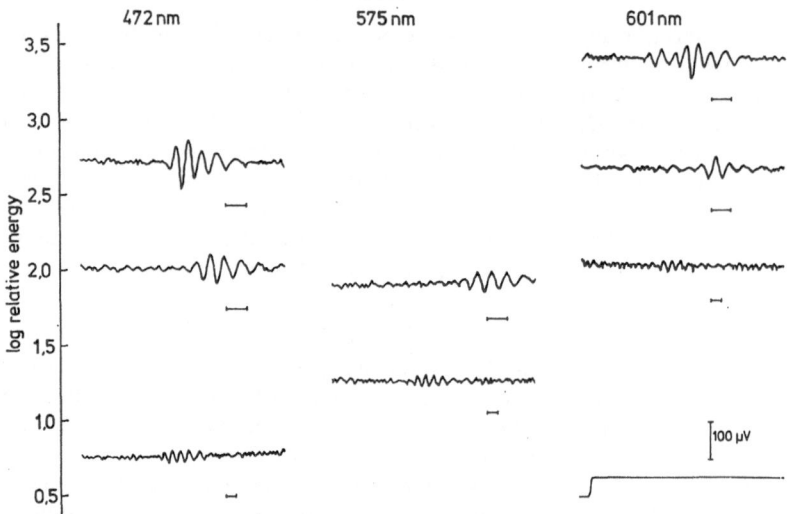

Fig. 1. FRP's at single stimuli (100 msec). Dark adapted human eye. Monochromatic light 472 nm (left), 575 nm (middle) and 601 nm (right). The logarithm of the relative test energy is given far left. The vertical position of the starting points of the records correspond to the relative test energy used. Sweep speed: 10 msec/cm or 20msec/cm. The horizontal bars below each trace correspond to 10 msec. Vertical bar: 100 μV. Bottom trace: stimulus marking at 10 msec/cm sweep speed.

Results

Fig. 1 shows records of FRP's evoked by 472 nm (left), 575 nm (middle) and 601 nm (right) test lights of rising luminance. The ordinate represents the relative test energy. The least energy to evoke FRP's is needed at 472 nm. In the records taken at 601 nm potentials appear with latencies shorter than those measurable at 472 nm. These potentials are a sign of photopic activity. In such cases conventional broadband records show an x-wave, according to Motokawa & Mita (1942) & Adrian (1945).

In Fig. 2 the amplitude of the b-wave (filled symbols) and the amplitudes of the second FRP (open symbols) recorded at 472 nm (■, □), 575 nm (▲, △) and 601 nm (●, ○) are plotted against the logarithm of the relative energy of

200

the test light. As far as the b-wave and the FRP_2 are concerned, less energy is needed with the shorter test wavelength to evoke the b-wave or FRP_2.

Fig. 3 shows relative spectral sensitivity values obtained by the method of constant response (SCHEIBNER & SCHMIDT, 1969). The criterion was an amplitude of 60 μV for the b-wave and 30 μV for the FRP's. The values agree well with the CIE scotopic luminosity function. Values could not be obtained for more than 3 wavelengths in a single session, because the stimulus interval of 90 sec

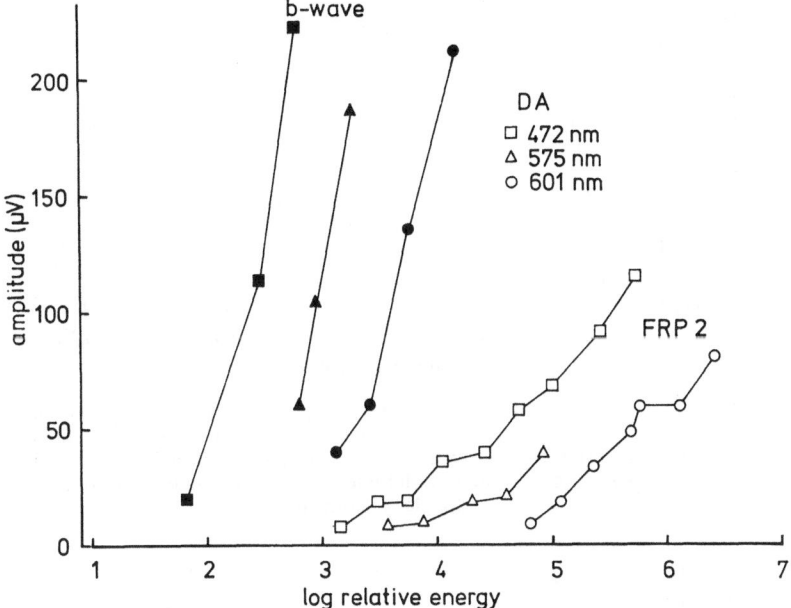

Fig. 2. The amplitudes (ordinate) of the b-wave (filled symbols) and of the second FRP (open symbols) are plotted versus the logarithm of relative energy of the test light (abscissa) at 472 nm (■, □), 575 nm (▲, △) and 601 nm (●, ○). Dark adapted human eye. Single stimuli. Single experiment.

limited the number of the test flashes during the available time of one hour. When the time interval between the stimulus onset and the peak of an FRP is plotted versus the logarithm of the relative test energy, as in Fig. 4, it can be shown that the time of this interval is shorter at the shorter wavelength, which indicates a higher relative spectral sensitivity in response to stimuli of shorter wavelengths.

DISCUSSION

The spectral sensitivity values presented here of FRP's obtained from records of the dark adapted human eye lead to the conclusion that FRP's are generated by the scotopic retinal elements when the eye is dark adapted. ADAMS & DAWSON (1971) concluded from their luminosity functions obtained from averaged FRP's recorded under photopic, mesopic and scotopic conditions that FRP's are

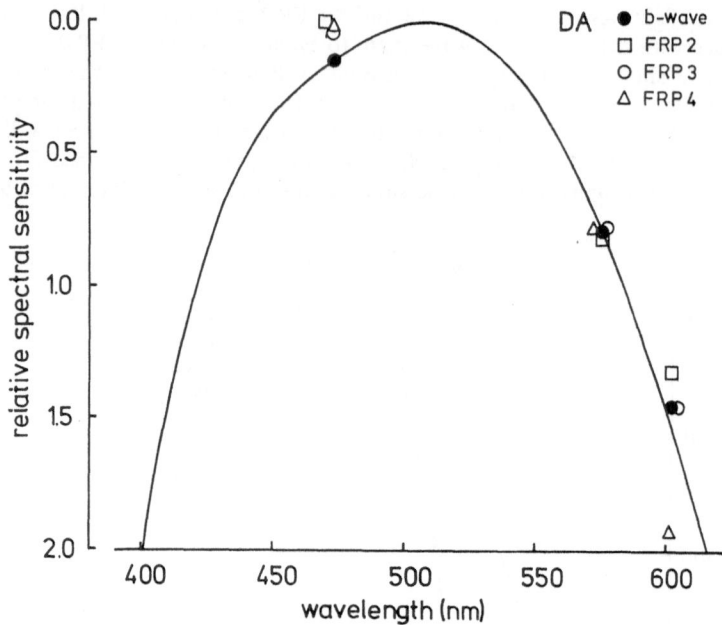

Fig. 3. Relative spectral sensitivity values obtained by the method of constant response from records of the dark adapted human eye at single stimuli. Amplitude criterion for the b-wave: 60 μV, for FRP's: 30 μV. b-wave: filled symbols; FRP's: open symbols. Solid line: CIE scotopic luminosity function. Single experiment.

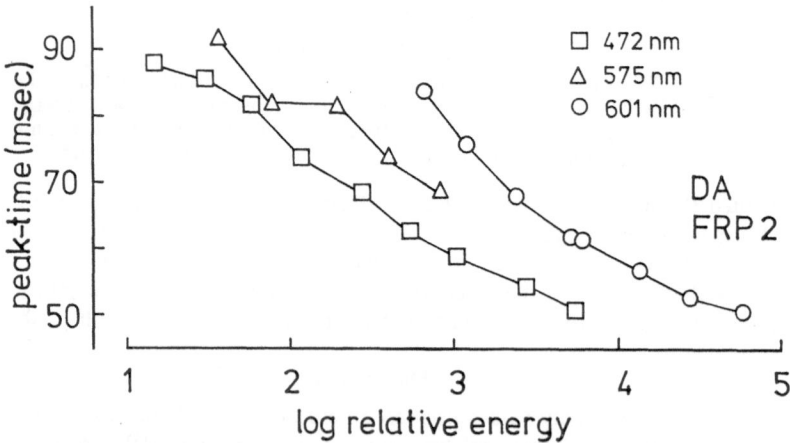

Fig. 4. The time interval between stimulus onset and the peak of the second FRP (ordinate) is plotted versus the relative spectral energy of the test light (abscissa) at 472 nm ($\square$), 575 nm ($\triangle$) and 601 nm ($\bigcirc$) test light wavelength. Dark adapted human eye. Single stimuli. Single experiment.

primarily of photopic origin. These authors stimulated the dark adapted human eye with weak flashes at a repetition rate of one per 5 sec. It seems likely that the repetition rate used by the above authors at the luminance selected was too high and that the flashes changed the state of adaptation during the experiment. The results of ALGVERE & WESTBECK (1972) suggest that consecutive flashes greatly influence the mechanism generating the FRP's.

KOZAK (1971) assumed that the FRP's are the result of activity in feedback loops involving lateral inhibition. The results shown here would imply that the lateral inhibitory activity of the dark adapted human retina is driven by the scotopic retinal elements.

The mechanisms generating FRP's and wavelets in the human ERG has been regarded by BORNSCHEIN & GOODMAN (1957) and JACOBSON et al. (1968) as being independent from the mechanisms generating the b- or a-wave. KOZAK's hypothesis (1971) could explain this independence. In spite of this independence, the dualism of the human retina is reflected by the FRP's if suitable stimulus conditions are chosen.

REFERENCES

ADAMS, K. C. & DAWSON, W. W. Fast retinal potential luminosity functions. *Vision Res.* 11: *1135–1146* (1971).

ADRIAN, E. D. The electric response of the human eye. *J. Physiol.* 104:*84–104* (1945).

ALGVERE, P. & WESTBECK, S. Human ERG in response to double flashes of light during the course of dark adaptation: A Fourier analysis of the oscillatory potentials. *Vision Res.* 12:*195–214* (1972).

BORNSCHEIN, H. & GOODMAN, G. Studies of the a-wave in the human electroretinogram. *A.M.A. Arch. Ophthal.* 58:*431–437* (1957).

DAWSON, W. W. & STEWART, H. L. Signals within the electroretinogram. *Vision Res.* 8:*1265–1270* (1968).

JACOBSON, J. H., HIROSE, T. & POPKIN, A. B, Independence of the oscillatory potential, photopic and scotopic b-waves of the human electroretinogram. The Clinical Value of Electroretinography. ISCERG Symposium Ghent 1966, pp. 8–20 (Karger, Basel/New York 1968).

JONES, A. E., FAIRCHILD, D. D. & SPYROPOULOS, P. Frequency analysis of the electroretinogram. 1969 Spring Meeting Opt. Soc. Amer. *J. opt. Soc. Amer.* 59:*511* (1969).

KOZAK, W. M. Electroretinogram and spike activity in mammalian retina. *Vision Res.* Suppl. Nr. 3, pp. *129–149* (Pergamon Press, 1971).

MOTOKAWA, K. & MITA, T. Über eine einfachere Untersuchungsmethode und Eigenschaften der Aktionsströme der Netzhaut des Menschen. *Tohoku J. Exp. Med.* 42:*114–133* (1942).

SCHEIBNER, H. & SCHMIDT, B. Zum Begriff der spektralen visuellen Empfindlichkeit, mit elektroretinographischen Ergebnissen am Hund. *Albrecht v. Graefes Arch. Klin. exp. Ophthal.* 177:*124–135* (1969).

SCHEIBNER, H. Personal communication (1970).

LUMINANCE RESPONSES TO PATTERN REVERSAL

H. SPEKREIJSE, O. ESTÉVEZ & L. H. VAN DER TWEEL*

(*Amsterdam*)

INTRODUCTION

The stimuli used in many spatial contrast studies were accompanied by overall changes in luminance (for a review see ESTÉVEZ & RÉMOND, 1972). This implies that the responses to these stimuli might have been a mixture of components to (a) changes in spatial contrast and (b) changes in luminous flux. In reality the situation seems to be even more complicated. The response is not merely an algebraic sum of (a) and (b), but the existence of one change may influence the response to the other change (SPEKREIJSE, VAN DER TWEEL & ZUIDEMA, 1973). To overcome this problem methods of spatial contrast stimulation were employed in which the total luminous flux remained constant in time. Although spatial contrast responses can be isolated in this way, it should be realized that even in this situation a luminance response may be produced. This complication seems especially important for the evaluation of the ERG's to spatial contrast variation. Such ERG's were first measured by RIGGS, JOHNSON & SCHICK, (1964) and are also studied concurrently with the VER's by ARMINGTON, CORWIN & MARSETTA, (1971). RIGGS introduced this stimulus to avoid stray-light so as to minimize scotopic response components.

STIMULUS

Our spatial contrast stimulus is formed by the reflecting and transparent elements of a patterned mirror. The intensities of the two sets of elements are set by two fluorescent tube light sources which can be modulated independently (for a full description see SPEKREIJSE, 1966; VAN DER TWEEL & SPEKREIJSE, 1968). In this paper the results of square wave and sine wave modulation are presented and for various reasons (VAN DER TWEEL & SPEKREIJSE, 1973) a checkerboard pattern is preferred as spatial contrast stimulus.

If both sets of checks are modulated equally and in counterphase the total amount of light falling on he eye remains constant. However, the spatial contrast stimulus differs depending on the mean intensities of the two sets of checks:

a. *Pattern reversal* (Fig. 1a) is obtained when both sets of checks have the same mean intensity. The "bright" and "dark" checks interchange rhythmically at twice the temporal modulation frequency. Hence only response components which are even multiples of the stimulus frequency can be obtained regardless their luminance or contrast origin.

b. *Appearnace-disappearance* (Fig. 1b) is achieved by adjusting the intensities of the two sets of checks in such a way that they are equal during half the stimulus period. The checkerboard pattern first appears then disappears to leave a blank field once during each stimulus cycle.

---

*Laboratory of Medical Physics, University of Amsterdam.

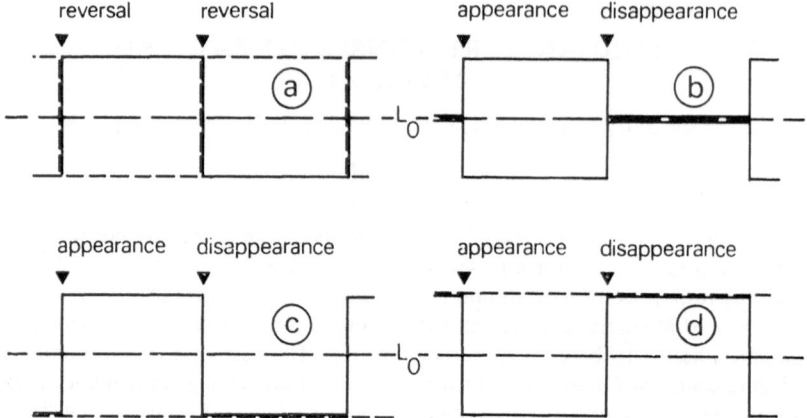

Fig. 1. Various modes of spatial contrast stimulation. In conditions a and b the luminous flux remains constant, in c and d the net luminance of the stimulus changes rhythmically.

Sometimes it is useful to modulate only one light source, in which situation the net luminance of the stimulus changes rhythmically. In the appearance-disappearance situation two conditions can be distinguished:

c. *Appearance of pattern at luminance increase* (Fig. 1c)
d. *Appearance of pattern at luminance decrease* (Fig. 1d)

RESULTS AND DISCUSSION

The VER's in the bottom row of Fig. 2 establish directly that the occipital responses have a spatial contrast origin, because in conditions c. and d. similar responses are obtained, although the luminance component in the stimulus shifts 180° in phase. Hence the relevant parameter for these VER's is the change in spatial contrast and not the change in luminance. The situation for the ERG is quite different to the situation for the EP. The simultaneously recorded ERG's in Fig. 2c and d follow the luminance component, because the ERG shifts 180° in phase.

If no spatial contrast component were present in the ERG, then one would expect at first sight that condition (a)—where the overall luminous flux remains constant—would not give an ERG at all. Therefore the ERG's to bar pattern reversal, described by RIGGS et al. (1964), would seem to have a spatial origin. However, condition (a) will only result in a zero luminance response if the system is linear. Then the responses of the two sets of checks will cancel (Fig. 3a). If on the other hand, the response to the modulation of either set of checks is already distorted then a luminance response to counterphase stimulation might be found (Fig. 3b). The amplitude of this response depends on the size of the spatial summation fields preceding the distorting stage. If the checks exceed the summation fields, the response, consisting of only even harmonics should

206

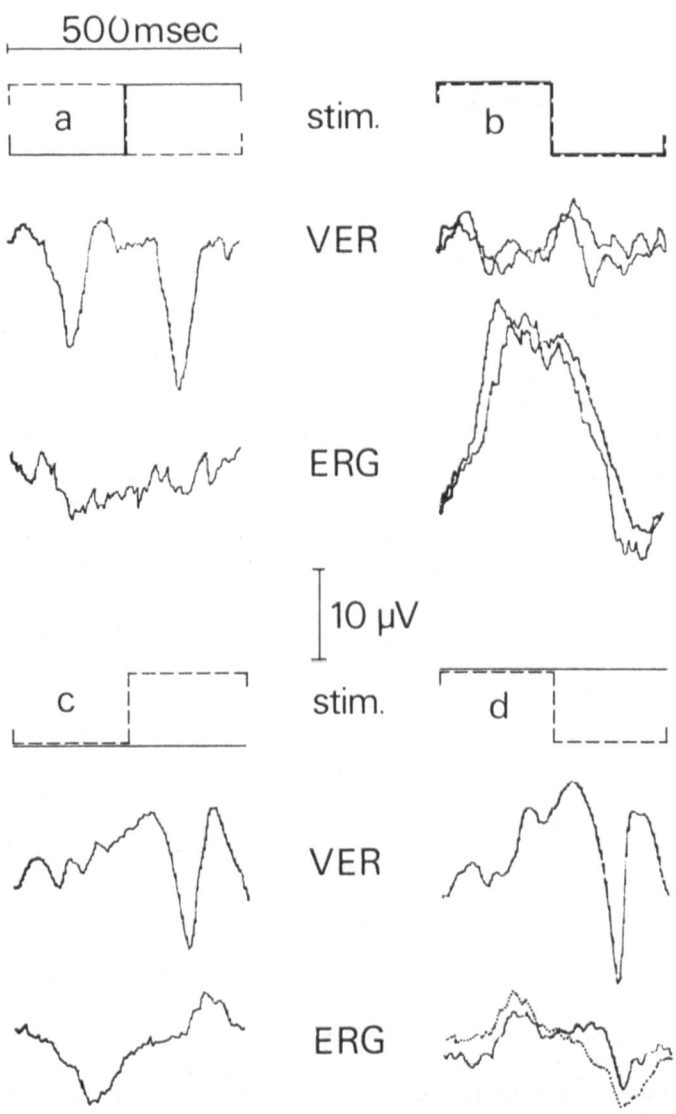

Fig. 2. VER's and simultaneously recorded ERG's to four stimulus conditions:
a. pattern reversal by counterphase modulation of the two sets of checks;
b. homogeneous field stimulation by in-phase modulation of the checks;
c. appearance of pattern at luminance increase;
d. appearance of pattern at luminance decrease. After a shift of 180°, the ERG of condition c is superimposed (dashed curve) on the ERG of condition d.
Left eye stimulation; 6° checkerboard with 15′ checks; VER from inion-ear derivation; mean luminance 50 asb; modulation depth 50%. The figure results from one single session. The single recordings were confirmed one by one in separated experiments.

model

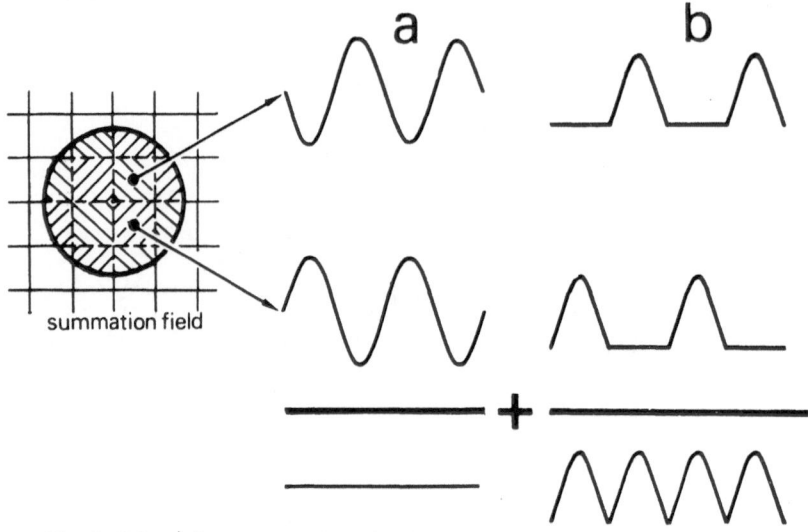

Fig. 3. Schematic representation of retinal modes of summation of responses generated by two sets of counterphase modulated squares of a checkerboard pattern.

Column a shows that no response will be obtained in the case that the spatial summing of the two counterphase signals occurs preceding a distorting stage. *Column b* demonstrates that the summed response consists of even harmonics in the case that retinal interaction takes place after a distorting element, in this example a rectifier.

resemble the contribution of the even harmonics in the response elicited by an unpatterned stimulus field.

The data in Fig. 4 and 5 demonstrate that indeed the ERG to (checker-board) pattern reversal is mainly caused by such luminance distortions. Fig. 4a shows the ERG of an 8° field square wave modulated with a modulation depth of 90%. Fig. 4b gives the same response but the trigger of the averager has been shifted half the period; i.e. the response is shifted 180° in phase. As would be expected, summation of both responses results in a symmetrical response (Fig. 4c). Such a symmetrical response of course consists only of even har- minics. In Fig. 5 this response is compared with the response to a checkerboard reversal stimulus. To make comparison easier and to decrease the duration of the experiment the averager was triggered twice per period; hence only even harmonics remain in the average. As can be seen, the shape and latency of both responses are similar. This holds irrespective of stimulus frequency. Therefore most if not all of the ERG to high contrast pattern reversal can be considered as the net result of the addition of responses to luminance increase and decrease.

In a number of cases a spatial contrast contribution in the cortical evoked response to a contrast stimulus with constant luminance flux is beyond doubt.

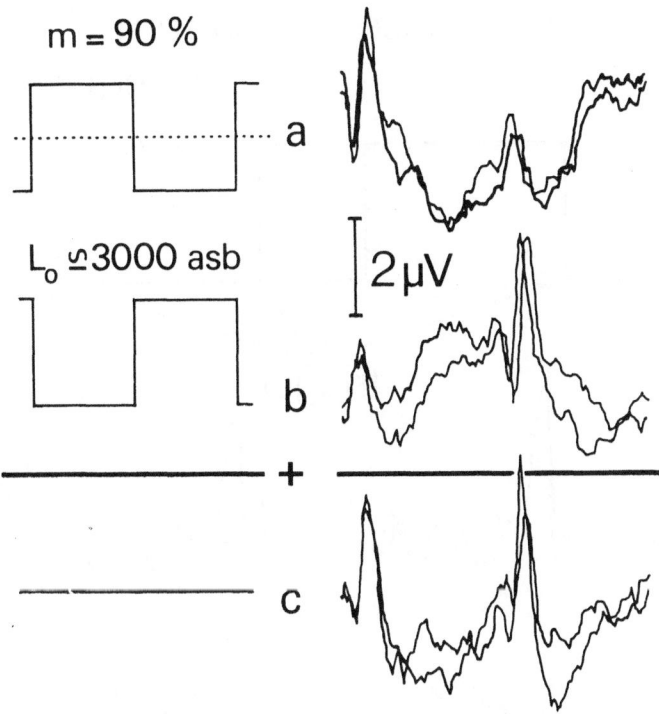

Fig. 4. ERG's to a 8° field, square wave modulated with a modulation depth of 90%. Figs. a and b give ERG's to the same stimulus but with the trigger of the averager at either the increase (Fig. a) or at the decrease (Fig. b) of the luminance stimulus. Fig. c gives the summed response of a and b.

Whether also an appreciable luminance contribution is present, will be revealed by controls, as outlined in this paper. Such controls are indicated whenever the response tends to symmetry and also when coarse, high contrast, patterns are needed as is often the case in studies of deteriorated vision. The fruitfulness of these controls has already been demonstrated in the judgement of the cortical potentials in monkey to patterned stimuli (PADMOS, HAAIJMAN & SPEKREIJSE, 1973).

The experiments reported in this paper may have implications for concepts about spatial contrast and luminance processing in the visual system. The apparent lack of a spatial contrast component in the ERG indicates that the contrast pathway separates from the luminance pathway after the structures that generate the ERG. Regarding possible depressing effects of lateral interactions on the response to homogeneous field stimulation, the finding that counterphase checkerboard and homogeneous field ERG's (Fig. 5) are practically identical in size and shape, is rather surprising. Lateral interactions seem not to play an important role up till the last stage that contributes to the ERG.

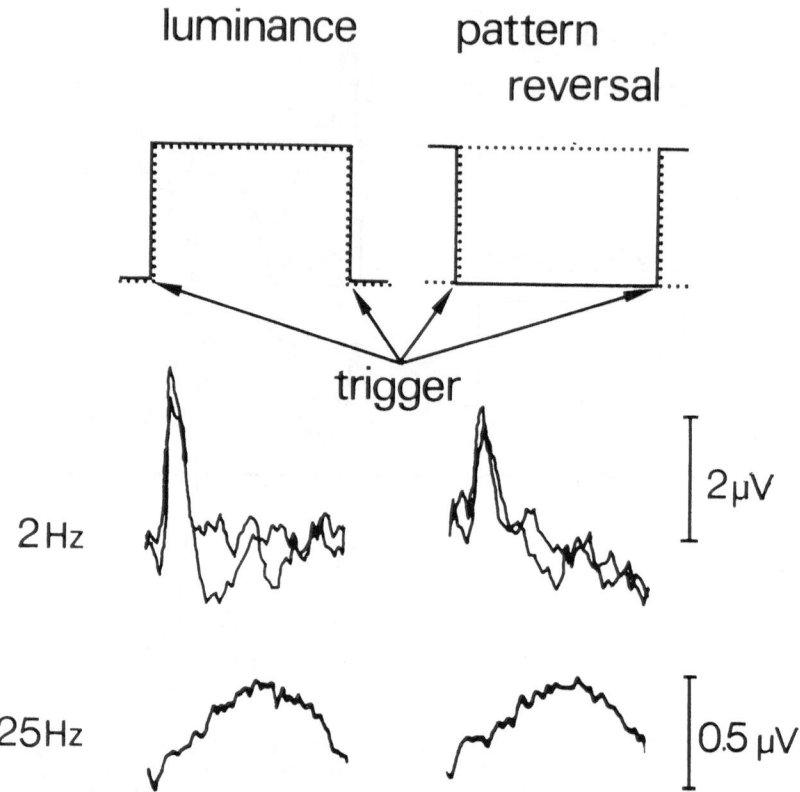

Fig. 5. ERG's to luminance modulation and pattern reversal. The averager is triggered twice per period. Identical responses are obtained irrespective stimulus frequency. Mean luminance is 3000 asb; modulation depth is 90%; checksize 60'. The stimulus field extends 8° and is surrounded by a steady field of equal luminance to minimize stray-light.

ACKNOWLEDGEMENTS

We are indebted to Mr. A. B. DE GRAAFF of the lighting design and engineering center of Philips, Eindhoven and to Mr. P. TH. I. PIREE of the fluorescent tube research center of Philips, Rozendaal for providing the fluorescent tubes with the required properties of brightness and rise time (<2 msec). Part of this work was supported by the Organization of Health Research (TNO), The Hague.

REFERENCES

ARMINGTON, J. C., CORWIN, T. R. & MARSETTA, R. Simultaneously recorded retinal and cortical responses to patterned stimuli. *J.O.S.A.* 61; *1514–1521* (1971).
ESTÉVEZ, O. & RÉMOND, A. ed.: Report on Program and Future in spatial contrast research. Trace (1972).
PADMOS, P., HAAIJMAN, J. J. & SPEKREIJSE, H. Visually evoked cortical potentials to patterned stimuli in monkey and man. *Electroenceph. clin. Neurophysiol.* (1973 in press).

RIGGS, L. A., JOHNSON, E. P. & SCHICK, A. M. L. Electrical responses of the human eye to moving stimulus patterns. *Science* 144: *567*– (1964).

SPEKREIJSE, H. Analysis of EEG responses in man evoked by sine wave modulated light. Thesis Univ. of Amsterdam Publ.: Dr. W. Junk, The Hague (1966).

SPEKREIJSE, H., VAN DER TWEEL, L. H. & ZUIDEMA, T. Contrast evoked responses in man. *Vision Res.* (1973: in press).

VAN DER TWEEL, L. H. & SPEKREIJSE, H. Visual Evoked Responses. In: The Clinical Value of Electroretinography Karger, Basel/New York (1968).

VAN DER TWEEL, L. H. & SPEKREIJSE, H. Psychophysics and electrophysiology of a rod-achromat. ISCERG-Symp., Los Angeles, 1972. This volume pp. 163–173.

ELECTROPHYSIOLOGICAL EQUIPMENT FOR TOTAL AND LOCAL RETINAL STIMULATION

G. H. M. VAN LITH*, J. MEININGER* & G. W. VAN MARLE*

(*Rotterdam*)

INTRODUCTION

A xenon flash is generally used to evoke electric responses of the visual system. When built in the ordinary lamphouse with a diffuser in front, the light mostly subtends a visual angle of about 30°. Such equipment has its disadvantages, the most important being, that the retina is only partly illuminated directly by the image of the diffuser. This part will have a high illumination. The rest of the retina will have a lower illumination, as it is illuminated indirectly by stray light. This stray light illumination is lower the farther away it is from the image of the lamp. As a result the response obtained is a mixture of high illuminated and low illuminated retinal fields (BERSON et al., 1968). Under such circumstances measurement of latency time and peak time makes no sense.

Another disadvantage is that when using a background illumination for light adaptation, the lamphouse has to be placed in front of the background. This will cast a shadow on the retina. So in light adaptation both stimulus and adaptation produce an unequal illumination of the retina.

A much better method is to use a hemisphere which is totally illuminated by test light and adaptation light (BERSON et al., 1968). The Ulbricht principle teaches that if one small part of a white diffuse globe is illuminated, the whole globe lights up equally at the inside by light scatter. Care should be taken that the patient does not see the light sources.

As we regularly apply local stimulation of the fovea for clinical purposes, we wanted to have the possibility to stimulate the retina totally and foveally with the same equipment. A difficult problem was how to present one small light spot in the hemisphere without lighting up the whole hemisphere by light scatter. The solution to this problem is the presentation of the local stimulus outside the plane of the hemisphere.

TECHNICAL DESCRIPTION

Fig. 1 presents the ball-stimulator in front view. The xenon lamp at the top of the globe, at position B, illuminates an opaque milky glass in the plane of the hemisphere. This causes a total and equal illumination of the whole inner wall. Colour filters and grey filters can be shifted between the xenon lamp and the milky glass.

---

* Eye Clinic, Medical Faculty, Rotterdam, The Netherlands.

213

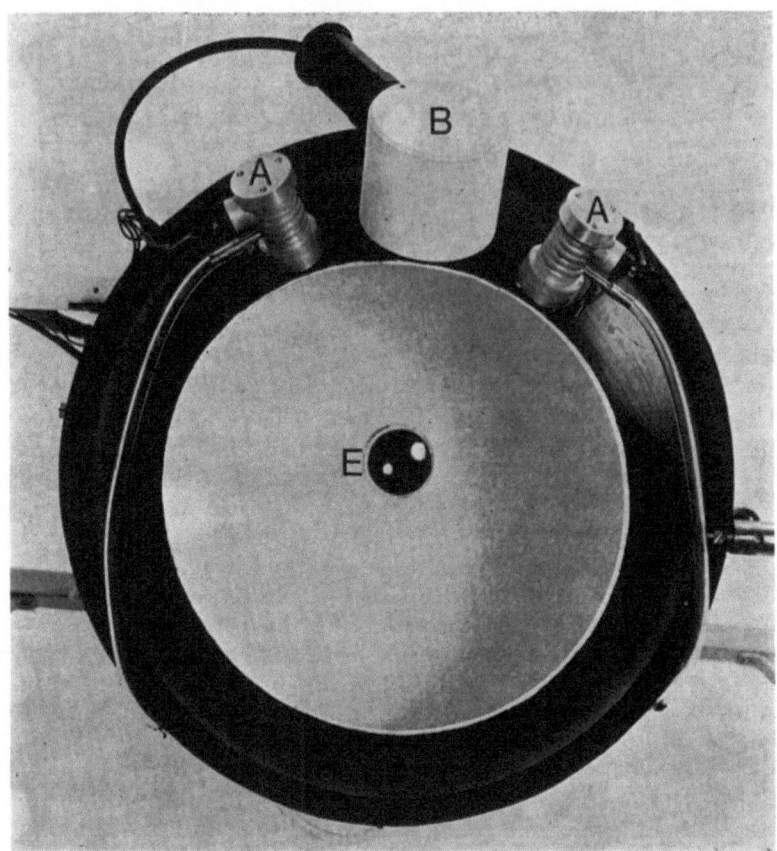

Fig. 1. Front view of the ball-stimulator. A. Halogen lamps for the background illumination. B. Xenon lamp for the total retinal stimulation. E. Lens of the optical system for the local stimulation.

For the local stimulation a xenon lamp illuminates a milky glass situated outside the plane of the globe and in focus of a lens (7.5 Dpt). Both xenon lamp and milky screen are placed in a black tube at the back of the globe (C, Fig. 2). The lens is placed in the plane of the globe (E, Fig. 1). From the lens an almost parallel beam goes to the subject's eye. As this parallel beam is directed into the gap of the globe, so that it does not touch the inner surface, light scatter is avoided. Only some reflection comes from the subject's face. If the local stimulus had a luminance of 10 asb, measured at a frequency of 30 Hz, we found only a luminance by light scatter at the inner side of the ball of less than 0.001 asb, which is 0.1 per cent. This is negligible, as with local stimulation a background illumination at the photopic level is always used.

The local stimulus, too, can be varied in luminance and colour by filters between lamp and diffuser. Moreover, the visual angle of the stimulus field

214

can be altered by means of diaphragms, shifted between the lens and the wall of the globe. Generally we use a 10°, 5° and 2.5° stimulus field. For the fixation a cross is made in the middle of the lens. For eccentric stimulation the subject has to look at small spots at the inner side of the ball.

The adaptation light is supplied by the two halogen lamps (A, Fig. 1). They

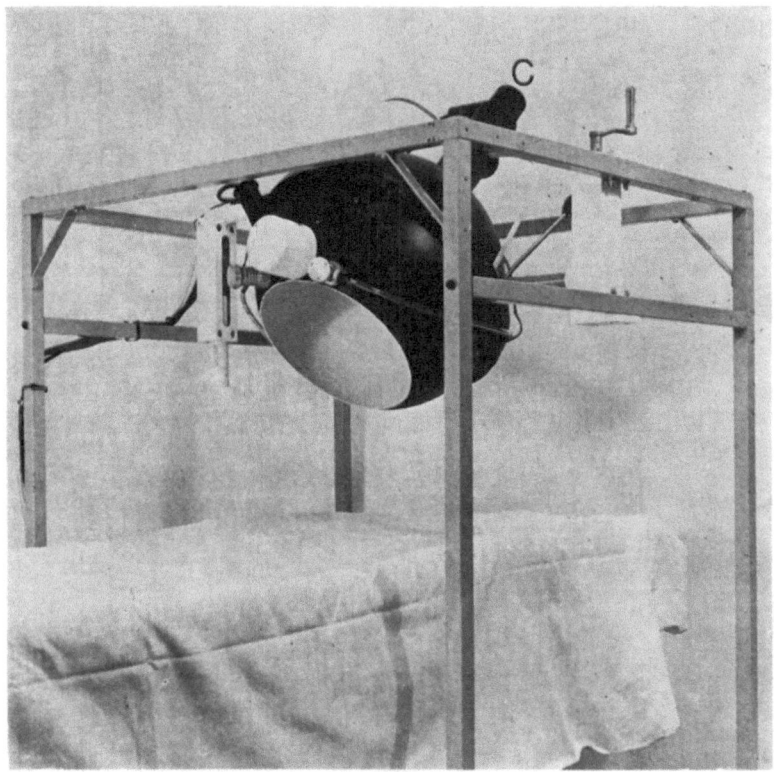

Fig. 2. Ball-stimulator in its frame. C. Black tube with the xenon lamp and opaque milky screen for the local stimulation.

provide a total, equal and steady illumination of the globe of maximally 1.000 asb. Halogen lamps and ball are air-cooled with fresh air.

RESULTS

Fig. 3 represents the ERG responses of the rod and the cone system with total retinal stimulation. A Henkes contact lens electrode has been used. The rod responses have been evoked in the dark adapted state. Relative luminance 0 refers to a xenon flash of 1 Joule. Luminance is lowered with neutral density filters. Flash frequency is 1 per second. Nine responses have been averaged with a

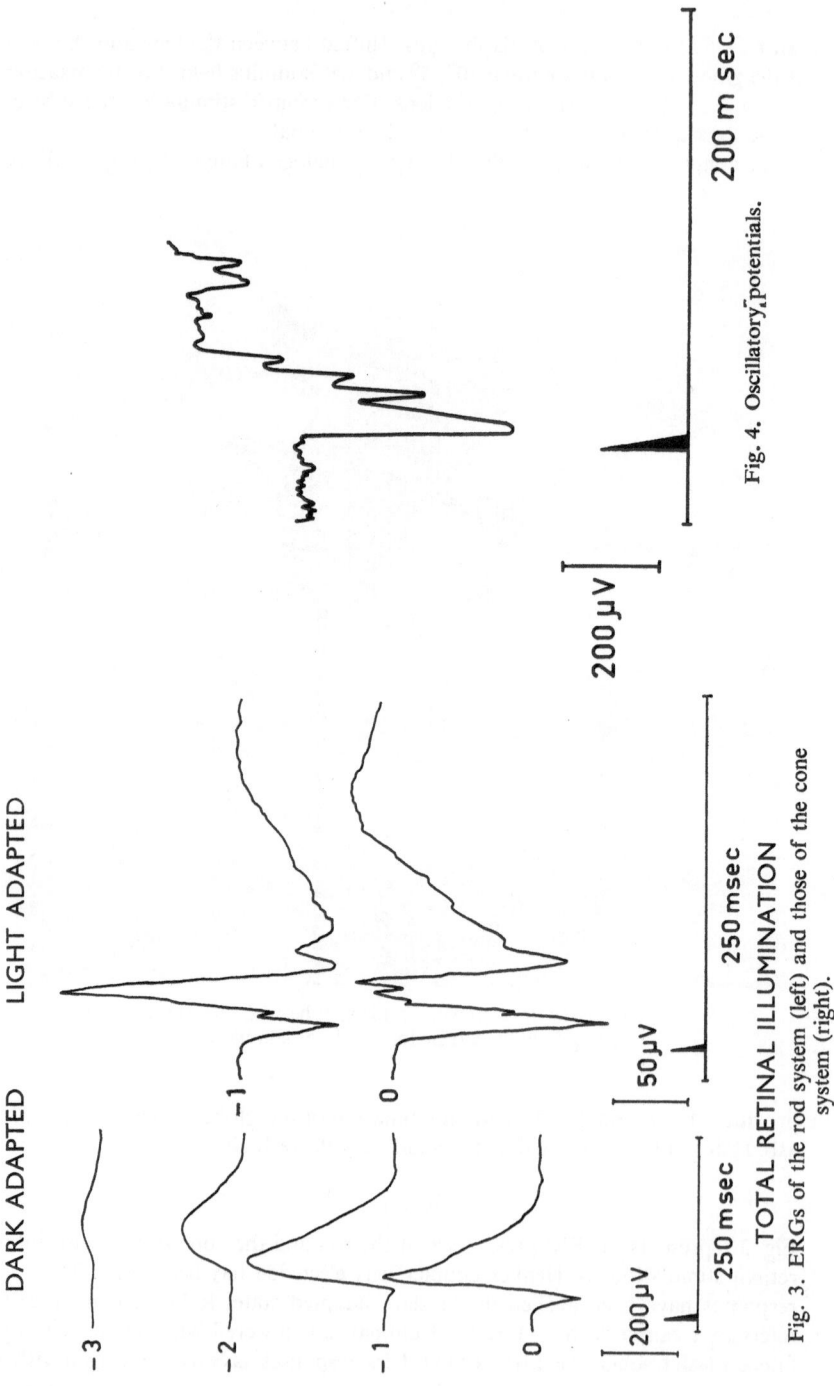

216

DARK ADAPTED   LIGHT ADAPTED

TOTAL RETINAL ILLUMINATION

Fig. 3. ERGs of the rod system (left) and those of the cone system (right).

Fig. 4. Oscillatory potentials.

CAT-computer. Cone responses have been made with a blue background and white flashes in a frequency of 4 per second. Ninety responses have been averaged.

Fig. 4 shows a recording of the oscillatory potentials. They have been evoked with a single flash of 10 Joule in the dark adapted state and photographed from the screen of an oscilloscope with a polaroid camera.

The local responses of the cone system in ERG and VER are shown in Fig. 5. The recordings on the left side have been made with central stimulation; those

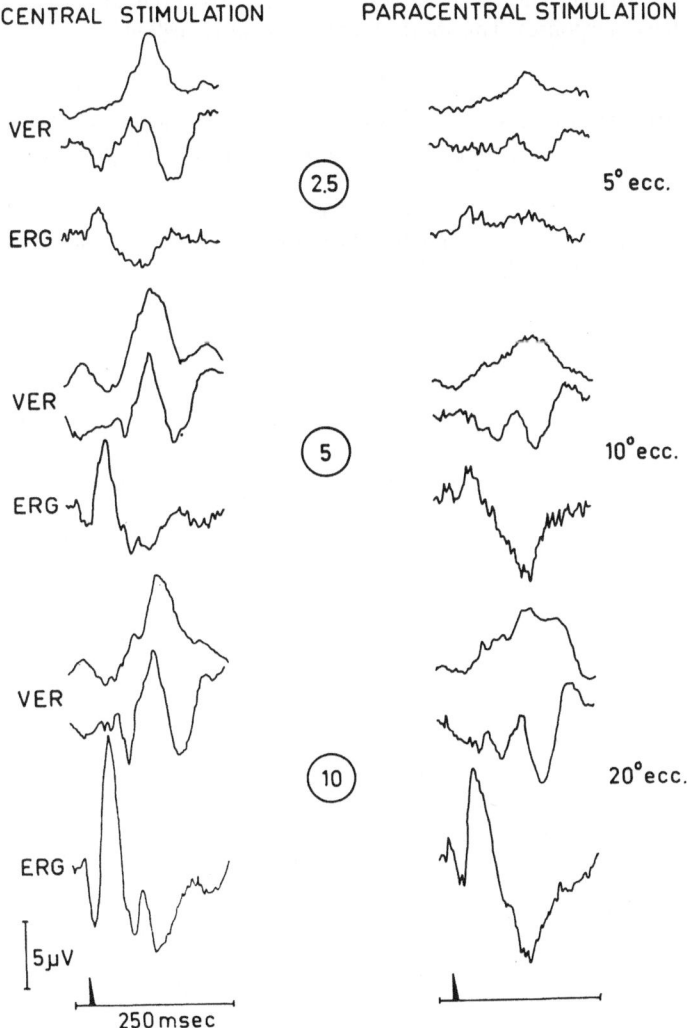

Fig. 5. ERGs and VERs in central and paracentral stimulation with stimulus fields of 2.5° (upper curves), 5° (middle) and 10° (lower curves).

on the right side with eccentric stimulation. The responses have been evoked with a 2.5°, 5° or 10° stimulus. For the eccentric stimulation the 2.5° field has been presented at 5° eccentricity; the 5° field at 10° eccentricity; and the 10° field at 20° eccentricity. With a frequency of 4 flashes per second, 350 responses have been averaged. The lower curve of each pair of VERs has been recorded from the occipital cortex (3 cm above the inion in the midline) to the earlobe; the upper curve also in the midline from 1.5 cm to 3 cm above the inion. Both ERG and VER, but particularly the ERG, increase regularly when the stimulus field is enlarged. The eccentric stimulation reveals, even at 5° eccentricity, much lower responses. This means that stray light is negligible.

Summary

A ball-stimulator is presented with which both total and local retinal stimulation can be given. With a strong blue background light the rod system can be suppressed.

REFERENCE

Berson, E. L., Gouras, P. & Gunkel, R. D. Rod responses in retinitis pigmentosa, dominantly inherited. *Arch. Ophthal.* 80:*58* (1968).

218

SLOW POTENTIALS OF ERG IN
HEMERALOPIA CONGENITA

P. HEILIG, A. THALER & H. BORNSCHEIN*

Since 1952, when SCHUBERT & BORNSCHEIN published the electroretinographic results of a subject with congenital night blindness, the specific anomalies of the ERG in these cases are well known: a-wave and x-wave are recordable, but the scotopic b-wave is completely absent. Up to now slow potentials of ERG were not studied in this form of night blindness.

THE SUBJECT

An eight years old girl, was sent to the clinic for examination with the diagnosis 'tapetoretinal degeneration.' There was no family history of ocular abnormalities.** Ophthalmological examination revealed no abnormal findings besides hemeralopia and slightly reduced visual acuity (o.d. = o.s.: 6/10). The dark adaptation curve, obtained with the Goldmann-Weekers adaptometer using ganzfeld stimulation resulted in a slightly (0,5 log units) elevated cone threshold and a markedly elevated final threshold of nearly 3 log units above the value which is reached by normals. These findings are in good agreement with the results of KRILL & MARTIN. They found that in inherited forms of night blindness there is, besides the fault in scotopic function, a defect in photopic function, too.

METHODS

The methods of electrophysiological examination comprised electrooculography and electroretinography with special regard to the slow potentials of the ERG. The EOG was performed after the method of ARDEN et al., using direct coupled amplifiers (Tektronix 3A9 in RM 565). Retinal luminance during the light phase was $3,5 \times 10^4$ td. The ERG was recorded under general anaesthesia. The routine ERG examination included a series of single flash stimuli of different intensities of white and red light (Schott neutral density filters and red filter RG_2) produced by a Grass photostimulator. The potentials were picked up by Echte/ Papst electrodes and recorded by an inkwriter (Mingograf 34). After light adaptation ($3,5 \times 10^4$ td over 10 minutes) an ERG recovery curve of one eye was performed (HEILIG & THALER). Finally, slow potentials of the ERG were examined in the other eye after it was dark adapted over a period of 30 minutes. The light source, a xenon arc lamp (150 V) in connection with a mechanical shutter produced a stimulus of intense white light (3×10^4 lx at the contact glass electrode) lasting over 10 seconds. In this special recording direct coupled amplification was used. Pupils were dilated by atropine.

* II. Eye Clinic and Institute of General and Comparative Physiology, University of Vienna.
** The mother of the girl was also examined: We could not find any pathological changes. Her dark adaptation was normal.

In accordance with the electrooculographic results of CARR et al. in a case of heritable nightblindness of Schubert-Bornschein's type, the EOG of the girl displayed a normal dark/light ratio of 204. The normal EOG supports the diagnosis of an essential night blindness. A pathological EOG could be the sign of an oligosymptomatic form of retinopathia pigmentosa. AUERBACH observed progression in 10 percent of 95 cases of congenital night blindness, and he agreed with FRANÇOIS, who emphasized that numerous cases of seemingly stationary night blindness might be in fact tapetoretinal degenerations without

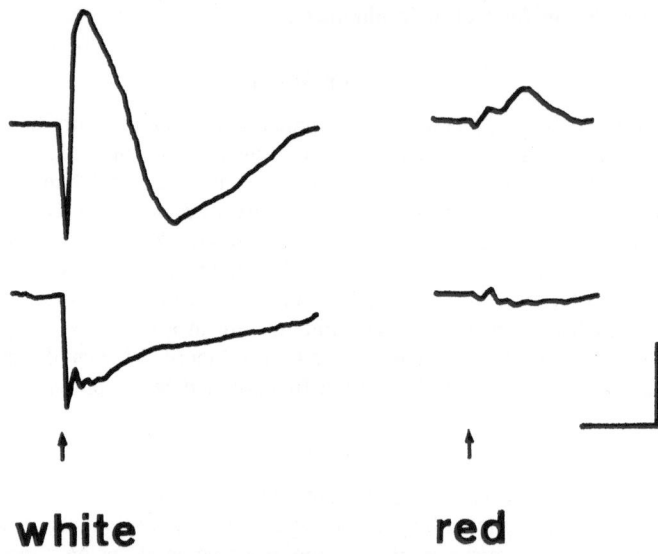

white   **red**

Fig. 1. upper row: normal ERG
lower row: ERG of the presented case, same stimulus conditions
white: maximal Grass intensity
red: Grass intensity 12, Schott filter RG₂
calibration: 100 μV, 100 msec

clinical symptoms other than night blindness. It should be noted, however, that there are other forms of congenital night blindness with a pathological EOG (FRANÇOIS et al., CARR et al., KRILL & MARTIN)

Routine ERG examination displayed the typical pattern as described by SCHUBERT & BORNSCHEIN (Fig. 1). The a-wave is of normal shape and amplitude; an x-wave, clearly discernible in its short latency, is present; but the scotopic b-wave is completely absent. The red light stimulus elicited an isolated x-wave. The photopic flicker ERG (30 Hz) is within normal limits and the flicker fusion frequency is normal. Oscillatory potentials are absent.

The recovery curve of the a-wave showed a normal increase of amplitude. The positive wave increased during the first minute of dark adaptation and then

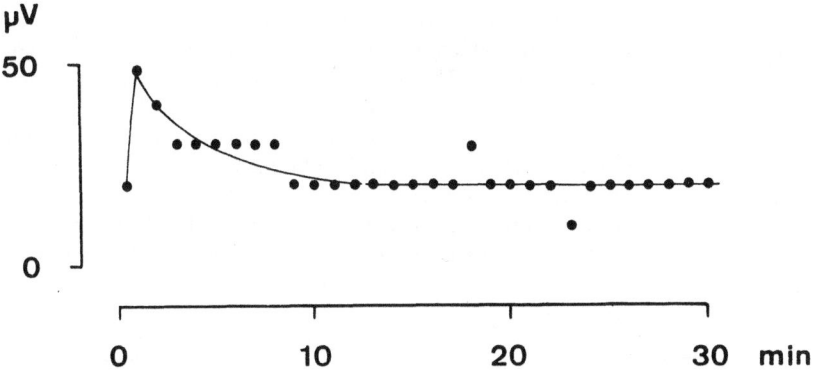

Fig. 2. ERG recovery curve of the x-wave in the presented case.

decreased gradually up to the approximately 10th minute, remaining constant up to the 30th minute. (Fig. 2). (GOODMAN & BORNSCHEIN, AUERBACH et al.).

The long lasting xenon light stimulus elicited an a-wave and a small x-wave, followed by a deep slow cornea-negative potential instead of the c-wave (Fig. 3). This negativity is terminated by a positive off-effect. The lowest point of the slow cornea-negative deflection is reached after about 2 seconds, whereas a normal c-wave evoked under the same stimulus conditions attains its maximum after 6–7 seconds.

DISCUSSION

NOELL (1954) stated that the c-wave is independent of the electrical events of retinal excitation. There is no doubt, therefore, that the negative slow potential of ERG in congenital night blindness (Schubert-Bornschein's type) is not a

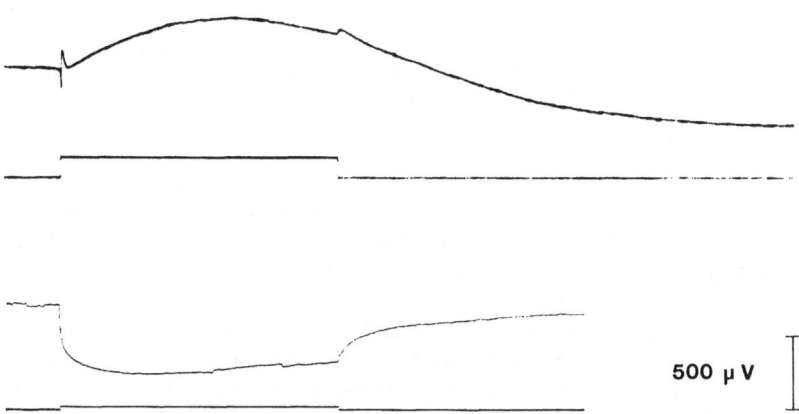

500 µ V

Fig. 3. upper trace: normal slow potentials in human ERG
lower trace: cornea negative slow potential in the presented case, note x-wave, same stimulus conditions.
stimulus duration: 10 seconds.

consequence of the lack of b-wave. In one of our experiments ischemia of a cat's retina was caused by accidental loss of blood. ERG-recording displayed a small a-wave and a preserved c-wave. The b-wave, however, was lacking. This result supports the supposition of the c-wave's independence from the b-wave. (Fig. 4)

Both EOG and c-wave are related in their association with the pigment epithelium, although divergent results can be obtained.

In the presented case, a normal EOG is accompanied by a pathological c-wave. It can be assumed, therefore, that the c-wave and the light induced increase of the standing potential are occurring at different points. (NOELL 1959, STEINBERG

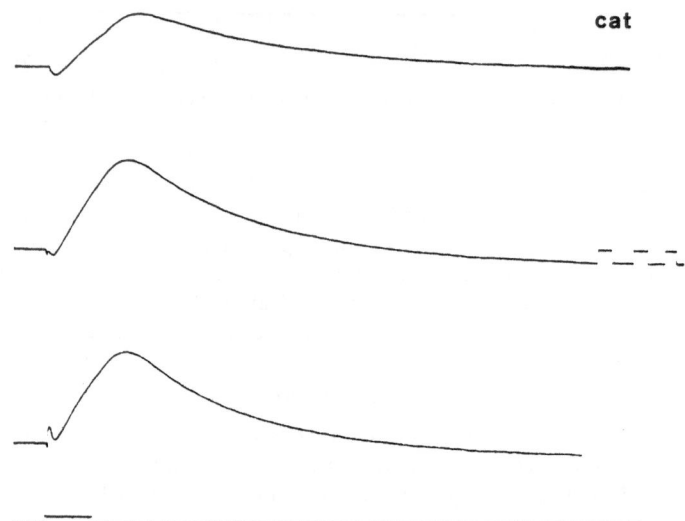

Fig. 4. upper trace: lack of b-wave and preserved c-wave in ischemic retina
traces below: successive recovery of the b-wave following intravenously
application of plasma expanders
duration of white xenon stimulus: 1 second
calibration: 200 μV

et al., GOURAS & CARR.) This assumption is affirmed by our results of electro-physiological examination in a case of fundus flavimaculatus. The EOG was pathological due to the abnormality of the pigment epithelium (KLIEN & KRILL); the ERG, however, was normal due to the practically normal function of the retina. Recording of slow potentials resulted in a preserved c-wave.

Cornea-negative slow potentials of ERG can be obtained experimentally after destruction of the pigment epithelium. (NOELL 1954). On the other hand, damage of the peripheral receptor cell and its connections with the pigment epithelium by the phenothiazine NP 207 (piperidylchlorophenothiazine) results in a slow cornea-negative potential, too, (MEIER-RUGE, HEILIG), and destruction of the entire retina by ischemia is followed by a similar electrophysiological phenomenon (BÖCK & BORNSCHEIN).

There is no evidence of a defect in the pigment epithelium in congenital night blindness. Histologically (Babel) and biomicroscopically the pigment epithelium was found to be entirely normal. In reflectometric studies a normal amount of rhodopsin and a normal regeneration rate in congenital night blindness was found (Carr et al.). Also, the normal EOG indicates that there is no obvious defect in the pigment epithelium of the presented patient.

Although in light microscopic studies (Babel) the retina of the hemeralope was found to be normal, a submicroscopic defect is probably responsible for the functional troubles: The absence of the b-wave is a symptom of a defect in the retina and cannot be explained by a fault in the pigment epithelium. A defect in transmission of excitation from receptor cell to the following retinal elements (e.g. bipolar cells, Müller fibers) could result in a failing b-wave. The negative slow potential of ERG might be caused by a disturbed interaction between receptor and pigment epithelial cells. The reduced visual acuity and the elevated cone threshold of subjective dark adaptation could be explained by a defect associated with the photopic receptor system. The a-wave in the ERG of the presented case could indicate good receptor function. After the previous considerations, however, it must be supposed that the retinal defect in congenital night blindness of Schubert-Bornschein's type can be found somewhere in relation with the receptor system and its connections.

All these considerations will remain essentially hypothetical until there is a better understanding of the nature and origin of electrophysiological phenomena in the eye.

Summary

Recording of slow potentials of ERG in a case of congenital night blindness of Schubert-Bornschein's type resulted in a slow cornea negative potential. Attempts are made to localize the retinal defect responsible for the functional abnormalities in this form of night blindness.

REFERENCES

Auerbach, E., Godel, V. & Rowe, H. An electrophysiological and psychophysical study of two forms of congenital night blindness. *Invest. Ophth.* 8:*332–345* (1969).

Babel, J. Constatations histologiques dans l'amaurose infantile de Leber et dans diverses formes d'héméralopie. *Ophthalmologica* 145:*399–402* (1963).

Böck, J. & Bornschein, H. Electrophysiological and histological aspects of retinal ischemia. *Trans. Ophthal. Soc. U.K.* 91:*399–403* (1971).

Carr, R. E., Ripps, H., Siegel, I. M. & Weale, R. A. Rhodopsin and the electrical activity of the retina in congenital night blindness. *Invest. Ophth.* 5:*497–507* (1966).

François, J., Verriest, G., de Rouck, A. & Dejean, C. Les fonctions visuelles dans l'héméralopie essentielle nougarienne. *Ophthalmologica* 132:*244–257* (1956).

François, J., de Rouck, A. & Verriest, G. L'électrooculogramme dans l'héméralopie essentielle. *Ann. Oculist.* 204:*1035–1046* (1971).

Goodman, G. & Bornschein, H. Comparative electroretinographic studies in congenital night blindness and total colour blindness. *Arch. Ophth.* 58:*174–182* (1957).

Gouras, P. & Carr, R. E. Light induced DC response of monkey retina before and after central retinal artery interruption. *Invest. Ophth.* 4:*310–329* (1965).

Heilig, P. & Thaler, A. Minimum duration of dark adaptation in clinical ERG. in: Wirth, A.: Symposium on electroretinography. Proc. VIIIth Symp. of ISCERG 1970 Pisa. Pacini Pisa 331–338 (1970).

HEILIG, P., HEISS, W.-D., HOMMER, K., HOYER, J. & THALER, A. Elektrophysiologische Untersuchungen einer experimentellen Phenothiazinretinopathie. 15. Jahreshauptvers. d. Österr. Ophth. Ges. Baden 1972.

KLIEN, B. A. & KRILL, A. E. Fundus flavimaculatus. Clinical, functional and histopathological observations. *Am. J. Ophthal.* 64:*3–23* (1967).

KRILL, A. E. & MARTIN, D. Photopic abnormalities in congenital stationary night blindness. *Invest. Ophth.* 10:*625–636* (1971).

MEIER-RUGE, W. Die medikamentöse Retinopathie. Thieme Stuttgart (1967).

NOELL, W. K. The origin of the electroretinogram. *Amer. J. Ophthal.* 38:*78–93* (1954).

NOELL, W. K. The visual cell: Electric and metabolic manifestations of its life process. *Amer. J. Ophthal.* 48:*347–370* (1959).

SCHUBERT, G. & BORNSCHEIN, H. Beitrag zur Analyse des menschlichen Elektroretinogramms. *Ophthalmologica* 123:*396* (1952).

STEINBERG, R. H., SCHMIDT, R. & BROWN, K. T. Intracellular response to light from the cat's pigment epithelium: origin of the c-wave of the electroretinogram. *Nature* 227:*728–730* (1970).

224

ELECTROPHYSIOLOGICAL EXAMINATIONS IN A FAMILY Ah WITH AUTOSOMAL DOMINANT RETINITIS PIGMENTOSA

KITETSU IMAIZUMI, RIHEI TAKAHASHI,
SHIN-ICHIRO IMAIZUMI & KOJI MITA

(*Morioka, Japan*)

INTRODUCTION

It is well known that all varieties of hereditary transmission may occur in retinitis pigmentosa. Although most of the cases of retinitis pigmentosa are inherited as an autosomal recessive trait some rare cases are inherited as an autosomal dominant trait. We have recently encountered a family with the latter type of inheritance. Our examinations were performed on six members of the family through six successive generations. Among the six members three cases were confirmed as affected individuals, and three others were thought to have early manifestations of retinitis pigmentosa.

MATERIALS AND METHODS

One member of the first generation (Ah 2), one of the second (Ah 4), and two of the third (Ah 11) have been presumed to be affected individuals according to their histories. In the present study, a female of the fourth generation (Ah 12), two males of the fifth generation (Ah 15, 16), and a male (Ah 18) and two females (Ah 19, 20) of the sixth generation were examined clinically and electrophysiologically.

Clinical testing included dark adaptation by means of Goldmann-Weekers's adaptometer, scotometry by a Bjerrum's scotometer, perimetry with Förster's and Goldmann's perimeters, and color perception using Ishihara's pseudoisochromatic plates and the Tokyo Medical College color test charts. These were performed for each subject.

A brief description of the recording methods will be given for the ERG's and EOG's in this paper, since the details have been given elsewhere (IMAIZUMI, 1969). ERG's were recorded by use of an oscilloscope (VC-7) with light stimulation provided by a xenon photostimulator (MSP-1) with intensities of 2 and 40 joule for the scotopic ERG and 80 joule for the photopic ERG. When necessary, the ERG's were added 20 times by a computer (ATAC 501-10). EOG's were recorded every minute during 30 minutes of dark adaptation and 15 minutes of light adaptation (1,000 lux) after 15 minutes pre-light adaptation. Responses were registered by a pen recorder (WI-260) after being amplified by a preamplifier (APB-20) and a direct coupled amplifier (AD 3-2). These electronic instruments were all made by Nihon Kohden Kogyo Co. Ltd.

For fluorescein fundus angiography a Topcon TRC-F3 was used, and pictures were taken every minute after an injection of 5cc of 10% sodium fluorescein.

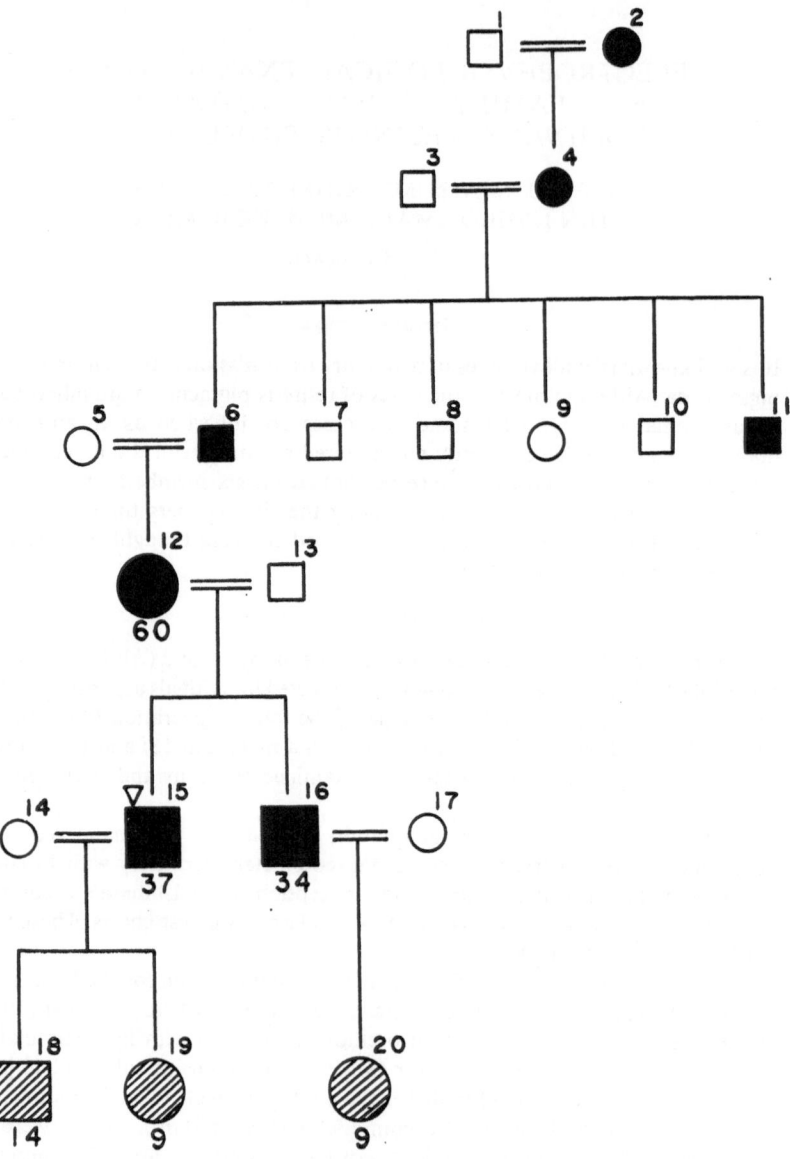

Fig. 1. Pedigree Ah.

1. *Typically affected cases:*

Table I indicates clinical data on the three members of the family; Ah 12, 15 and 16 in the fourth and fifth generations, who were diagnosed as typically affected members. Disorders of their visual functions such as visual acuity, visual fields and dark adaptation threshold, were remarkable. Ophthalmoscopically, their fundi showed the typical appearance of retinitis pigmentosa. On electrophysiological examination, the ERG's were non-recordable in both scotopic and

Table I. *Clinical findings in family* Ah.

Case	Age	Sex	Side	Visus	Visual Field Förster	Goldmann	Scotoma	Dark Adapt.	Color Sense	Fundus
Ah 12	60	F	R	(0.4) Myopia	White(+)	not test.	+	5.3	norm.	Typical ret.
			L	0.5 (n.c.)	Blue (+)		+	3.1	norm.	Pigmentosa o.u.
Ah15	37	M	R	s.l.	unmeas.	unmeas.	unmeas	7.0	unmeas.	Typical ret.
			L	s.l.				7.0		Pigmentosa o.u.
Ah16	34	M	R	0.08(n.c.)	White(+) 10°	not test.	+	5.3	abnor.	Typical ret.
			L	0.2 (n.c.)	o.u.		+	5.6	abnor.	Pigmentosa o.u.
Ah 18	14	M	R	1.5 (n.c)	W. B. norm.	normal	−	1.8	norm.	Dirty periph.
			L	1.5 (n.c)	W.norm. B. (+)	normal	−	2.5	norm.	
Ah 19	9	F	R	(0.2) Myopia	W.(+)15° B.(+)	depression	+	night blind	norm.	Depigmentation Pigmentation Tapetalrefrex
			L	(0.3) Myopia	o.u.		−	blind.	norm.	
Ah 20	9	F	R	(0.4) Myopia	W(+)20°	not test.	−	3.5	norm.	Depigmentation Tigeroid dirty Periph.
			L	(0.4) Myopia	B(+)30° o.u.	not test.	−	3.2	norm.	

Table II. ERG *and* EOG *in family* Ah.

Case	Age	Sex	Side	ERG Scotopic b-P(40)	Oscill-P	Type	Photopic b-P	Type	EOG d	Q	Type
Ah 12	60	F	R	−	−	non record.	−	non record.	80	1,17	flat
			L						220	1,90	subn.
Ah 15	37	M	R	−	−	non record.	−	non record.	10	1,02	flat
			L						15	1,01	flat
Ah 16	34	M	R	−	−	non record.	−	non record.	20	1,02	flat
			L						30	1,02	flat
Ah 18	14	M	R	186	O₁(O₂₋₃₄)	subn.	76	subn.	365	2,07	norm.
			L						325	2,08	norm.
Ah 19	9	F	R	60 Computer (+)	−	subn.	20	subn.	not test.	not test.	not test.
			L								
Ah 20	9	F	R	174	O₁ O₂₋₃₄	subn.	not test.	not test.	140	1,47	subn.
			L						120	1,38	subn.

227

photopic conditions, and the EOG's were considerably depressed. From these results, these three cases can be confirmed as affected individuals.

2. *Cases of the early disease involvement:*

The next three subjects were cases determined to be individuals in the early stages of retinitis pigmentosa.

The first case, Ah 18, a 14-year-old male, did not have any complaints. He was examined at the occasion of his father's regular visit to our clinic.

As shown in Fig. 2a, his fundus did not show any abnormal findings.

With fluorescein fundus angiogram studies (Fig. 2b), however, a characteristic appearance of a number of disseminated small fluorescent spots were observed in background fluorescence.

Except for a slight elevation of the dark adaptation threshold in his left eye, the clinical tests involving visual acuity, visual fields and color perception were normal (Table 1, Fig. 3).

Electrophysiologically, deteriorations of the b-wave in both scotopic and photopic conditions, and of oscillatory potentials were detected (Table 2, Fig. 4). In contrast to the depressed ERG, the EOG of this case was preserved intact, as shown in Fig. 5.

The second case, Ah 19, a 9-year-old female, is the younger sister of Ah 18. She has been complaining of hemeralopia since she was 5 years old. As shown in Fig. 2c, a tapetal-like reflex was seen in the posterior pole, and pale, tigroid and dirtily turbid appearance was seen at the equatorial portions of her fundus where depigmentation changes and small deposits of pigment were observed. The abnormality of the fundus of this case was more severe than that of her brother. The dark adaptation tests were not performed because of failure to obtain her co-operation. Perimetry using a Goldmann instrument revealed apparent depression in her visual fields with a ring scotoma.

In an examination of fluorescein angiography, characteristically abnormal findings were observed at the late stages of background fluorescence, resulting in increased visibility of the choroidal vessels (Fig. 2d). At the periphery, the background fluorescence formed a mottled appearance and remained persistently for a longer time than normal. These fluorescein angiographic findings resemble those of patients with retinitis pigmentosa.

Electrophysiologically, only a very small positive deflection was recorded by a conventional recording method under general anesthesia (upper half of Fig. 6). However, when the ERG's were treated with an adding technique by the computer, then each ERG component became recognizable in both scotopic and photopic conditions, as shown in the lower half of Fig. 6. An EOG test was not performed, unfortunately, because the subject was not old enough for the examination.

The third case, Ah 20, is a 9-year-old female who is the cousin of the last two persons. She began to notice blurring in her vision for the past year. It was interesting to note that no abnormalities were found when she was examined four years ago.

228

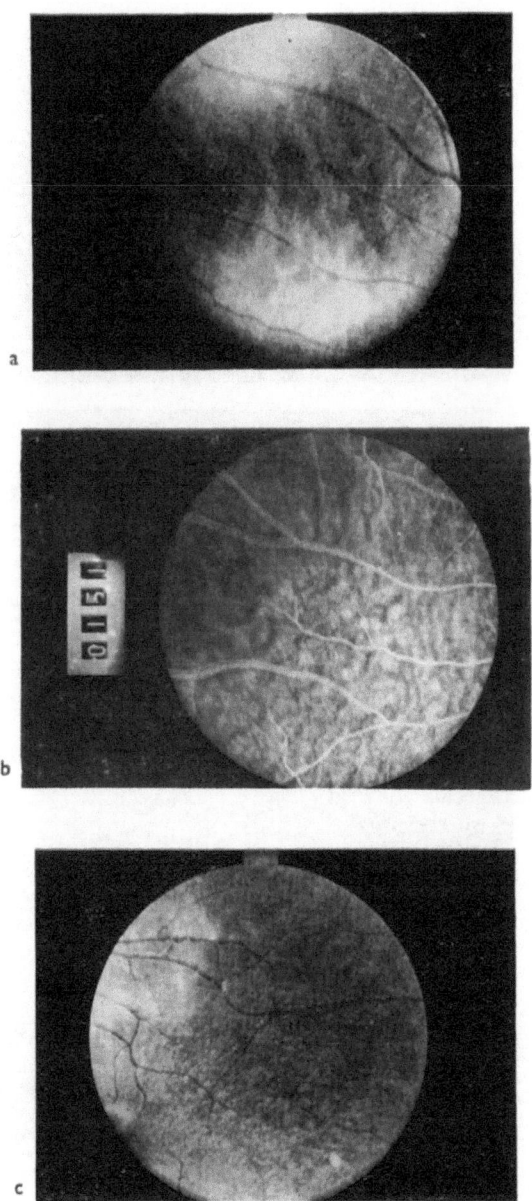

Fig. 2. Fundus photographs. a: Peripheral fundus color picture of left eye in Ah 18. b: Peripheral fluorescein angiograph of left eye in Ah 18. c: Peripheral fundus color picture of left eye in Ah 19. d: Fluorescein angiograph of right posterior pole in Ah 19. e: Peripheral fundus color picture of left eye in Ah 20. f: Peripheral fluorescein angiograph of left eye in Ah 20.

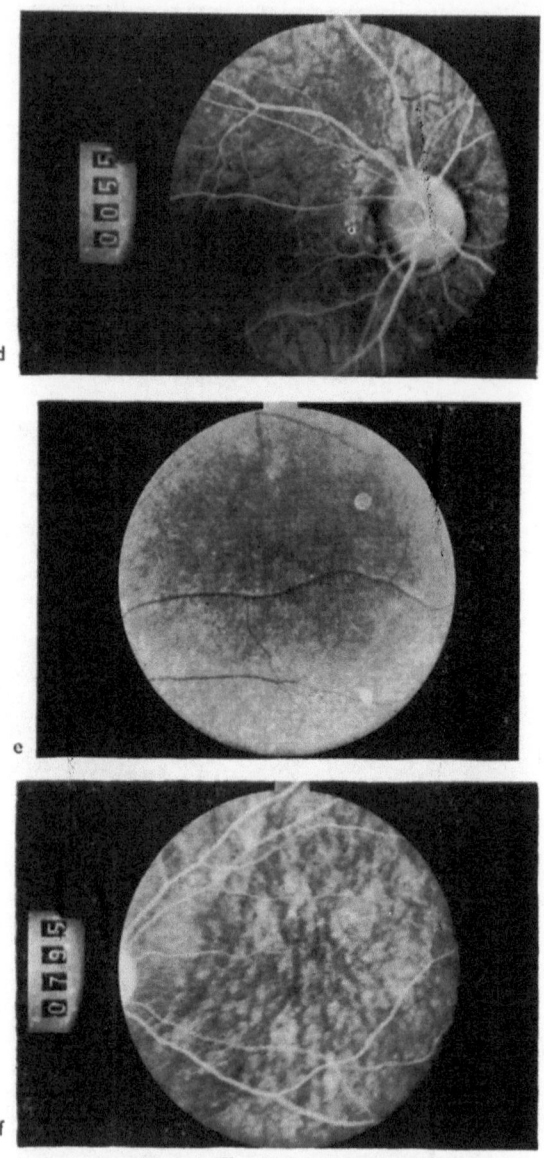

Fig. 2. (*continued*).

The equatorial portions of her fundus were tigroid and dirtily opaque with scattered depigmentation-like flecks as shown in Fig. 2e.

Fluorescein angiography (Fig. 2f) showed large and small fluorescence spots disseminated in the mottled background fluorescence. These fluorescence spots seemed to correspond to the position of the depigmentation-like flecks observed

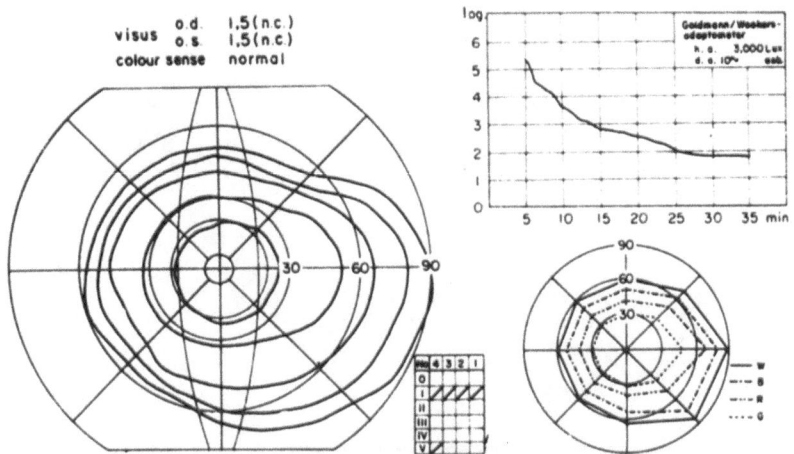

Fig. 3. Visual fields and dark adaptation curve of Ah 18.

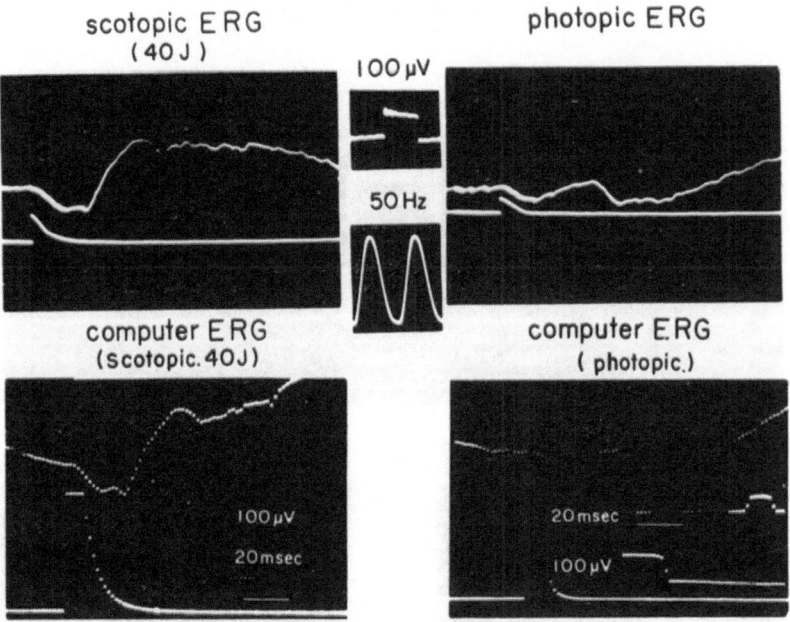

Fig. 4. Scotopic and photopic ERG from Ah 18.

with an ophthalmoscope. Delayed disappearance of the choroidal fluorescence was also noted in this case.

Constriction of the blue isopter was observed in perimetry by using a Förster's perimeter. A slight elevation of dark adaptation threshold was also recognized (Table 1).

231

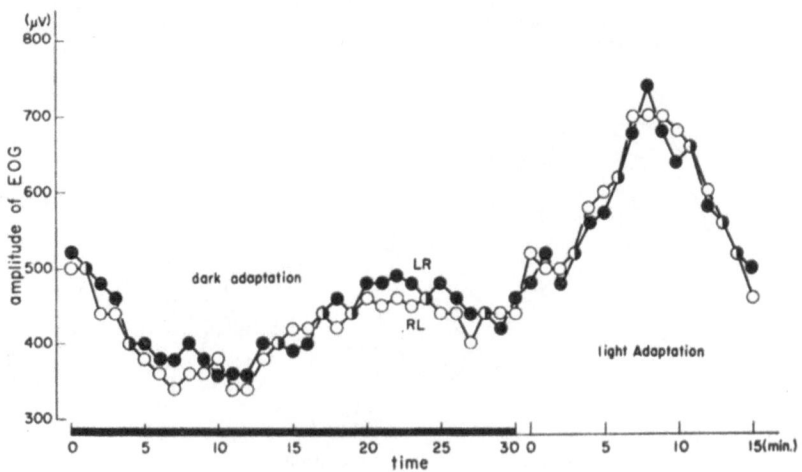

Fig. 5. EOG time curve of Ah 18.

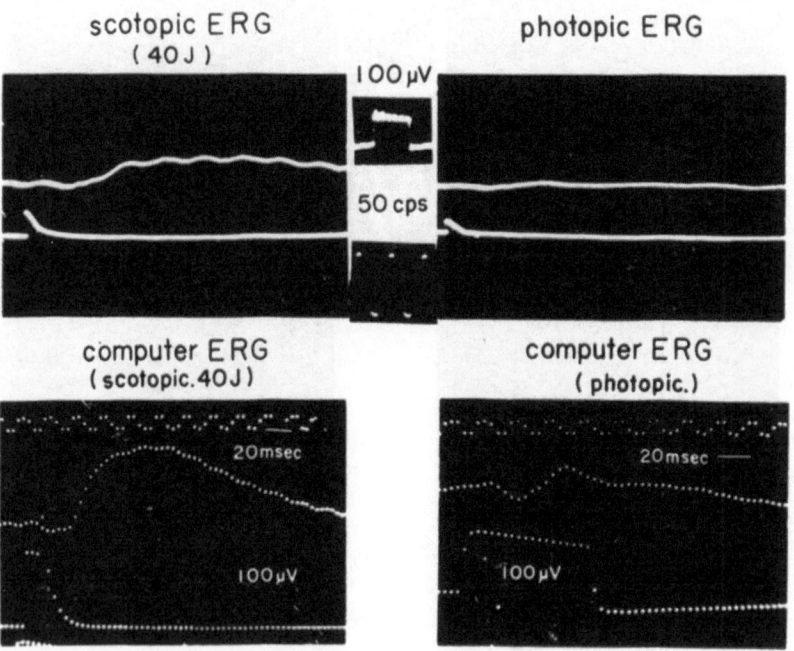

Fig. 6. Scotopic and photopic ERG from Ah 19.

232

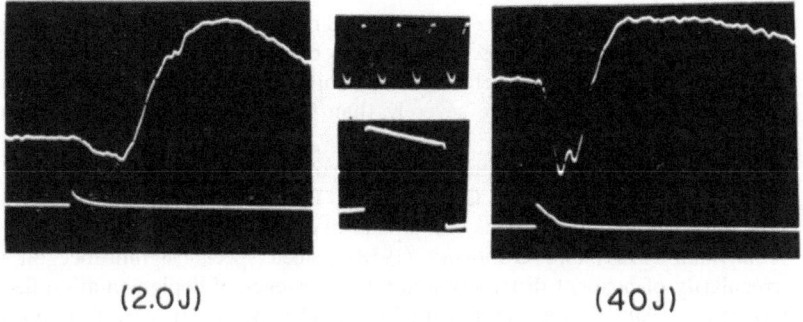

(2.0J) (40J)

Fig. 7. Scotopic ERG from Ah 20.

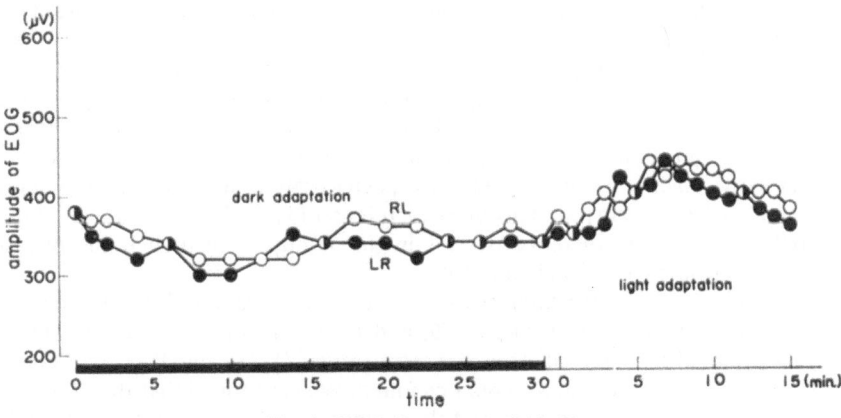

Fig. 8. EOG time curve of Ah 20.

A subnormal type ERG was obtained from this case (Table 2, Fig. 7). A EOG of this case was also of a subnormal type (Table 2, Fig. 8).

DISCUSSION

It is well known that the symptomatic features of dominantly inherited retinitis pigmentosa are relatively mild, with a slow progression, and the prognosis is not severe (FALLS, 1950; FRANÇOIS, 1961; DUKE-ELDER, 1967; KOBAYASHI, 1959; FRANCESCHETTI & DIETERLE, 1957; KOBAYASHI, 1969; FALLS & COTTERMAN, 1948; CRICK, 1955). Electrophysiologically, relatively well preserved ERG's especially photopic ERG (GOODMAN & GUNKEL, 1958; RUEDEMAN, 1959; GOURAS & CARR, 1964), have been reported on such cases by FRANÇOIS (1958), GOODMAN (1958), RUEDEMANN (1959), GOURAS (1964) and BERSON (1968), even though the fundi showed a typical appearance of retinitis pigmentosa. However, there is a report by BERSON (1968) of a case in a family with dominant transmission that showed an abnormal ERG despite having nearly normal fundus findings. In this study, non-recordable ERG's were detected in both scotopic and photopic conditions.

233

GOURAS (1964) and BERSON (1968) reported moderately depressed EOG's from dominantly inherited families. EOG's from our cases were more severely affected than those reports. Therefore, this family seemed to be one whose retinal functions were affected more severely than usual in a dominantly inherited family.

There are few reports on fundus findings of the early stages of retinitis pigmentosa, but FALLS (1948), CRICK (1955), FRANÇOIS (1958) and KOBAYASHI (1969) have noted the presence of a tapetal-like reflex as a sign of early changes. KOBAYASHI (1969) and GOODMAN (1958) placed special significance on the irregularity of pigment distribution and the existence of depigmentation flecks. GOODMAN (1958), GOURAS (1964) and BERSON (1968) have stressed the point that cases with a dominant form of early retinitis pigmentosa show an elevation in the dark adaptation threshold and an abnormality in the scotopic ERG in spite of the mild changes in the fundi.

GOURAS (1964) proposed that cases of early stages of retinitis pigmentosa featured less severe fundus changes, slight impairment of visual fields, preserved ERG, and a slight elevation of dark adaptation threshold. According to these criteria pointed out by GOURAS, our three cases seemed to be in the category of the early stages of this disease. However, deteriorations in the ERG, even in the photopic ERG, were found in our cases. It is considered that these deteriorations reflect the severity of retinal lesions in this family, even though the disease was transmitted as a dominant trait.

With reference to the findings of fluorescein angiogram in the early stages of retinitis pigmentosa, GELTZER (1969) and KRILL (1970) stated that no abnormality could be observed. However, HYVÄRINEN (1971) and WENSTEIN (1971) reported that subtle changes could be found. We have found that the combined use of fluorescein angiography and electrophysiological tests constitutes the best method for detecting retinitis pigmentosa in its early stages, and may serve to clarify the pathogenesis of this disastrous disease.

SUMMARY

Clinical and electrophysiological examinations were carried out on 6 members in a family (Family Ah) with retinitis pigmentosa. It was confirmed that 3 members of them were typically affected individuals and the other 3 members had the early stages of this disease. It was also disclosed from the family pedigree and the results of the examinations that this family was transmitting the character as an autosomal dominant trait.

The 3 individuals, who were determined as the typical cases, showed a typical fundus appearance, markedly disturbed visual functions, non-recordable ERGs and flat type EOGs.

The other 3 individuals, who were diagnosed as having the early stages of the diease, showed a slight abnormality in their fundi, subtle change in fluorescein angiography, a slight elevation of dark adaptation threshold and abnormal EOG's.

234

REFERENCES

BERSON, E. L., GOURAS, P. & GUNKEL, R. D. *Arch. Ophth.* 80:*58* (1968).
CRICK, R. P. *Brit. J. Ophth.* 39:*312* (1955).
DUKE-ELDER, S. System of Ophthalmology, Vol. X, Herry Kimpton (1967).
FALLS, H. F. *Trans. Amer. Acad. Ophth.* 54:*617* (1950).
FALLS, H. F. & COTTERMAN, C. W. *Arch. Ophth.* 40:*685* (1948).
FRANCESCHETTI, A. & DIETERLE, P. *Bibl. Ophth., Basel,* 48:*161* (1957).
FRANÇOIS, J. *Arch. Ophth.* 59:*88* (1958).
FRANÇOIS, J. Heredity in Ophthalmology, C. V. Mosby Co. (1961).
GELTZER, A. I. & BERSON, E. L. *Arch. Ophth.* 81:*776* (1969).
GOODMAN, G. & GUNKEL, R. D. *Am. J. Ophth.* 46:No. 3, Pt. II, *142* (1958).
GOURAS, P. & CARR, R. E. *Arch. Ophth.* 72:*104* (1964).
HYVÄRINEN, L., MAUMENEE, A. E., KELLY, J. & CANTOLLINO, S. *Am. J. Ophth.,* 71:*17* (1971).
IMAIZUMI, K. *Acta Soc. Ophth. Jap.* 73:*2347* (1969).
KOBAYASHI, F. *Acta Soc. Ophth. Jap.* 63:*3839* (1959).
KOBAYASHI, M. Genetics in Ophthalmology, Kanehara Co. (1969).
KRILL, A. E., ARCHER, D. & NEWELL, F. W. *Am. J. Ophth.* 69:*826* (1970).
RUEDEMANN, A. D. JR. *Trans. Amer. Acad. Ophth.* 63:*141* (1959).
RUEDEMANN, A. D. JR. & NOELL, W. K. *Am. J. Ophth.,* 47:No. 1, Pt. II, *564* (1959).
WENSTEIN, G. W., MAUMENEE, A. E. & HYVÄRINEN, L. *Ophthalmologica,* 162:*82* (1971).

SECTORAL RETINOPATHIA PIGMENTOSA. INVOLVEMENT OF THE RETINA AND PIGMENT EPITHELIUM AS REFLECTED IN BIOELECTRIC RESPONSE

A. THALER, P. HEILIG & H. SLEZAK*

(*Vienna*)

ABSTRACT

Opinions differ with regard to the extent of involvement of the background of the eye in sectoral retinopathia pigmentosa. In a series of different forms a new understanding could be obtained by electrophysiological examinations, especially with the EOG.

In sectoral retinopathia pigmentosa there are two groups which are clearly separated. One type was described by VUKOVICH (1959): Ophthalmoscopically, a sector of the retina is free of pigmentation and the fields are partly preserved. The elevated threshold of dark-adaptation and the extinguished ERG prove that this form belongs to the diffuse tapetoretinal degenerations.

The other type differs from that of VUKOVICH (1959) by the preserved ERG (HOMMER 1959). With the diagnosis of this type of sectoral retinopathia pigmentosa two questions arise: First: Is the sector of retinal background, which is free of pigmentation, indeed healthy? Second: Will it be spared from pigmentary degeneration forever, or will the disease finally spread out all over the fundus?

In 1949, RUBINO (1949) pointed out that the field defect in sectoral retinopathia pigmentosa is larger than would be expected from the pigmented area, as seen ophthalmoscopically. This incongruity was interpreted to be a sign of a progressive course. On the other hand, in cases of sectoral retinopathia pigmentosa, which seem to remain unaltered over years, field defects and pigmented areas do not correspond. The first ERG examinations resulted in normal amplitudes and could not give information concerning the extent of retinal involvement. Because of the apparently normal ERG and the normal dark-adaptation curve HOMMER (1959) assumed, that the retina is partly involved. More recent exact statistical evaluations (HOMMER & WOHLZOGEN 1970) resulted in a reduction of ERG-amplitudes to less than 50%.** BERSON's (1971) normal implicit time of scotopic ERG in sectoral retinopathia pigmentosa is in accordance with HOMMER & WOHLZOGEN's (1970) results. Nevertheless KRILL's (1970) fluorescein studies showed a mottled hyperfluorescence in an area greater than the pigmented retinal sectors. This symptom indicates a fault in the pigment epithelium much more widespread than that in the retina. Localization and extent of retinal

---

* Eye-Clinic, University of Vienna, Director: PROF. DR. J. BÖCK.
** Because of the remaining portion of ERG they assumed that the sector of the retina, which is free of pigmentations, is not involved.

changes in sectoral retinopathia pigmentosa vary from case to case. Therefore, the results may differ. The cases which we are presenting can be classified according to the extent of retinal pigmentation. The series of manifestations range from forms with narrow pigmented retinal sectors and ones in which the lower half of the retina is involved, up to those in which only a narrow sector remains unaffected. All of these manifestations are located in the midperiphery of the

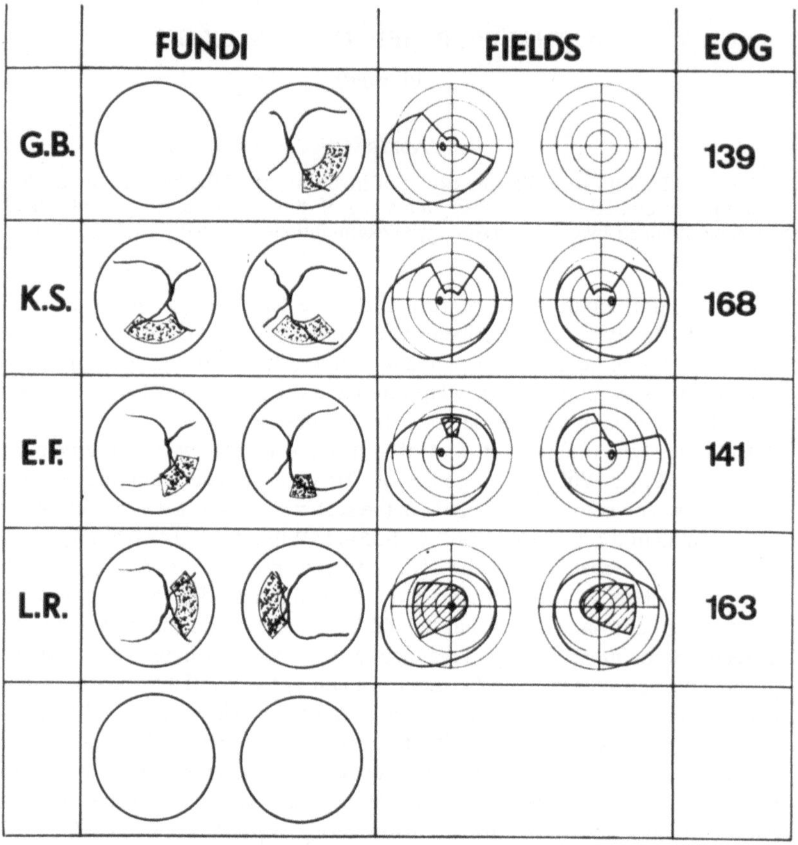

	FUNDI	FIELDS	EOG
G.B.			139
K.S.			168
E.F.			141
L.R.			163

Fig. 1

retina. They are variations of equatorial retinopathia pigmentosa. According to our observations, an inverse sectoral retinopathia pigmentosa also exists.

In one patient (G. B.) with a detachment of the retina in the right eye the bone corpuscle-like pigmentations are limited on the lower temporal quadrant of the left eye. The visual field of the left eye shows a defect of the nasal upper quadrant. Two more patients (K. S., E. F.) have narrow sectoral pigmented areas in the lower parts of the fundi and wedge-shaped field defects. One patient (L. R.) shows bone corpuscle-like pigmentation in the midperiphery nasal of the discs. The field defects correspond to the pigmented retinal areas. In all these patients

238

integral dark-adaptation curves are normal. The ERG amplitudes are subnormal. All electrooculograms but one are pathological, one is subnormal (Fig. 1).

The next four patients we took together in one group because of their very similar findings (M. H., F. E., L. P., P. S.). The bone corpuscle-like intraretinal pigmentations are spread semicircularly in the midperiphery of the lower halves of the fundi. The vessels of the lower parts of the retina are narrow. The visual fields show loss of the upper halves. The integral dark-adaptation curves are normal. The ERG-amplitudes are subnormal. The EOG is pathological in all

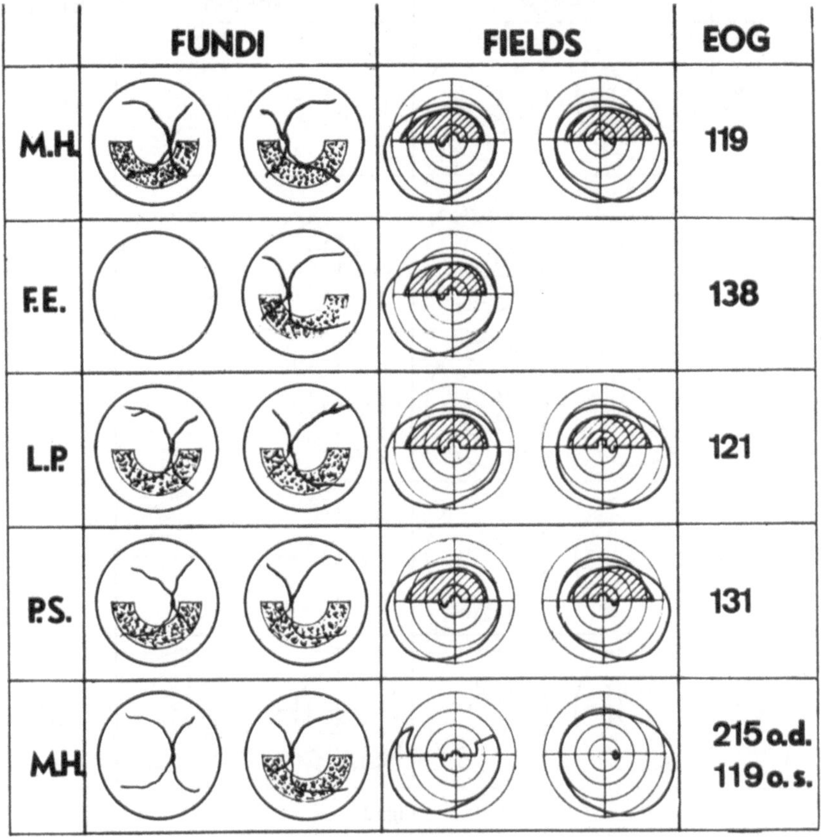

	FUNDI	FIELDS	EOG
M.H.			119
F.E.			138
L.P.			121
P.S.			131
M.H.			215 a.d. 119 a.s.

Fig. 2

four patients. One of these cases was examined by HOMMER (1959) 13 years ago, one 9 years and one 8 years ago. The results of that time are in accordance with the recent ones. This leads to the assumption that the tapetoretinal degeneration came to a standstill in these patients. Though, because of a very slow progression, this period might be too short. Also, in these cases the field-defects are slightly larger than would be expected in relation to the extent of the retinal pigmentations (Fig. 2).

239

In one patient (M. H.) (THALER, HEILIG & SLEZAK 1972) the pigment deposits are to be found only in the lower half of the eyeground of the left eye. The disc is pale and the vessels of the lower parts of the left fundus are more narrow than those of the upper parts. There is a loss of the upper half of the visual field of the left eye. Disc, vessels and periphery of the right eye are without pathological findings. The integral dark-adaptation curve is normal. The amplitudes of ERG

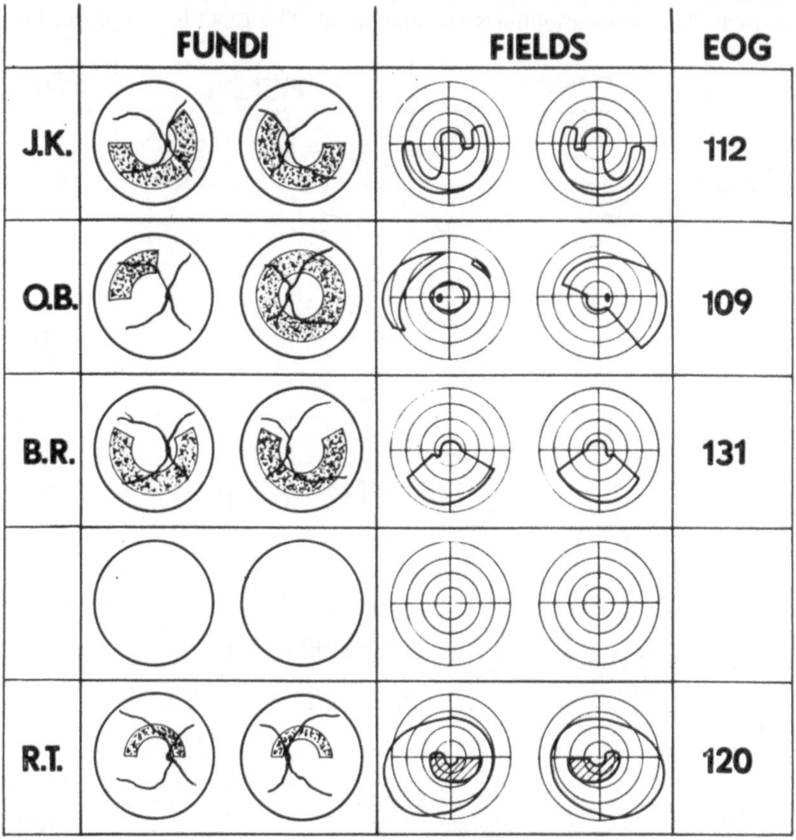

	FUNDI		FIELDS		EOG
J.K.					112
O.B.					109
B.R.					131
R.T.					120

Fig. 3

of the left eye are, on an average, 30% smaller than the amplitudes of the right eye. The EOG of the right eye is normal, that of the left eye is pathological. (Fig. 2).

A young man of 21 (R. T.) is suffering from a form of tapetoretinal degeneration which has not been described up to now. The retinal changes are not located in the midperiphery, but they are placed on the posterior pole and near the disc. The intraretinal pigmentations are located in a semicircular fashion in the upper half of that area. Fields show an intracentral semicircular scotoma. The integral dark-adaptation curve is normal. In ERG the a- and b-waves are subnormal, a

240

little x-wave and a reduced flicker response is recordable. In this case the EOG is also pathological. (Fig. 3).

In three patients (J. K., O. B., B. R.) the pigmentations are distributed from the lower half to the upper parts of the retina as described by LISCH (1955) in his elder patients. The field defects extend over the lower half. The integral dark-adaptation curves are normal. The ERG-amplitudes are subnormal and in one case almost extinguished. The EOG is pathological in all these patients. (Fig. 3).

In spite of the great number of cases of sectoral retinopathia pigmentosa known up to now, very seldom has an electrooculographic examination been carried out. As far as we know, only GRAHAM reported a pathological EOG in one case and KRILL found a patient with a narrow sector of pigmental deposits in the retina to have a subnormal EOG.

From the extent of the primarily involvement of the background in sectoral retinopathia pigmentosa conclusions can be drawn regarding the prognosis of the disease. We tried to get additional information about the extent of the disease by electrooculographic examinations. In tapetoretinal degenerations the EOG is usually affected, even when no signs of a heredodegeneration can be found yet by means of ERG (ARDEN et al. 1962). Accordingly, we could expect that in sectoral retinopathia pigmentosa the EOG would be pathological if the disease is expanding over a greater part of the background than it would correspond to the extent of the pigmented retinal area. On the other hand, the EOG would be expected to be normal, if the tapetoretinal degeneration is limited to the pigmented sector of the fundus, in accordance with an old occlusion of a branch of retinal vessels (ARDEN et al., 1962; GLIEM, 1968; HELLEMANN & BASTIEN, 1968). In occlusion of the central artery the EOG is pathological. In old occlusions of branches of the retinal artery the EOG is normal. If the tapetoretinal degeneration is limited to a sector of the background—in accordance to occlusions of arterial branches—this would not be sufficient to cause a pathological EOG. In all cases of sectoral retinopathia pigmentosa we could examine, a pathological EOG was recordable. Therefore, we have to conclude that the disease has spread over the limits of the sector with the intraretinal pigment deposits. It has yet to be clarified whether the pathological EOG is caused by damage to the sensory retina or to the pigment epithelium. The increase of the standing potential in light is reduced not only by an isolated fault of the retina, which means the absence of retinal inductance, (as for example in occlusion of the central vessels or in detachment of the retina), but also by an exclusive disturbance in the pigment epithelium, (as for example, in fundus flavimaculatus), which can be responsible for a low dark-light ratio.

Biomicroscopically, no damage is seen in the retina of the unpigmented area in sectoral retinopathia pigmentosa. The preserved part of the fields, as well as the practically normal integral dark-adaptation and the remaining portion of ERG point out that the morphologically normal appearing sector of the retina has a good function, and, therefore, the pathological EOG is not caused by a fault in the retina. Therefore, we may suppose that the pathological EOG in these cases is caused by functional problems in the pigment epithelium, as in fundus flavimaculatus (KLIEN & KRILL 1967). This supposition is affirmed by changes

241

of this tissue which are transcending the limits of the pigmented sector of the retina and which can be seen biomicroscopically and in fluorescein angiographic examinations.

The initial question, i.e. whether the sector free of retinal pigmentation is healthy or not, can be answered as follows: The pathological EOG and the biomicroscopical findings show that more than the pigmented sector is affected by the disease. The question relating to the prognosis cannot be answered yet. On the one hand, in three of our cases function and clinical morphology remained constant over about 10 years. On the other hand, examinations of affected families and follow ups of affected patients proved that in some cases the disease was progressive. (LISCH, 1955; KÜPER, 1960; ZIV & DUNPHY, 1964; KLIER, 1965; FLEDELIUS & SIMONSEN, 1970; KRILL, 1970.)

Lastly we should consider, if in sectoral retinopathia pigmentosa the pathological EOG and the biomicroscopical findings support the supposition that primarily the pigment epithelium and secondarily the retina is involved. If this turns out to be correct, the same assumption should be valid for diffuse retinopathia pigmentosa. Up to now the theory of a primarily defect of the neural epithelium in tapetoretinal degeneration is favored.

REFERENCES

ARDEN, G. B., BARRADA, A. & KELSEY, J. H. New clinical test of retinal function based upon the standing potential of the eye. *Brit. J. Ophthal.* 46:*449–467* (1962).

BERSON, E. L. & HOWARD, J. Temporal aspects of the ERG in sector retinitis pigmentosa. *Arch. Ophthal.* 86:*653–665* (1971).

FLEDELIUS, H. & SIMONSEN, S. E. A family with bilateral symmetrical sectoral pigmentary retinal lesions. *Acta Ophthal.* 48:*14–22* (1970).

GLIEM, H. Das Elektro-Okulogramm bei Gefäßerkrankungen der Netzhaut. "Advances in Electrophysiology and -pathology of the Visual System." G. Thieme Verlag Leipzig 77–82 (1968).

GRAHAM, M. V. Bilateral symmetrical sectoral pigmentary lesion of the retina. *Brit. J. Ophthal.* 47:*682–686* (1963).

HELLEMANN, I. & BASTIEN, A. EOG in cases of thrombosis of the vena centralis retinae. "Advances in Electrophysiology and -pathology of the Visual System." G. Thieme Verlag Leipzig 83–87 (1968).

HOMMER, K. Elektroretinographische Untersuchungen bei sektorenförmiger tapetoretinaler Degeneration. Sitzung der Ophthalmologischen Gesellschaft in Wien (9.6.1958). *Klin. Mbl. Augenheilk.* 134:*437* (1959).

HOMMER, K. Das ERG bei sektorenförmiger Retinitis pigmentosa (Retinopathia pigmentosa). *A.v. Graefes Arch. Ophthal.* 161:*16–21* (1959).

HOMMER, K. & WOHLZOGEN, F. X. The size of ERG amplitudes as an aid to the differential diagnosis of sectorial retinitis pigmentosa. in WIRTH, A.: Symposium on electroretinography, Proc. VIIIth ISCERG Symp., Pacini Pisa 216–221 (1970).

KLIEN, B. A. & KRILL, A. E. Fundus flavimaculatus. Clinical, functional and histopathological observations. *Am. J. Ophthal.* 64:*3–23* (1967).

KLIER, A. Zur Kenntnis der sektorenförmigen Retinopathia pigmentosa. *Klin. Mbl. Augenheilk.* 147:*361–365* (1965).

KRILL, A. E., ARCHER, D. & MARTIN, D. Sector retinitis pigmentosa. *Amer. J. Ophthal.* 69: *977–987*, (1970).

KRILL, A. E., ARCHER, D. & NEWELL, F. W. Fluorescein angiography in retinitis pigmentosa. *Am. J. Ophthal.* 69:*826–835* (1970).

KÜPER, J. Familiäre sektorenförmige Retinitis pigmentosa. *Klin. Mbl. Augenheilk.* 136:*97–102*, (1960).

LISCH, K. Segmentäre tapetoretinale Degeneration. *Forschung und Praxis* 10:*54–58* (1955).

RUBINO, A. Alcuni rilievi sui reperti perimetrici nella degenerazione pigmentaria retinica. *Giorn. Ital. Oftal.*, 2:*417–426* (1949).

THALER, A., HEILIG, P. & SLEZAK, H. Chlorochinretinopathie und einseitige sektorenförmige Pigmentdegeneration der Netzhaut. 15. Jahreshauptversammlung der Österreichischen ophthalmologischen Gesellschaft (1972).

VUKOVICH, V. Das Elektroretinogramm bei Retinitis pigmentosa mit bitemporalem Gesichtsfeldausfall. *A.v. Graefes Arch. Ophthal.* 161:*27–31* (1959).

ZIV, B. & DUNPHY, E. Pigmented retinal arteries in retinitis pigmentosa. *Amer. J. Ophthal.* 57:*132–133* (1964).

243

ELECTROPERIMETRY

H. E. HENKES & G. H. M. VAN LITH*

(*Rotterdam*)

INTRODUCTION

Since the registration of electric responses of the visual system following small local stimuli of the retina became practicable, the next logical step was trying to use these local responses for clinical purposes, viz. for the determination of the retinal sensitivity in the visual field. In 1966 BEINHOCKER et al. introduced the term electroperimetry for such an examination. Their electroperimeter was made up of a hemisphere in which, in fixed positions, a number of flash lights were built in.

Presently, 6 years later, neither the Copenhaver apparatus nor any other instrument is in use clinically, and the interest in this project seems to have been greatly reduced. We assume that the reason for this lies in the many problems which were encountered in 1966 and which were not worked out sufficiently at that time to guarantee a successful attempt in clinical electroperimetry. As a number of problems have been solved, it seems worthwhile to revitalize the whole issue. Our approach thus far will be reported, and the many physiological and technical problems we were faced with will be discussed. We shall not deal with the technique of how to get real local responses avoiding stray light responses. This has been reported extensively by BRINDLEY & WESTHEIMER (1965), ARDEN & BANKES (1966), and ARMINGTON (1968).

PROCEDURE

The 90° blue background consists of 6 fluorescent tubes (Philips, 20 Watt, colour 34), in front of which a diffuser and a blue filter are placed. The illumination at the plane of the cornea amounts to 2.000 lux without and 150 lux with the blue filter.

The stimulus is provided by the projection of a beam of a Xenon arc (Leitz XBO 150-1) on white discs, placed in front of the adapting field. Luminance, colour, duration and area of the stimulus can be varied. White light was always used, the maximum luminance amounting to log 3.0 cd/m².

The ERG was registered with a contact lens electrode and a reference electrode at the ear lobe, while bipolar leads over the occipital lobe were used for the VER. After amplification (time constant 0.3, high frequency filter 75 cps) the responses are averaged (CAT Mnemotron 400B) and recorded with an X-Y plotter.

RESULTS

The first question to be discussed is which electrical response of the visual system should be used as a criterion, the ERG or the VER. From literature it

---

* Eye Clinic, Medical Faculty, Rotterdam, The Netherlands.

is known that the VER is considered to be a projection of the central foveal area (VAN HOFF et al., 1966; ARMINGTON, 1968; DEVOE et al., 1968; VAN LITH & HENKES, 1970). If this is true, electroperimetry by means of the VER is not feasible.

Fig. 1a represents the photopic retinal and cortical responses of a 4° light stimulus, presented foveally and at 5° and 12° eccentricity. It appears that the amplitudes both of ERG and VER decrease, going from the fovea to the periphery. If, however, the stimulus field presented outside the fovea is enlarged,

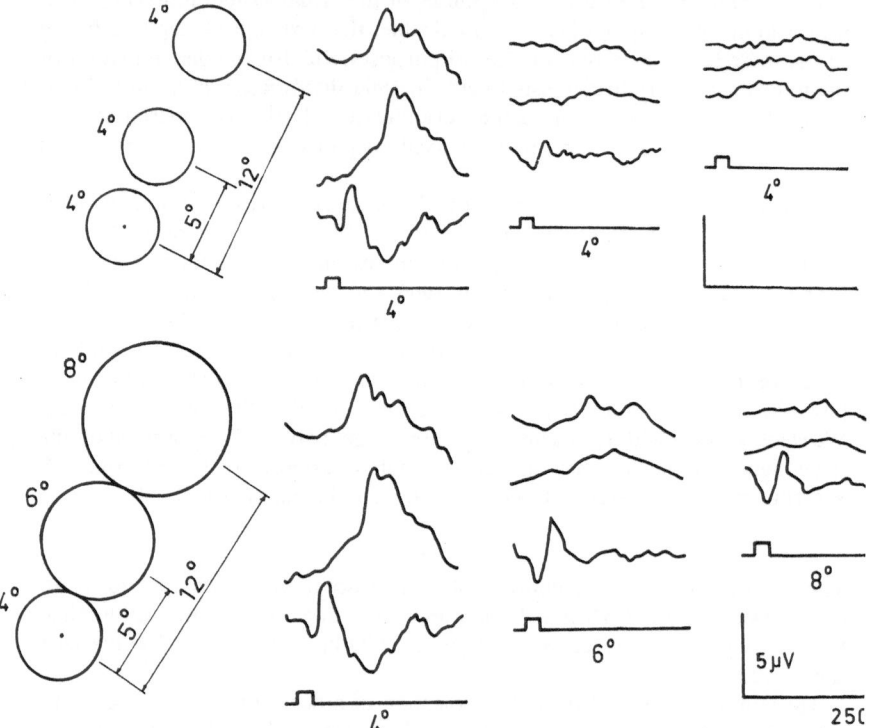

Fig. 1. ERG and VER of a 4° stimulus, presented foveally and at 5° and 12° eccentricity (a), and ERG and VER of a 4°, 6° and 8° stimulus, presented respectively at the fovea and again at 5° and 12° eccentricity (b). The 4° field, marked with a black point in the centre, has been fixed. Background blue, stimulus white log 1.5 cd/m², frequency 4 stimuli per second, 500 responses averaged.

it appears that retinal responses of about equal height as those derived from the fovea, can be recorded (Fig. 1b). A 4° stimulus, foveally presented, produces an ERG of about the same height as a 6° stimulus, presented at 5° eccentricity, or as an 8° stimulus, presented at 12° eccentricity.

Although under these experimental conditions the ERGs are comparable in height, the VERs become smaller as the stimulus is moved to the periphery.

246

These peripheral responses are too small to be registered, which is also the case when the stimulus field is enlarged to 15° or 20°. This means that at the moment the VER is not suitable for electroperimetry. Using the local ERG response as a criterion for the retinal sensitivity one should record the responses of the rod system and those of the cone system separately. ARMINGTON (1968), VAN LITH & HENKES (1968) followed by JACOBSON et al. (1969) demonstrated that under photopic conditions the amplitude of the local ERG depends on the number of cones stimulated. At the top of Fig. 2 the cone density, taken from ØSTERBERG (1935), is drawn. The responses, both of a 5° and a 10° stimulus field, projected in one meridian are given below. According to cone density, the responses are higher in the fovea than in the periphery.

In trying to measure local rod responses, it appears that the rod responses neither show a relationship with the rod density nor with retinal sensitivity under scotopic conditions (VAN LITH & HENKES, 1972). The reason for this may be that the ERGs recorded do not represent a response of the receptors themselves. Moreover, the rods, more than the cones, converge into the bipolar and ganglion cells. An advantage in using the cone system for electroperimetry is that it has a direct linkup with the psychophysical clinical perimetry.

As the local ERGs of the cone system are highest in the fovea and lowest in the periphery, the problem in electroperimetry will not be how to measure the sensitivity of the central area, but how to measure the sensitivity of the retinal periphery. Therefore, we firstly have to determine the stimulus conditions under which a reasonable response can be obtained from the retinal periphery. It is logical that we have to keep the stimulus field as small as possible, since the smaller the test field the more precise will be the method. A large local cone response is obtained when the luminance of the background, the adaptive field, is kept low. This is limited, however, by the requirement that stray light responses have to be avoided and that if low stimulus frequencies are used, rod activity has to be suppressed. A large local retinal response can also be obtained by increasing the luminance of the stimulus. The necessity to avoid stray light responses will again be a limiting factor.

A blue background instead of a white one and a white stimulus instead of a red one will also help obtain a large cone response. A blue background suppresses the rods just as much as a white background does. However, blue light spares the cones more than white light does, as it suppresses only the blue cones. Fortunately enough blue cones are relatively few in number as compared with the number of green and red cones. On the other hand, a white stimulus light has the advantage of triggering all the cones, while red light, which is generally used, leaves the green cones relatively undisturbed.

The stimulus time also influences the height of a local cone response, as is shown in Fig. 3. A stimulus of 10 msec reveals a much higher response than a stimulus of 1 msec. An electronic flash, not shown in the figure, will also produce a smaller response than the 10 msec response. This is the result of the temporal summation of the cones. As BEST (1957) demonstrated, further lengthening of the stimulus duration makes no sense. He found that on the photopic level a 100 msec response is smaller than a 10 msec cone response.

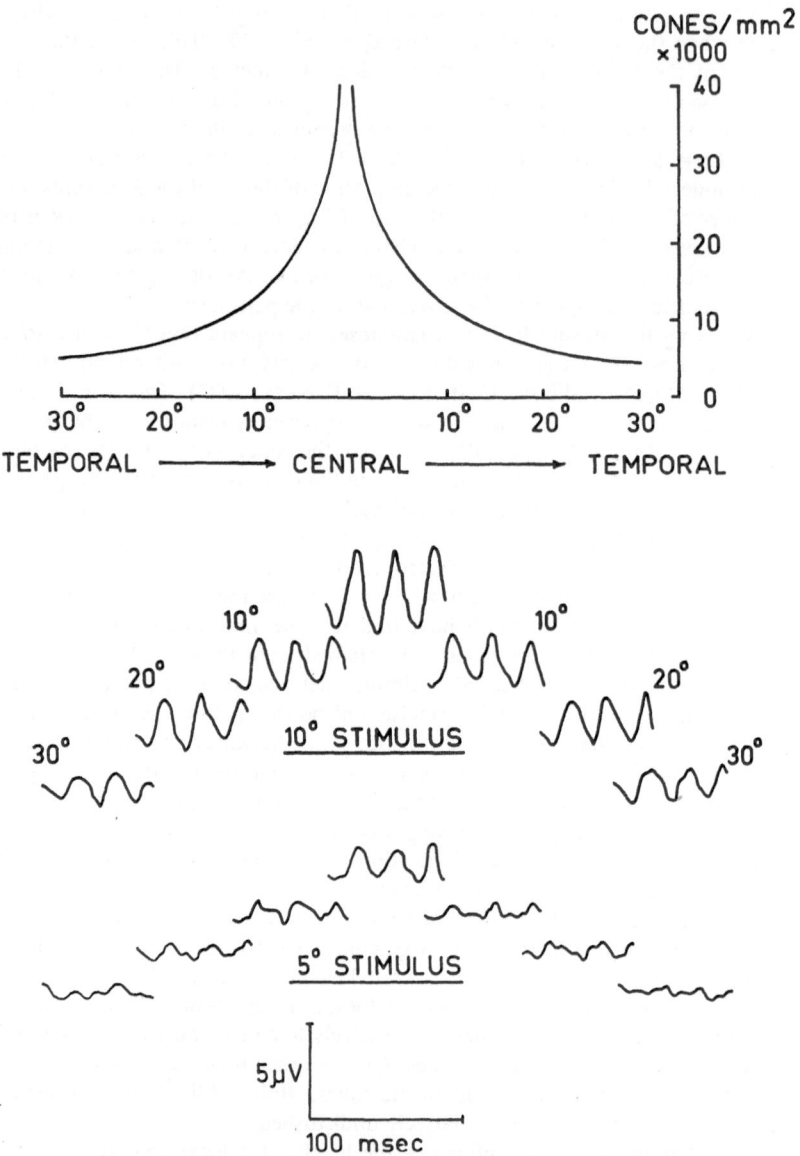

Fig. 2. a. Cone density curve (ØSTERBERG, 1935). b. ERGs after 10° and 5°
stimulation. Stimulation began on the temporal side of the retina at 30°
eccentricity, moving on to the centre in steps of 10° and returning to the
temporal side again. Stimulus conditions as in Fig. 1, except for the
frequency, 40 stimuli per second.

248

The last, but most predominant and crucial problem for a successful electro-perimetry, is the examination time. To be able to test a great many retinal fields we have to reduce recording and registration time as much as possible. Physiologically, this can be done by choosing such stimulus conditions that the highest electrical signal possible is obtained. A high electrical signal or a reasonable

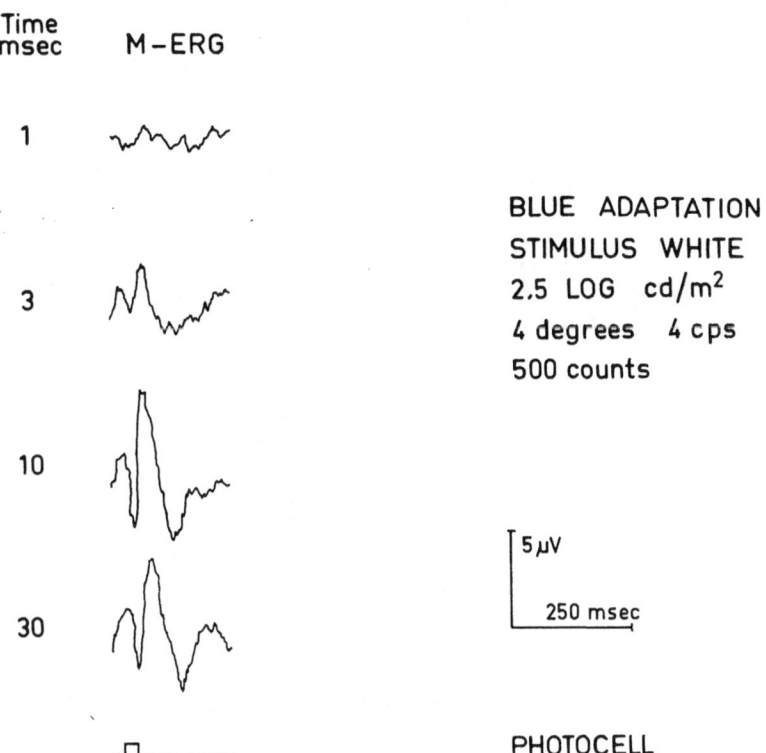

CONSTANT LUMINANCE RESPONSE

Fig. 3. ERGs of a foveally presented 4° stimulus. Stimulus time varies from 1 to 30 msec. Other stimulus conditions as in Fig. 1.

signal-to-noise ratio means that when using averagers we need less summation time. These stimulus conditions, achieving a high response, have already been discussed. Another way to shorten registration time using averagers is to increase the stimulus frequency, provided that the response does not become much smaller. This was determined experimentally. A 10° stimulus, foveally presented and at a 20° eccentricity in the temporal part of the visual field appears to remain of about the same height when the stimulus frequency is increased up to 40 stimuli per second. Therefore, a frequency of about 30–40 stimuli per

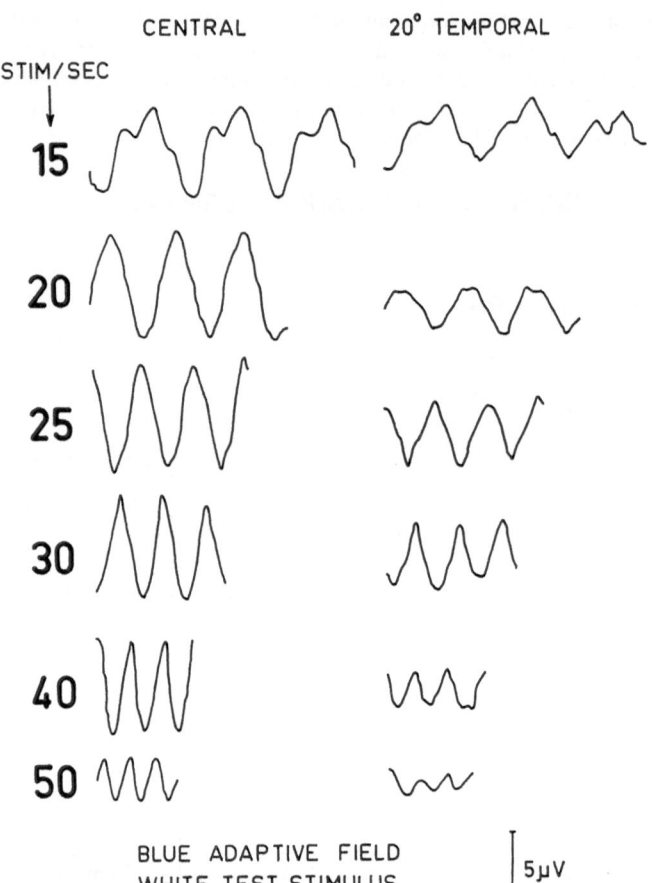

CENTRAL   20° TEMPORAL

STIM/SEC

15

20

25

30

40

50

BLUE ADAPTIVE FIELD
WHITE TEST STIMULUS

5μV

Fig. 4. Influence of the stimulus frequency on the ERGs of a 5° stimulus, presented foveally (on the left) and 20° eccentricity (on the right) in the temporal part of the visual field. Other stimulus conditions as in Fig. 1.

second is the most favourable one to use. An additional advantage of this frequency is that the rod system does not contribute anymore to the response, which makes the level of the adaptive luminance less critical.

DISCUSSION

Having performed the experiments to determine the conditions with which the best response could be obtained, we were convinced that electroperimetry is feasible. We were sceptical, however, if such an electroperimetry could become a useful clinical examination. With an averager and X-Y plotter as a recording system we needed 10 to 15 minutes to determine retinal sensitivity in one meridian only. Moreover, the smallest stimulus field with which measurable responses could be obtained was 5 degrees. At least a faster recording system had to be found, which will be reported in the next paper (VAN LITH & HENKES, 1973).

SUMMARY

For electroperimetry the ERG is more suitable than the VER. Moreover, the ERG of the cone system is a better criterion than that of the rod system. In order to keep the registration time short, stimulus conditions must be chosen with which the highest local response can be obtained. In our set-up a blue background was used in combination with a white stimulus of 20 msec. Until now the smallest field with which recordable responses from the retinal periphery could be obtained amounted to 5 degrees. Registration time can further be shortened by increasing the stimulus frequency.

REFERENCES

ARDEN, G. B. & BANKES, J. L. K. Foveal electroretinogram as a clinical test. *Brit. J. Ophthal.* 50:*740* (1966).
ARMINGTON, J. C. The electroretinogram, the visual evoked potential, and the area-luminance relation. *Vision Res.* 8:*263* (1968).
BEINHOCKER, G. D., BROOKS, P. R., ANFENGER, E. & COPENHAVER, R. M. Electroperimetry. *Trans. Bio-med. Engin. BME*-13:*11* (1966).
BEST, W. & BOHNEN, K. Über den 'off-Effekt' im Elektroretinogramm des Menschen. *Graefes Arch. Ophthal.* 158:*568* (1957).
BRINDLEY, G. S. & WESTHEIMER, G. The spatial properties of the human electroretinogram. *J. Physiol. Lond.* 179:*518* (1965).
DEVOE, R. G., RIPPS, H. & VAUGHAN, H. G. Cortical responses to stimulation of the human fovea. *Vision Res.* 8:*135* (1968).
HOF, M. W. VAN., HOF-VAN DUIN, J. VAN. & RIETVELD, W. J. Enhancement of occipitocortical responses to lightflashes in man during attention. *Vision Res.* 6:*109* (1966).
JACOBSON, J. H., KAWASAKI, K. & HIROSE, T. The human electroretinogram and occipital potential in response to focal illumination of the retina. *Invest. Ophthal.* 8:*545* (1969).
LITH, G. H. M. VAN. & HENKES, H. E. The local electric response of the central retinal area. 6th ISCERG Symposium, 1967 Erfurt, p. 163. Leipzig, Thieme (1968).
LITH, G. H. M. VAN. & HENKES, H. E. The relationship between ERG and VER. *Ophthal. Res.* 1:*40* (1970).
LITH, G. H. M. VAN. & HENKES, H. E. Receptor density, ERG and VER. 8th ISCERG Symposium, 1970 Pisa, p. 133. Pisa, Pacini (1972).
LITH, G. H. M. VAN. & HENKES, H. E. Local scotopic responses in ERG and VER. 9th ISCERG Symposium, 1971 Brighton, p. 273. New York, Plenum Press, (1972).
LITH, G. H. M. VAN., HENKES, H. E. & MARLE, G. W. VAN. Electroretinotopography (ERTG). This volume.
ØSTERBERG, T. Topography of the layer of rods and cones in the human retina. Copenhagen, Besck, (1935) (*Acta Ophthal.*, suppl. 6).

ELECTRORETINOTOPOGRAPHY (ERTG)

G. H. M. VAN LITH, H. E. HENKES & G. W. VAN MARLE*

(*Rotterdam*)

In the foregoing paper the physiological circumstances which are to succeed in electroperimetry have been discussed (HENKES & VAN LITH 1973). Now the technical possibilities to register the retinal sensitivity as quickly and reliably as possible will be dealt with.

Local ERG responses obtained with stimuli of less than 10° are too small to be recorded with the ordinary amplifiers (EEG machines, oscilloscopes). Averaging is necessary. Presently, averagers like the CAT (Mnemotron 400B) are generally used in combination with an X-Y plotter. Such a system, however, is too slow to make electroperimetry successful. We needed 10–15 minutes to examine retinal sensitivity in one meridian with stimuli of 10° or 5° in steps of 10° or 5° over an angle of 90°.

Time can be saved, at least for the patient, when a tape-recorder is used and averaging and plotting of data is done afterwards. The disadvantage, however, is clear. The results or failures cannot be seen directly. Moreover, one needs rather expensive equipment. The same applies to the memory core of a computer instead of the slow X-Y plotter. A much cheaper and far more simple method is to photograph the averaged records directly from the screen of the oscilloscope using a polaroid camera. The plotting of data with the X-Y plotter is then avoided. This method is one of those used in our laboratory.

A better and faster system, more suitable to electroperimetry, seems to be the lock-in amplifier. Such an apparatus has the characteristics of a selective amplifier. It indicates continuously the electric activity of a certain frequency. FRICKER (1971) in the U.S.A. and PADMOS and VAN NORREN (1971, 1972) in The Netherlands, introduced this kind of selective amplification in electro-ophthalmology. FRICKER in order to detect small responses in patients with retinitis pigmentosa, PADMOS and VAN NORREN to determine spectral sensitivity curves. A great advantage of the lock-in amplifier is that it indicates the electric activity, representing retinal sensitivity, continuously and directly. However, the time-saving obtained is at the expense of information, viz. the wave form. The actual response is no longer seen, but this is not necessary, for perimetry means only the determination of retinal sensitivity. Another advantage is that even flicker ERGs with a peak-to-peak amplitude of 0.1 μV can be detected from the noise level.

PROCEDURE

Adaptation light and test light were the same as described in the foregoing paper (HENKES & VAN LITH, 1973). Moving of the stimulus was done with a provisional set-up. The signal, only the ERG, was led off with a Henkes contact lens electrode, the neutral electrode being at the ear-lobe.

* Eye Clinic, Medical Faculty, Rotterdam, The Netherlands.

Signal processing was obtained with two lock-in amplifiers. Since the amplifiers are controlled by the stimulus frequency (input signal), they only detect electric activity of this special frequency in the output signal (flicker-ERG). Since the phase relation between stimulus and the ERG can vary, it is preferable to use two lock-in amplifiers with a 90° phase difference between one another. We used a PAR lock-in amplifier, model 126 provided with a pre-amplifier model 117, and a lock-in amplifier model 127. The output signal, obtained in two components, has to be summed up according to the function $A = VA_x^2 + A_y^2$ to get the full signal amplitude (PADMOS & VAN NORREN, 1972).

The signal is recorded with a two channel X-time writer. One channel registers the amplitude, the other the phase-angle. The latter did not alter much in the present experiments, as a constant luminance of background and stimulus was used. Therefore only the amplitude of the signal is presented in the figure. Band pass of the pre-amplifier was 10–1000 Hz, while the stimulus frequency was 40 Hz. The time constant of the lock-in systems representing the integration of the analysers amounted to 10 seconds.

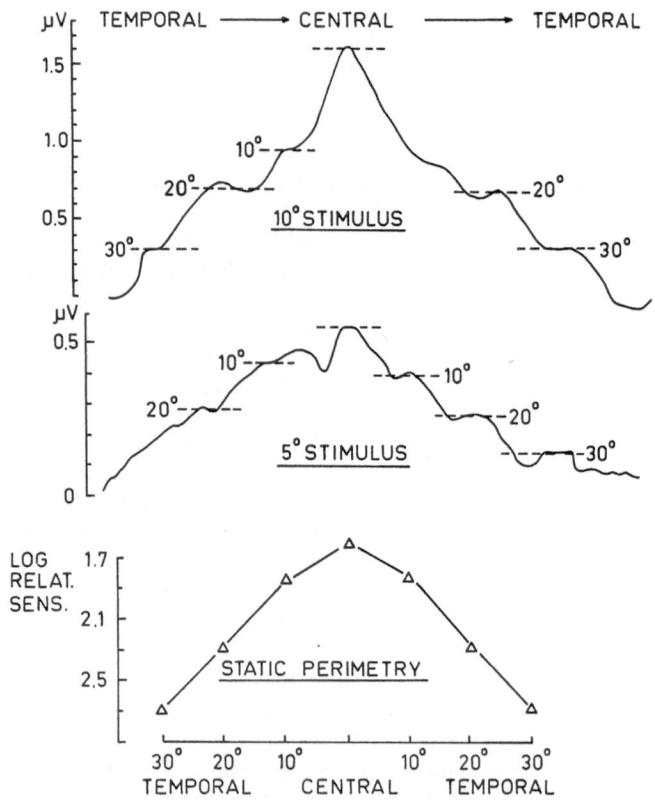

Fig. 1. Recordings of the lock-in amplifier obtained after 10° and 5° stimulation. Below the results of static perimetry in the same subject.

254

Figure 1 represents the curves, directly recorded via the lock-in amplifier with an X-time writer. Stimulation began on the temporal side of the retina at 30° eccentricity, moving on to the centre in steps of 10° and returning to the temporal side again. The horizontally dashed lines indicate that a steady potential level was reached; the stimulus was then moved on to the next place. It is important to mention that each curve has been obtained in 4–5 minutes. The amplitude of the flicker-ERG can be directly seen.

The height of the response i.e. the amplitude of the flicker-ERG increases to the center (fovea) and according to the cone density. There is also a resemblance between the height of the response and the psychophysical sensitivity curve, obtained by static perimetry, as shown below. The 10° stimulation produces a clear response, while the 5° stimulation creates a much smaller one. Even at 30° eccentricity, however, a small electric response can be registered.

The set-up with which these recordings have been made was a very primitive one. The subject had to move his eyes, while the stimulus remained in the same place. Our team is now developing, with the aid of the Delft Institute of Technology, a special stimulator for the electroperimetry. In its intermediate stage of development we constructed, what might be called a contraption, with which we could examine patients. The stimulus could be moved, although only along a straight line, in the horizontal meridian. The advantage was that the eyes could be held quietly in a fixed position.

The recordings of Figure 2 have been made with this stimulator on a normal subject. For the two curves at the top of the figure the stimulus was moved in steps of 5° from the nasal side of the visual field to the temporal side. The two lower curves have been obtained by moving the stimulus from the temporal side to the nasal side. Each experiment has been done twice. The vertical bars indicate the moment the stimulus is moved. Some 10–20 msec later a steady state level of electric activity is reached, which is indicated by the horizontal dashes. The time to reach this level is determined by the time constant (analysis time) of the amplifier and probably by local retinal adaptation, too. In the center, at 0°, it takes more time to reach a steady state, possibly due to the high electric activity here.

The blind spot is not visualized. Either the stimulus of 5° is too large, or the fixation of the subject's eye is not stable enough. The temporal part of the visual field clearly shows, however, lower potentials than the nasal part. As this is the case both in the upper and the lower recordings, it reflects, in our opinion, a real retinal sensitivity difference. On examining more subjects, however, such a difference was not always observed, as can be seen in Fig. 3. Only the two upper curves indicate lower retinal activity at the temporal side. while the last subject (Lh) even shows the reverse.

Before going further into the development of a special stimulator we wanted to check the method in a few patients. The recordings of two patients are represented in Fig. 4 together with the recordings of a normal subject. Both patients show a macular degeneration. The patient with the relative scotoma has a lower than normal sensitivity foveally and parafoveally, while the patient with the absolute scotoma shows no sensitivity increase at all towards the center. In the latter the periphery seems to have a somewhat higher sensitivity than the center.

Discussion

The results obtained show that electroperimetry is not a fancy idea any longer, but may become a real examination technique. However, are we to go on calling

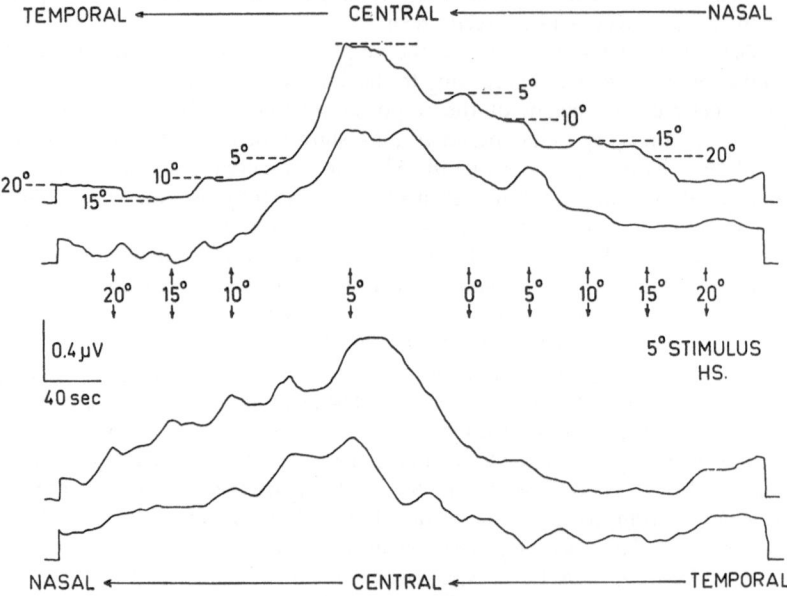

Fig. 2. Recordings of the lock-in amplifier after 5° stimulation. The recordings have to be read from right to left. The two upper curves have been made from nasal to temporal in the horizontal meridian, the two lower curves from temporal to nasal.

it electroperimetry? In comparison with static perimetry we only test a limited area of the retina with rather large stimulus fields. Because this method is at any rate a determination of the topographic sensitivity of the retina we will call it: "Electroretinotopography", for short ERTG. The term ERTG implies too, that the sensitivity is determined by means of the ERG.

At this moment we are not ready yet to introduce this method for clinical purposes. We need a well-constructed, versatile stimulator system with which the stimulus can be moved in an arc around the eye in variable steps. The meridian in which the stimulus is moved must be variable too. Using such a specially constructed stimulator we are sure that measuring time will be limited. For instance: a few minutes may perhaps suffice to test 90° of one meridian. We will limit ourselves to the central visual field of 90°, as such a limitation will simplify the construction of the stimulator and in our opinion, testing of the retinal periphery with this method is not very interesting.

256

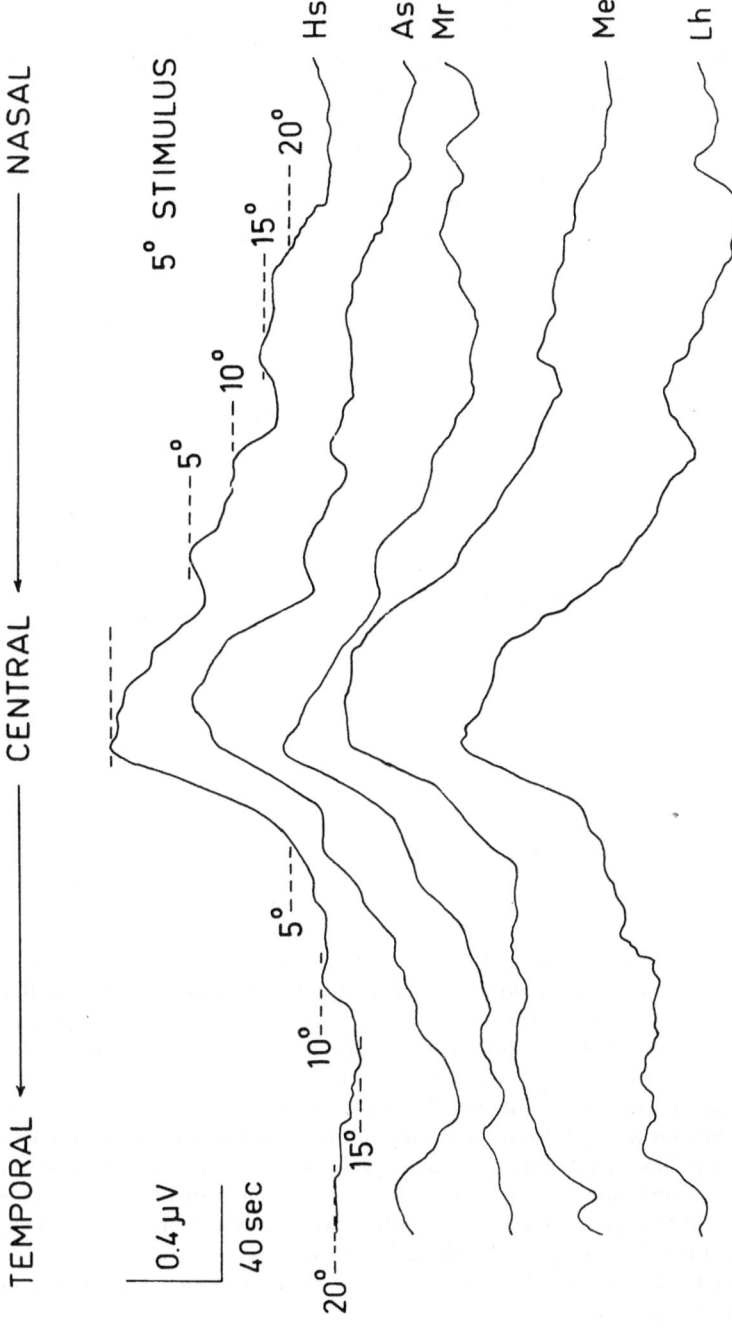

Fig. 3. Recordings of 5 normal subjects. Horizontal meridian.

257

At the moment a 5° stimulus is the smallest with which reasonable curves can be obtained. It is not ruled out that in future by choosing stimulus conditions carefully, the test field may become smaller. In the figures only stimulation up to 30° eccentricity can be seen. As cone density does not decrease considerably outside 30°, we may expect the response to remain about equal if the stimulus is moved further away into the periphery.

A great problem is the patient's cooperation and his ability to fixate. But the same problem exists in psychophysical perimetry. For this reason a further development in ERTG should not be stopped. In psychophysical perimetry

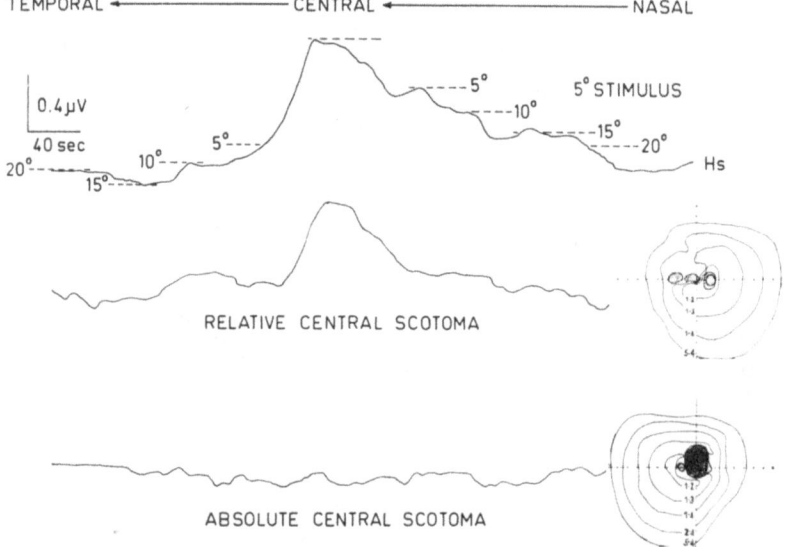

Fig. 4. Recordings of a normal subject (upper curve), of a patient with a relative central scotoma (middle) and of a patient with an absolute central scotoma. Horizontal meridian.

fixation is generally checked by the examiner himself using an optical system. This, of course, can be done in ERTG, too. Easier is the use of a small TV-camera and monitor. The sophisticated method, developed and reported by HACHE and co-workers (1972) at the 9th ISCERG Symposium at Brighton last year, may be promising. HACHE uses a servo-mechanism, which follows the eye movements. However, with a central scotoma, in which fixation is not centric, this method will fail. More promising in the distant future may be the testing of more than one meridian simultaneously. This can be done by using more than one lock-in amplifier in combination with a number of light stimuli presented to the eye at different frequencies. Scotomata can then be found easily in the ERTG-curves, provided the light stimuli cross the scotoma.

Our final conclusion is that the ERTG will become an accepted procedure in electro-ophthalmology.

258

SUMMARY

To succeed in electroperimetry a reasonable number of retinal fields will have to be tested. Averagers, like a CAT-computer, together with X-Y plotter are too slow. A better system seems to be lock-in amplifiers and X-time writers, registering directly and continuously the electric activity of the retina. The recordings presented in this paper have been made with such amplifiers. The stimulator was still provisional. The results obtained, however, encourage us to build a special apparatus for this purpose. We prefer the word electroretino-topography (ERTG) instead of electroperimetry, as the term ERTG expresses that the examination is done via the ERG.

REFERENCES

FRICKER, S. J. Application of synchronous detector techniques for electroretinographic studies in patients with retinitis pigmentosa. *Invest. Ophthal.* 10:*329* (1971).

HACHE, J. C., DUBOIS, P., BERTOLACCI, G., VETU, E. & MALVACHE, N. New method of stimulation for the study of photoreceptors. In: The visual system; Proceedings 9th ISCERG Symposium, Brighton 1971; ed. by G. B. Arden. p. 273. New York, Plenum Press (1972).

HENKES, H. E. & LITH, G. H. M. VAN. Electroperimetry; Proceedings 10th ISCERG Symposium, Los Angeles 1972. This volume. pp. 245–251.

PADMOS, P. & NORREN, D. VAN. Cone spectral sensitivity and chromatic adaptation as revealed by human flicker electroretinography. *Vision Res.* 11:*27* (1971).

PADMOS, P. & NORREN, D. VAN. The Vector voltmeter as a tool to measure ERG spectral sensitivity and dark adaptation; Report No. IZF 1972–4. Soesterberg, Institute for Perception RVO-TNO (1972).

THE PERFUSED MAMMALIAN EYE AS A PREPARATION FOR ELECTROPHYSIOLOGICAL STUDIES

GÜNTER NIEMEYER, M.D. & PETER GOURAS,* M.D.

(*Zurich and Bethesda*)

In studying local electroretinograms (ERG's) and especially intracellular responses within the retina, a particular mechanical stability is required. In mammalian eyes the nonpulsatile arterial perfusion of the whole globe represents a technique which reduces the movements of the retina to a minimum. It has been shown earlier that retinal function and neural transmission can be maintained in such a preparation for about 10 hours (GOURAS & HOFF, 1970). A relatively high flow rate and an accurate temperature control turned out to be important factors for a high sensitivity to light of both the ERG b-wave and single unit responses in different retinal layers. (NIEMEYER, 1973).

METHODS

A detailed description of the techniques will be published elsewhere (NIEMEYER). The setup for the perfusion of isolated eyes is shown diagrammatically in Fig. 1. The perfusate consists of oxygenated salt solution which contains calf serum. Hydrostatic pressure drives the heated perfusate through a fine tubing into the ophthalmociliary artery of the enucleated eye. This vessel supplies both the retinal and the choroidal circulation in the cat.

Gross electrodes on the cornea and on the posterior pole detect the corneal ERG; a glass micropipette is introduced through a scleral hole in the pars plana region and records the vitreal and intraretinal ERG, and subsequently single cell responses. The data are amplified and displayed on an oscilloscope or stored on magnetic tape.

An optical double beam system (right side of Fig. 1) provides facilities for stimulation and adaptation of the retina. A modified fundus camera presents the stimulus in a Maxwellian view, allowing simultaneously observation or photography of the region being stimulated. Fig. 2 shows a fluorescein angiogram of the central cat retina with the optic disc and the area centralis, both in the tapetum lucidum region.

India ink injections of the ophthalmociliary artery were used for localization of the area centralis and of the electrode position.

---

* From the Department of Ophthalmology, University of Zürich, Switzerland and the Section of Neurophysiology, Laboratory of Vision Research, The National Eye Institute, National Institutes of Health U.S. Department of Health, Education, and Welfare, Bethesda, Maryland, 20014.

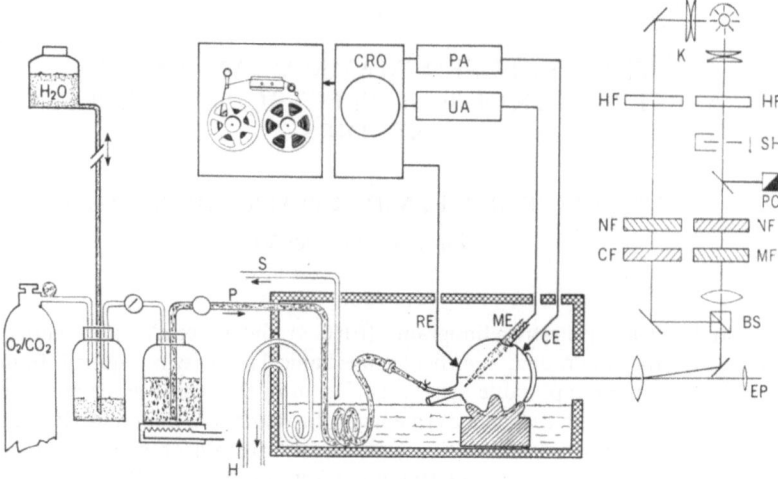

Fig. 1. Schema of a setup for the perfusion of isolated mammalian eyes. Left side, perfusion system; middle: eye chamber and electronics; right, optical stimulator. BS, beam splitter; CE, corneal electrode; CF, color filter; CRO, cathode ray oscilloscope; EP, eye piece of fundus camera; H, heating device; HF, heat filter; K, condenser; ME, microelectrode; MF, monochromatic filter; NF, neutral filter; P, perfusate; PA, preamplifier; PC, photocell; RE, reference electrode; S, suction, SH, electromagnetic shutter; UA, unity gain amplifier.

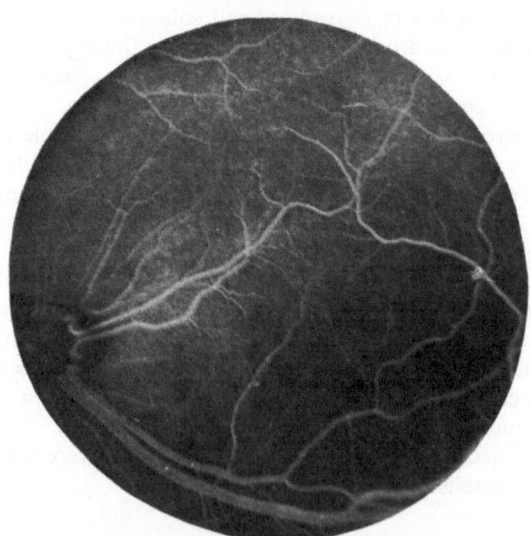

Fig. 2. Fluorescence angiogram of the central retina of a left cat eye. The area centralis is found about 3 disc diameters laterally and slightly above the optic disc within the tapetum lucidum, where there are no larger vessels.

The experiments presented here were carried out in the dark-adapted state. Light pulses of 10 to 200 msec duration have been applied in 1 to 10 second intervals.

All electrical responses were elicited with various monochromatic lights distributed over the range of the visible spectrum. Intensities from threshold to 3 to 5 logarithmic units above threshold were used; the maximal intensity of colored light was 1.98×10^3 ergs/cm²/sec for 575 nm.

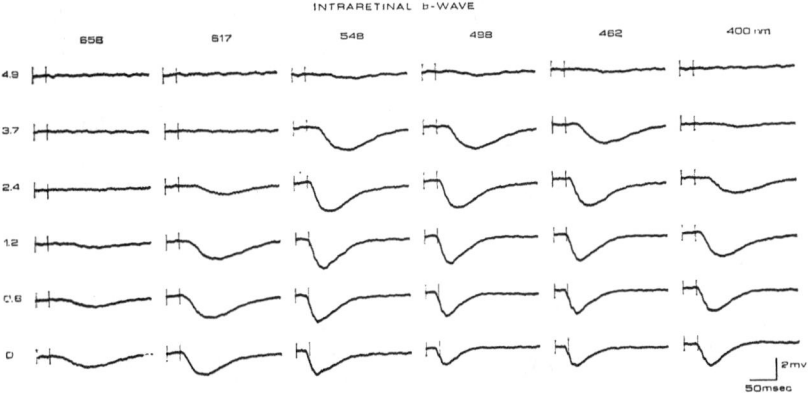

Fig. 3. Records of the intraretinal b-wave as a respose to a variety of brief monochromatic flashes of different intensity. The numbers on the left indicate the optical density of interposed neutral filters in logarithmic units. With bright light of this stimulus duration one sees the effect of adaptation in the lower-most records.

RESULTS

The ERG has been recorded from the cornea, the vitreous close to the inner limiting membrane and from various sites within the retina. The action spectra of these responses have been obtained by applying constant response criteria to the amplitude intensity functions for the various monochromatic stimuli. As an example Fig. 3 shows a series of intraretinal (inversed) b-waves as responses to brief pulses of monochromatic light. Fig. 4 shows an amplitude intensity function for the intraretinal b-wave which was recorded from the area centralis.

Fig. 5 shows an action spectrum from the corneal ERG b-wave in comparison to the one of the intraretinal b-wave originated in the area centralis. The dotted and the dashed curve represent the action spectra of the rod and the cone ERG, respectively, in the intact cat (replotted from DODT & WALTHER). In the dark-adapted perfused cat eye the cone action spectrum could be detected in the intra-retinal b-wave of the area centralis when high response criteria were applied. The corneal and the vitreal ERG never revealed spectral sensitivity of the cones in the dark-adapted state. This was found as well for the intraretinal b-wave recorded from the tapetal and from the tapetum-free periphery which always reflected the rod action spectrum (Fig. 6). Usually the threshold was higher in the tapetum free region.

18

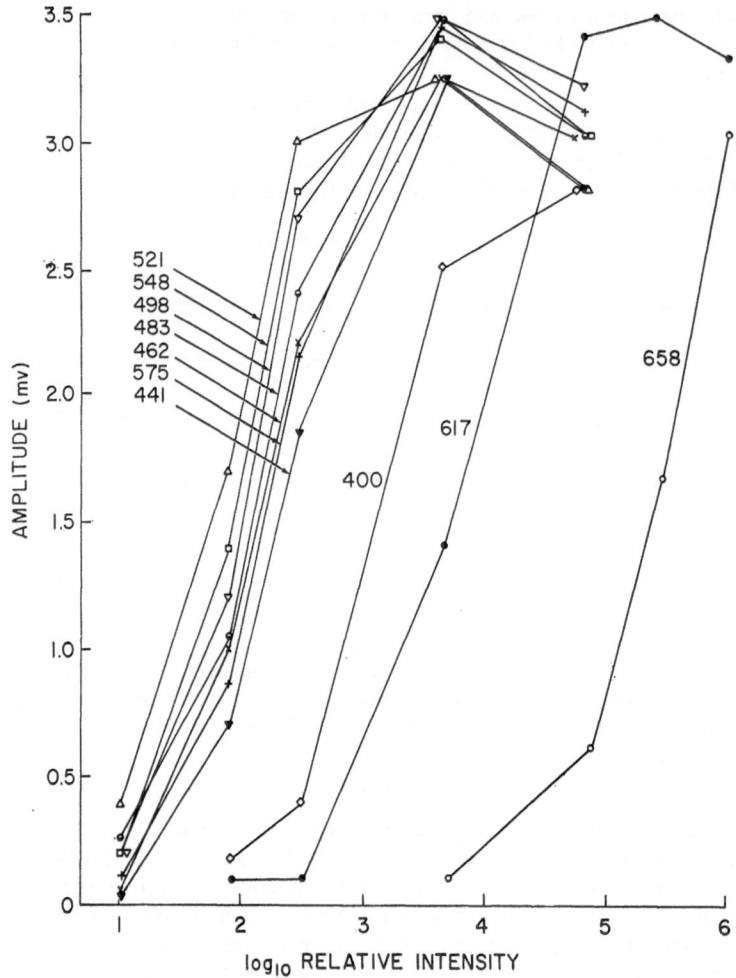

Fig. 4. Amplitude-intensity functions for a b-wave recorded intraretinally near to the area centralis. The numbers at the curves indicate the peak transmission of the narrow band interference filters in nanometers. Corrections for the different transmissivity of the various filters were applied in plotting the data.

Responses from retinal ganglion cells were easily obtained when fine glass micropipettes were inserted in the vicinity of the area centralis. Fig. 7 shows an example of spectral responses from a tonically responding ganglion cell (SAITO et al., 1970). The action spectra of this unit revealed cone characteristics when responses of 14, 22 or 44 spikes were used as criteria. The peak sensitivity was found at 550–560 nm, which is in agreement with the findings of DAW & PEARL-MAN (1969) in the cat's optic tract and lateral geniculate. Most retinal ganglion

264

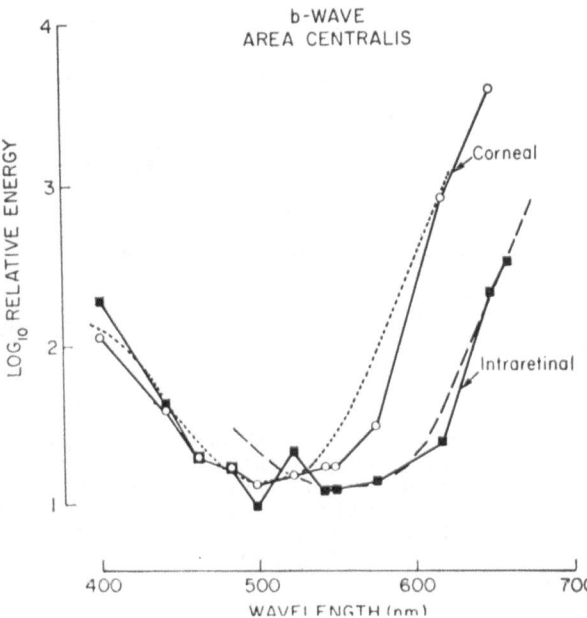

Fig. 5. The action spectra of the b-wave of the corneal ERG (○) and of the intraretinal b-wave, recorded from the area centralis (■) are shown. The dotted curve represents the action spectrum of the rod ERG, replotted from DODT and WALTHER (1958a), the dashed curve shows the action spectrum of the cone ERG of the intact cat, replotted from DODT & WALTHER (1958b). In the dark-adapted isolated cat eye only the intraretinal ERG could detect the cone action spectrum at suprathreshold response criteria in the longer wavelength range.

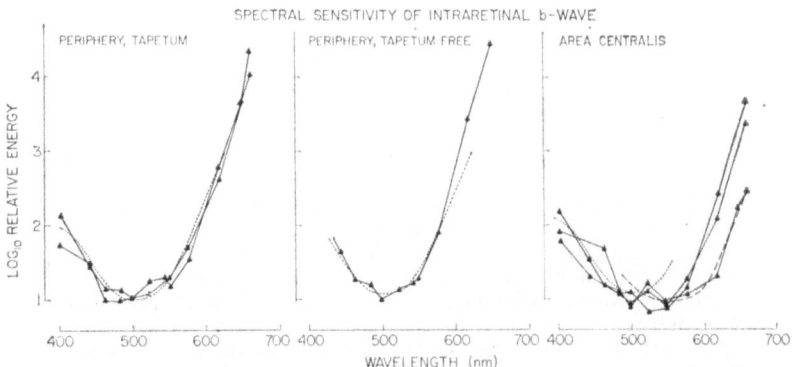

Fig. 6. The action spectra of the intraretinal b-wave recorded from two sites in the tapetal periphery, in the tapetum-free periphery and from 3 locations within the area centralis are compared. The dotted and the dashed curves represent the rod and cone action spectra respectively as mentioned in Fig. 5.

265

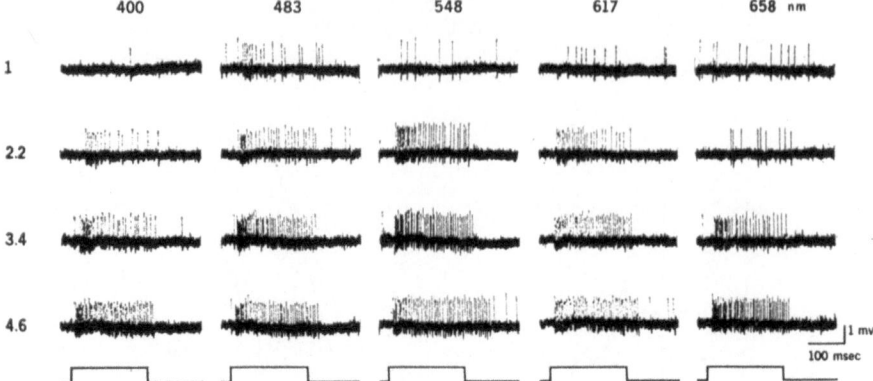

Fig. 7. Spectral responses from a single unit in the ganglion cell layer are shown. The stimulus was a 23° spot presented for 200 msec, as indicated on the bottom of each row, at 2 second intervals. The spectral sensitivity of this tonically responding unit revealed cone input, when 14, 22 and 44 spikes were taken as response criteria. The numbers on the left indicate the relative intensity in logarithmic steps.

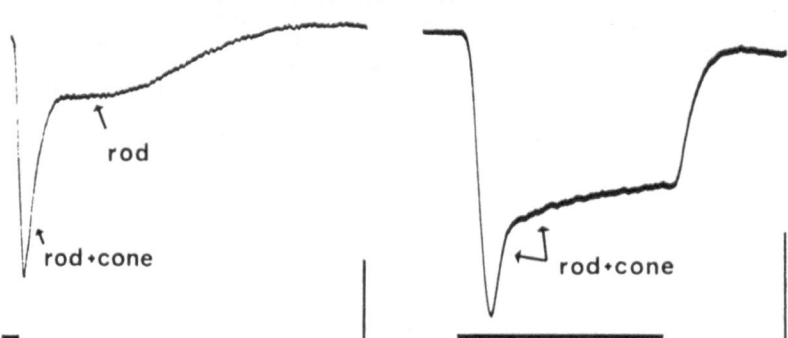

Fig. 8. S-potentials from the isolated perfused cat retina, which revealed both rod and cone input. A response to a 20 msec (left) and a response to a 200 msec light pulse (right) are shown. The wavelength of the stimulating light was 548 nm for the brief pulse and 400 nm for the longer pulse on the right side. The response to the brief stimulus consists of a fast and short hyperpolarization which is followed by a characteristic slow after-potential of a smaller amplitude. Spectral studies of the former revealed input from rods and cones whereas in the after-potential only the rod action spectrum could be detected. In the same unit a response to a longer pulse revealed rod and cone contribution in the initial transient hyperpolarization as well as in the plateau-like maintained phase. Calibration: vertical bars, 10 mv; horizontal bars, 20 msec (left) and 200 msec (right), indicating the stimulus duration.

cells showed rod input at threshold intensities, and at suprathreshold intensities cone input similar to the data of ANDREWS & HAMMOND (1970). Phasically responding on-and-off center ganglion cell units were found, but not further analyzed in this study.

In the inner nuclear layer S-potentials could be studied intracellularly for periods of up to 1 hour. These intracellular responses were always hyperpolarizing and superimposed on resting potentials of −20 to −40 mv. The recording site, a large spatial summation, the graded and the maintained correlation to the stimulus allowed the identification of these responses as S-potentials, generated in horizontal cells (KANEKO, 1970; STEINBERG & SCHMIDT, 1971).

Fig. 8 shows S-potentials from a single cell, which received input from rods and cones. The response to a brief stimulus (left in Fig. 8) shows a fast and short initial hyperpolarization which is followed by a slow after potential.

Whereas the initial deflection showed rod input at threshold, and at higher response criteria cone input, the after potential always showed the rod action

400   617nm

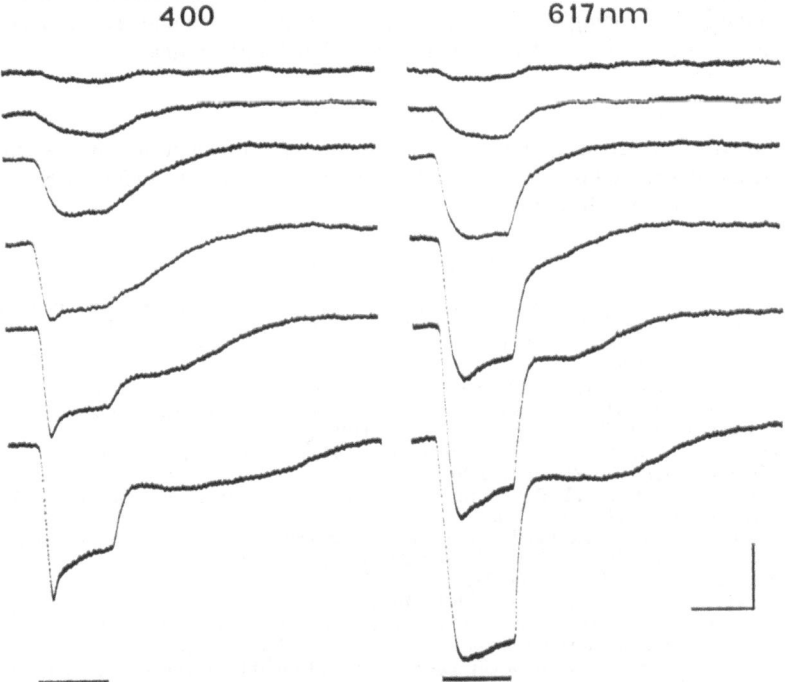

Fig. 9. S-potentials elicited by 200 msec light pulses of deep blue light (400 nm) and of red light (617 nm) of different intensities. The intensity increased from top to bottom in 0.6 steps of log. optical density. Notice the difference in shape of the suprathreshold responses to blue as compared to red light in the 3 lower traces. The after-potential described in Fig. 8 is also seen in this unit and appears to be more pronounced in the short wavelength responses. Calibration 200 msec and 10 mv.

267

spectrum in isolation. This was first observed by STEINBERG (1969). The right side of Fig. 8 shows an S-potential elicited by a 200 msec pulse of blue light. The initial peak and the maintained phase of the signal revealed rod and cone input. However, such "mixed units" show a different response shape under stimulation with long wavelength light (Fig. 9). This difference of spectral responses was found in most S-potentials in the frame of this work, which is discussed in detail in another publication (NIEMEYER & GOURAS).

Occasionally intracellular responses could be obtained in the pigment epithelium. The resting potential of these cells was −60 to −65 mv; the hyperpolarizing response to light had a characteristic slow time course. The amplitude as well as the peak time of those signals increased with the logarithm of the light intensity.

CONCLUSIONS

The isolated perfused cat eye represents a suitable preparation for electrophysiological testing at both the ERG and the single cell level. The sensitivity to light of this *in vitro* preparation remains stable over many hours and is comparable to the corresponding *in vivo* data. By means of spectral techniques rod and cone contributions can be detected in any given signal in the retina.

ACKNOWLEDGMENT

GÜNTER NIEMEYER, during part of this study, was supported by the Swiss National Science Foundation, and later by the National Eye Institute, National Institutes of Health, Bethesda.

REFERENCES

ANDREWS, D. P., & HAMMOND, P. Mesopic increment threshold spectral sensitivity of single optic tract fibres in the cat: cone-rod interaction. *J. Physiol.* 209:*65–81* (1970).

DAW, N. W. & PEARLMAN, A. L. Cat colour vision: one cone process or several? *J. Physiol.* 210:*745–764* (1969).

DODT, E. & WALTHER, J. B. Netzhautsensitivität, Linsenabsorption und physikalische Lichtstreuung. Der skotopische Dominator der Katze im sichtbaren und ultravioletten Spektralbereich. *Pflügers Arch.* 266:*167–174* (1958a).

DODT, E. & WALTHER, J. B. Der photopische Dominator in Flimmer-ERG der Katze. *Pflügers Arch.* 266:*175–186* (1958b).

GOURAS, P. & HOFF. M. Retinal function in an isolated perfused mammalian eye. *Invest. Ophthalmol.* 9:*388–399* (1970).

KANEKO, A. Physiological and morphological identification of horizontal, bipolar and amacrine cells in goldfish retina. *J. Physiol.* 207:*623–633* (1970).

NIEMEYER, G. submitted. *Vision Res.*

NIEMEYER, G. & GOURAS, P. submitted. *Vision Res.*

SAITO, H., SHIMAHARA, T. & FUKADA, Y. Four types of responses to light and dark spot stimuli in the cat optic nerve. *Tohoku J. exp. Med.* 102:*127–133* (1970).

STEINBERG, R. H. The rod after-effect in S-potentials from the cat retina. *Vision Res.* 9:*1345–1355* (1969).

STEINBERG, R. H. & SCHMIDT, R. The evidence that horizontal cells generate S-potentials in the cat retina. *Vision Res.* 11:*1029–1031* (1971).

SCOTOPIC SPECTRAL SENSITIVITY AND THE ABSORBANCE OF VISUAL PIGMENTS IN ISOLATED VISUAL CELLS AND IN THE INTACT RETINA

JAMES K. BOWMAKER*

(*Los Angeles*)

INTRODUCTION

In the study of scotopic spectral sensitivity and the absorbance of visual pigments, it has been generally assumed that the absorption properties of the visual pigments in the intact retina are the same as the absorption properties of the visual pigments when extracted into aqueous solution. Most data regarding the absorbance of visual pigments have been taken from extracts and these findings have been found to be in general agreement with scotopic function (GRANIT, 1947; DARTNALL, 1953; CRESCITELLI & DARTNALL, 1953). However, with more accurate determinations of the absorbance of visual pigments, a discrepancy between scotopic spectral sensitivities and the absorbance of the visual pigments in solution has become apparent, in that the scotopic spectral sensitivity is often found to be greater at longer wavelengths than would be suggested by the absorbance of the visual pigment. For example, in the human, the scotopic spectral sensitivity has a maximum at 497 nm (CRAWFORD, 1949) whereas the visual pigment, extracted in digitonin, has a maximum absorbance at 493 nm (WALD & BROWN, 1958). These discrepancies raise the question as to whether the assumption that the absorbance properties of visual pigments in solution are the same as the absorbance properties of the visual pigments in the intact visual cell is justified.

The absorbance of the visual pigments within the isolated outer segments of the visual receptor cells has been shown to be identical to the absorbance of the visual pigments in digitonin solution (DARTNALL, 1961; LIEBMAN & ENTINE, 1968). However, a number of investigations (ARDEN, 1954; BARER & SIDMAN, 1955; DOBROWOLSKI, JOHNSON & TANSLEY, 1955; RUSHTON, 1956; DENTON & WALKER, 1958; WALD & BROWN, 1958; DARTNALL, 1961; WALD, BROWN & GIBBONS, 1963; BAUMAN, 1967; DONNER & REUTER, 1969) have shown that the difference spectra of visual pigments in either suspensions of the outer segments of the visual cells, or in the retinae themselves, are displaced by as much as 20 nm towards the red, from the corresponding difference spectra obtained from solutions of the visual pigments. RUSHTON (1956) and DARTNALL (1959, 1961)

* This investigation was supported in part by a FIGHT FOR SIGHT Postdoctoral Research Fellowship, financed by FIGHT FOR SIGHT, INC., New York City, and aided by grant B-1509 from the Division of Research Grants and Fellowships, National Institutes of Health, U.S. Public Health Service.
Present address: Medical Research Council's Vision Unit, School of Biological Sciences, University of Sussex, Falmer, Brighton, BN1 9QY, England.

suggested that the red shift was due to photoproducts which were formed in the outer segments and which were different from the photoproducts formed in solution. These photoproducts absorbed within the visible region of the spectrum and had the effect of displacing the difference spectrum towards the red.

In all of these investigations, with the exception of those of WALD & BROWN (1958) and WALD, BROWN & GIBBONS (1963), hydroxylamine was not added to the suspensions of visual cells. Hydroxylamine, when added to extracts of visual pigments, has the useful property of converting the photoproducts of the pigment to retinal oxime, which absorbs maximally at about 365 nm, thus markedly reducing the possible distortion of the difference spectrum. If hydroxylamine has the same effect on suspensions of outer segments as it does on extracts, it should be possible to obtain difference spectra from suspensions of outer segments which are identical to those obtained from solutions of the visual pigments.

In this paper results are presented from experiments with Rana pipiens and Gekko gekko which show that the red shift, observed in the difference spectra obtained from suspensions of the visual cells, is due to photoproducts which can be removed with hydroxylamine. However, in the isolated intact retina there is a discrepancy between both the absorbance spectrum and the difference spectrum of the visual pigment in the intact retina and the absorbance of the pigment in solution, which cannot be the result of photoproducts. This difference in absorbance is correlated with the discrepancy found between scotopic spectral sensitivity and the absorbance of visual pigments in solution.

METHODS

The Rana pipiens and Gekko gekko were dark adapted, following which the eyes were removed and the retinae dissected out. Suspensions of the outer segments were obtained by the conventional method (DARTNALL, 1957) in 40% sucrose, buffered to pH 7.1 and hydroxylamine was added to the suspensions when required as a drop of a 0.1 M solution, also buffered to pH 7.1. For studies of the intact retina, the isolated retina was mounted receptor-side up in a small chamber on a piece of gauze and held in place with a washer fitted to the cover of the chamber. The retina was mounted with the whole chamber submerged in Ringer solution so that when finally arranged the retina was bathed in a small volume of Ringer, free of air bubbles. The chamber was then mounted in the spectrophotometer in such a way that the outer segments of the visual cells were orientated facing towards, and with the majority of cells parallel to, the spectrophotometer light beam.

The spectral absorbance of the preparations was measured using a Beckman DU spectrophotometer over the range 360–700 nm. To overcome the problem of light scattering in the preparations, a modified form of Dartnall's 'opal glass' method was used (DARTNALL, 1961). With this technique it was possible to obtain absorbance curves from suspensions of outer segments with a D_{min}/D_{max} of about 0.6 and from isolated retinae of about 0.32–0.40. The stability of the preparations during the measurement of the absorbance spectrum and the homogeneity of the preparations were tested in the usual way (DARTNALL, 1957, 1961).

270

1. *Rana pipiens.*

As shown in Fig. 1 (triangles) the absorbance spectrum of a suspension of frog rod outer segments was similar to the Dartnall nomogram for the absorbance of an extract of frog rhodopsin (Fig. 1, full line), at least at wavelengths above 500 nm. This is similar to the findings of DARTNALL (1961). To investigate the effect of hydroxylamine on the difference spectrum derived from bleaching a

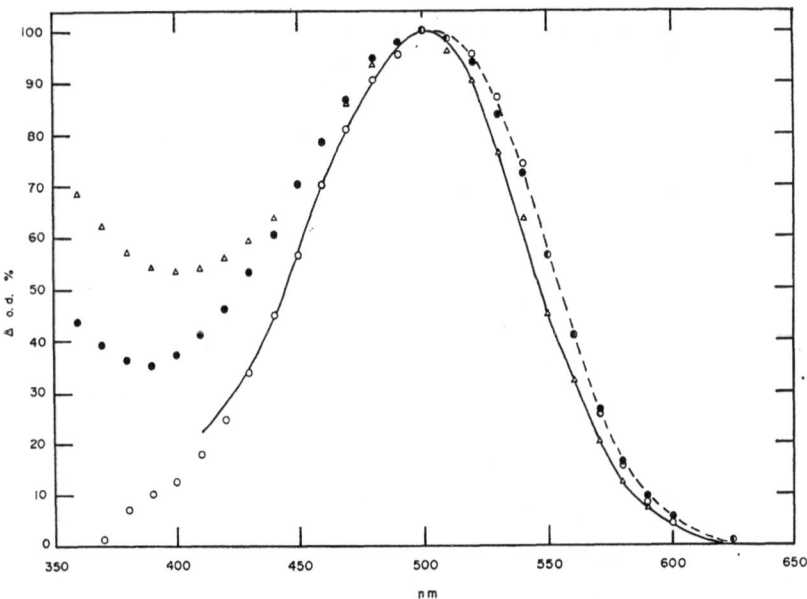

Fig. 1. Spectral absorbance curves and difference spectra for the intact retina and suspensions of outer segments of Rana pipiens. ●, absorbance curve (mean of 22) of the retina before bleach; ○, difference spectrum (mean of 22) obtained from the retina after bleach; △, mean absorbance curve of suspensions of outer segments before bleaching. Full line is the nomogram for frog rhodopsin in solution.

suspension of outer segments, the suspension was exopsed for 60 min to a bleaching light of 600 nm. The difference spectrum, resulting from this bleaching, indicated a maximum optical density loss at 512 ± 2 nm [Fig. 2, curve (a)], and a maximum density gain at 385 nm. Hydroxylamine was then added to the suspension and this produced a result such that the difference spectrum between the final absorbance, after adding hydroxylamine, and the initial absorbance of the suspension before bleaching had a λ max of 502 ± 1 nm [Fig. 2, curve (b)], with the maximum absorbance of the photoproducts displaced from 385 nm to about 370 nm, the position of retinal oxime.

The absorbance curve obtained from the isolated retina of the frog is shown in Fig. 1 (filled circles), each point being the mean obtained from experiments on

271

22 retinae. The curves were normalised by correcting the optical density at 650 nm to zero and bringing the maximum optical density in the region of 500 nm to 1.0. Each retina was bleached with 500 nm light for 90 sec and the absorbance again measured. The decay of the photoproducts of the visual pigment was followed until the absorbance of the retina became stable i.e. when all the transient photoproducts had been reduced, presumably to Vitamin A_1.

The mean difference spectrum (obtained from the 22 experiments), between the initial absorbance spectrum and the final absorbance of the retina after the

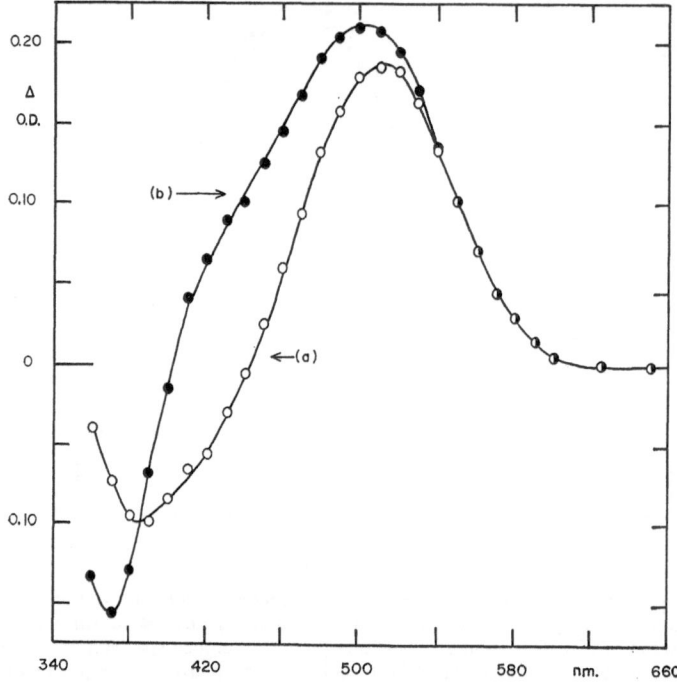

Fig. 2. Difference spectra obtained from bleaching a suspension of outer segments from Rana pipiens. Curve (a) without hydroxylamine; curve (b) after the addition of hydroxylamine to the bleached suspension.

bleach, was obtained (Fig. 1, open circles) and found to have a maximum change in optical density at 504–505 nm. Although the difference spectrum obtained from the isolated retina had a λ max only 2–3 nm further towards the red than the nomogram for frog rhodopsin, the right hand limb of the curve was displaced 4–5 nm towards the red and fitted relatively closely to the right hand limb of a nomogram for a pigment with a λ max at 506–507 nm.

In twelve of the 22 experiments the retinae were exposed to a second bleach with 500 nm light and the same procedure followed as before. The mean difference spectrum obtained from the second bleach is shown in Fig. 3 (filled circles) and compared with the mean difference spectrum derived from the first

272

bleach (Fig. 3, open circles). The second difference spectrum had a λ max at about 498 nm, but possessed a shape similar to that of the difference spectrum derived from the first bleach, in that the right hand limb of the second difference spectrum gave a reasonable fit to the right hand limb of the nomogram for a pigment absorbing maximally at 502–503 nm. The nomogram curves for $P502_1$ and $P498_1$ are shown in Fig. 3 for comparison.

To determine if the displacement of the right hand limb of the absorbance curve derived from the initial bleach was due to a second pigment absorbing

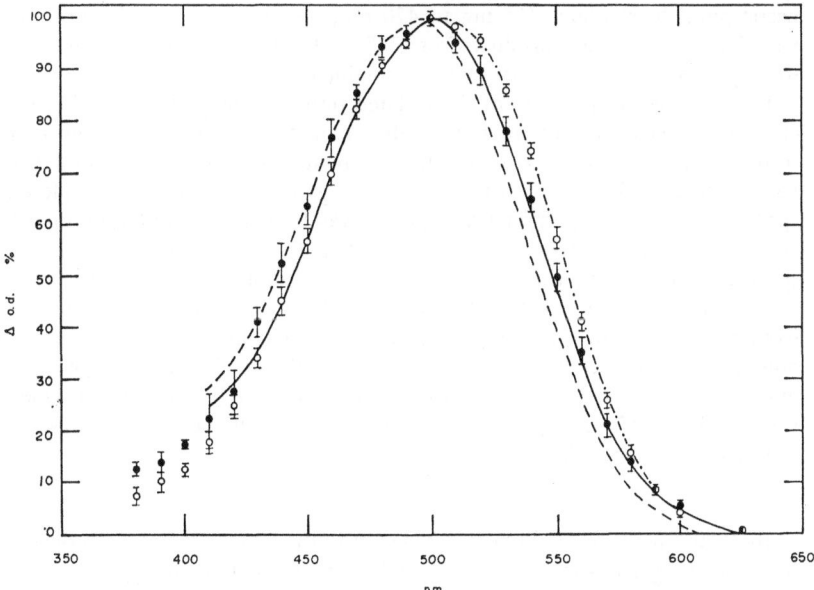

Fig. 3. Difference spectra from the first and second bleaches with 500 nm light of the isolated frog retina, with the maximum density losses brought to 100%. $\bigcirc$, difference spectrum from first bleach (mean of $22 \pm$ S.D.); $\bullet$, difference spectrum of second bleach (mean of $14 \pm$ S.D.). Solid line is the nomogram for $P502_1$ and dashed line is the nomogram with λ max of 498 nm.

further towards the red than the extractable $P502_1$, partial bleaching experiments were performed. However, as previously found in outer segment suspensions (BOWMAKER, 1972), only one photosensitive pigment could be detected. The difference between the difference spectra derived from the first and second bleaches of the retina was presumably due to the presence of isorhodopsin in the second difference spectrum, produced by isomerization of rhodopsin during the first bleach. This will be discussed later.

2. Gekko gekko

In extracts of gecko visual pigments, two visual pigments have been identified, $P521_1$ and $P478_1$ (CRESCITELLI, 1963). To study the effect of hydroxylamine on the difference spectrum of the $P521_1$, a suspension of gecko outer segments, free of hydroxylamine, was exposed for 60 min to light of 600 nm wavelength, which would not bleach the $P478_1$. This resulted in a decrease in the absorbance of the suspension above 450 nm, with a difference spectrum (Fig. 4B, triangles) having a λ max at 521 $\pm$ 1 nm, the same as that obtained from extracts (CRESCITELLI 1963). The photoproducts absorbed maximally at about 385 nm. Hydroxylamine was then added to the bleached suspension resulting in a change in absorbance from which a second difference spectrum was obtained. The second difference spectrum showed that, although hydroxylamine had the effect of shifting the isobestic point from about 455 nm to 420 nm, and of changing the maximum absorbance of the photoproducts from 385 nm to about 370 nm, it did not affect the λ max of the photopigment which remained at 521 nm.

The absorbance spectrum of the isolated retina of the gecko (Fig. 4A, filled circles) consisted of a broad peak with a maximum at about 500 nm and a secondary peak at about 410–420 nm, which was presumably due to the Soret band of haemoglobin. As with the outer segments, to obtain the difference spectrum of the $P521_1$, the isolated retina was bleached with 660 nm light for 10 min and the absorbance again measured (Fig. 4A, open circles). The difference spectrum derived from the bleach had a λ max of about 524–525 nm (mean of 7 experiments), but with the right hand limb of the curve displaced still further from the nomogram for $P521_1$ (Fig. 4B), so that it fitted more closely to the nomogram with a maximum absorbance at 528–529 nm. The product of bleaching absorbed maximally at about 390 nm, the position of retinal, and no evidence was noted either for any photoproducts other than retinal or for the conversion of retinal to Vitamin A_1.

DISCUSSION

In the experiments reported here, a red shift in the difference spectrum obtained from outer segment suspensions as compared with the difference spectra derived from extracts of the visual pigments was observed only in the frog. In Rana pipiens the 10 nm displacement to longer wavelengths of the difference spectrum derived from suspensions of outer segments was completely removed with the addition of hydroxylamine. Thus, as DARTNALL (1961) suggested, the red shift is due to photoproducts which, in suspensions, behave differently from those in solution. These photoproducts can be removed by hydroxylamine so that the difference spectra obtained from extracts and suspensions are identical.

In Gekko gekko no red shift was found in the difference spectrum obtained from outer segment suspensions, even though hydroxylamine had the effect of converting the photoproducts of retinal oxime. The lack of any shift to longer wavelengths in the suspensions is presumably due to the unusual visual pigment found in Gekko gekko, which, although it is a retinal based pigment, absorbs maximally at 521 nm. The photoproducts absorbing maximally at 385 nm would, therefore, have less effect on the difference spectrum of a 521 nm visual pigment than on a 502 nm visual pigment.

In the intact retina of Rana pipiens a displacement towards the red from the absorbance of the visual pigment in solution was seen in both the absorbance

274

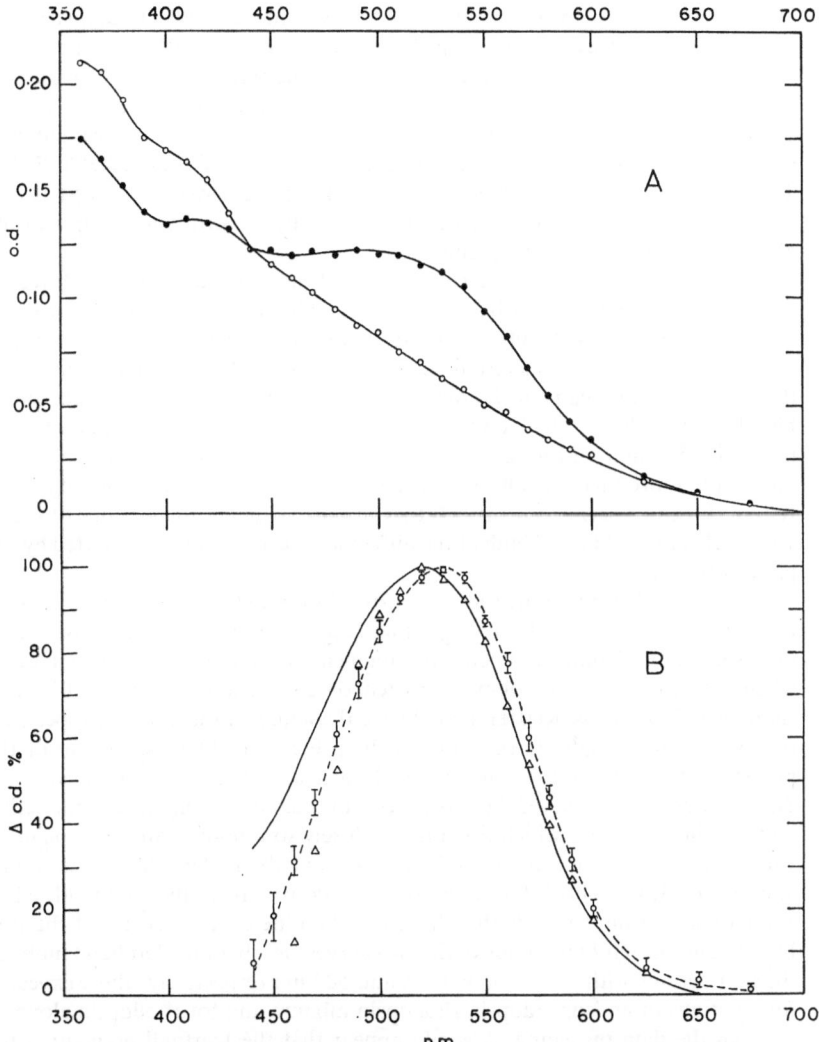

Fig. 4. Spectral absorbance curves and difference spectrum obtained from the isolated retina of Gekko gekko. A: Absorbance curves of the isolated retina; ●, before bleaching; ○, after bleaching with 660 nm light for 10 min. B: Difference spectrum derived from 660 nm bleach, with maximum density loss brought to 100%. ○, difference spectrum from the intact retina (mean of $7 \pm$ S.D.); △, mean difference spectrum from outer segment suspensions. Full line is the nomogram for P521$_1$.

spectrum and in the difference spectrum derived from a bleaching of the visual pigment in the intact retina. The displacement of the two curves from the Dartnall nomogram for frog rhodopsin $P502_1$ was identical which suggested that the displacement was not due to photoproducts which absorbed in the visible region of the spectrum and which remained in the retina, as these would have displaced the difference spectrum, but not the absorbance spectrum. Partial bleaching of the retina also demonstrated that the red shift was not caused by a second pigment absorbing further towards the red than the extractable $P502_1$. The absence of a second pigment is not surprising as LIEBMAN & ENTINE (1968) calculated that the red cones of the frog (with a $P575_1$) probably comprise only about 1 % of the total visual pigment.

In Gekko gekko the absorbance spectrum of the isolated retina was distorted primarily by the large Soret band of haemoglobin and so could not be used to determine whether a red shift, similar to that found in the frog, occurred in this species. The absorbance spectrum was also complicated by the small amount of the blue absorbing pigment. However, the difference spectrum obtained after a bleach with red light, which only affected the $P521_1$, did show a displacement of the right hand limb of the spectrum towards the red. It is unlikely that this was due to photoproducts as, although it appeared that retinal was not reduced to retinol, it can be seen from Fig. 4B that in outer segment suspensions of gecko visual cells, the right hand limb of the difference spectrum was not affected by the photoproducts.

A similar red displacement also occurred in the difference spectrum derived from the second bleach of the frog retina (Fig. 3). BRIDGES (1962) showed that in suspensions of outer segments the pigment remaining after a first bleach, when extracted with digitonin, consisted of 80 % rhodopsin and 20 % iso-rhodopsin. DONNER & REUTER (1969) gave the λ max of the difference spectrum obtained from a digitonin solution (in the presence of hydroxylamine) of the pigment left in the retina after a first bleach as 498–500 nm. However, the difference spectrum derived from the second bleach of the pigment in the retina had a right hand limb which fitted more closely to a nomogram for a pigment with a λ max of 502 nm, though it had a λ max at about 499–500 nm. As can be seen in Fig. 3, the whole difference spectrum derived from the second bleach is shifted about 5 nm towards the blue from the difference spectrum of the first bleach, and the left hand limbs of the two curves closely fit the left hand limbs of the nomograms with λ max of 498 nm and 502 nm respectively, those expected for solutions of an isorhodopsin-rhodopsin mixture and for rhodopsin alone.

From the data presented, it would appear that the Dartnall nomogram for visual pigments in solution, which can also be applied to suspensions of the outer segments of the visual cells, may not be applicable to the absorbance of the pigment in the intact retina and, therefore, that a direct comparison of scotopic spectral sensitivities with the absorbance of visual pigments in solution may not be justified when precise comparisons are required. The scotopic spectral sensitivity of the frog, as measured by GRANIT (see DARTNALL, 1953, Fig. 2), is indeed displaced towards the red from the absorbance of frog rhodopsin in solution and in Fig. 5 the spectral sensitivity data of GRANIT are compared with

276

the nomogram for $P502_1$ and with the difference curve of the visual pigment as measured in the intact retina. In the gecko a spectral sensitivity has been determined by using the fast component of the ERG (CRESCITELLI, 1965), and this had a λ max of about 520 nm, which could be correlated with the extractable $P521_1$, but the shape of the sensitivity curve does not resemble closely either the absorbance of the visual pigment in solution or in the intact retina. This is due, presumably, to the difficulty in isolating the spectral sensitivity of the $P521_1$ from that of the blue absorbing pigment.

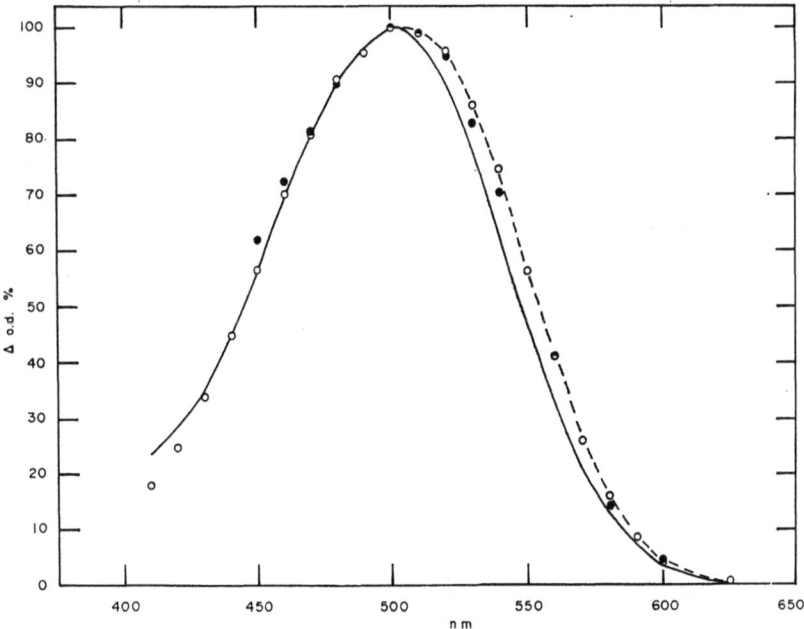

Fig. 5. Comparison of the scotopic spectral sensititivy of the frog with the difference spectrum of frog rhodospin in the intact retina. ○, difference spectrum of rhodopsin in the intact retina; ●, scotopic spectral sensitivity of the frog from Granit (see Dartnall, 1953); full line is the nomogram for $P502_1$.

The best documented scotopic spectral sensitivity is that of the human and it is determined to have a λ max of 497 nm (CRAWFORD, 1949). The λ max of the difference spectrum of extracts of human rhodopsin was first accurately determined by CRESCITELLI & DARTNALL (1953) and was found to be 497 $\pm$ 2 nm, in excellent agreement with the scotopic senstivity data. However, hydroxylamine was not used in this study. Later, WALD & BROWN (1958) measured the difference spectrum of human rhodopsin both in solution and in a sucrose suspension of outer segments. In the presence of hydroxylamine the λ max of the difference spectrum in solution was found to be 493 nm and in the suspension of outer segments to be at 500 nm. WALD & BROWN (1958) suggested that the 7 nm difference between the two results was an example of Kundt's rule, but they did

277

not test for the homogeneity of their suspension and there is the possibility of cone visual pigments causing the 7 nm displacement. The λ max of 493 nm for human rhodopsin in solution has since been confirmed by CRESCITELLI (personal communication).

If the similarity between the absorbance curve of the visual pigment, as measured in the intact retina of the frog, and the scotopic spectral sensitivity of the frog is extrapolated to human rhodopsin, the apparent discrepancy of 4 nm

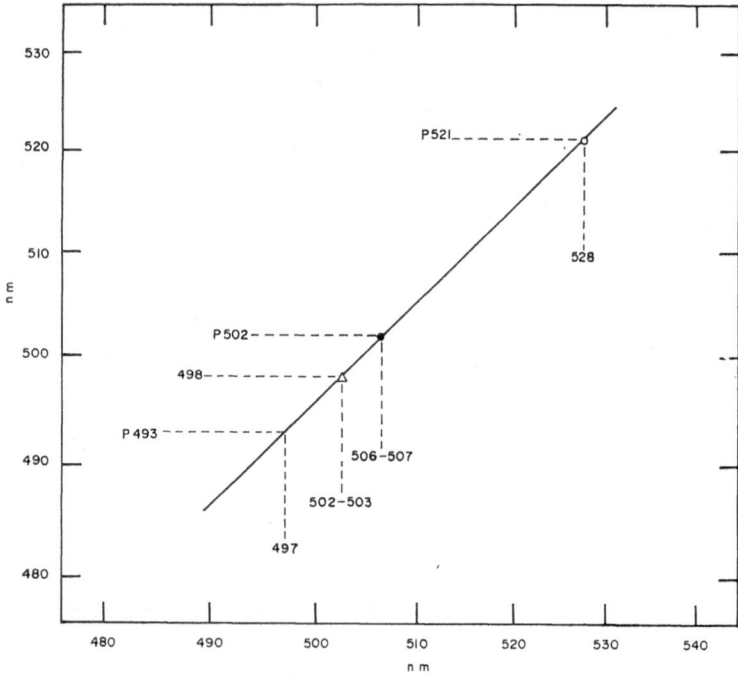

Fig. 6. Suggested relationship between the absorbance of visual pigments in solution and the absorbance of the pigments in the intact retina. $\bigcirc$, Gekko gekko with P521$_1$; $\bullet$, Rana pipiens with P502$_1$ and $\triangle$, rhodopsin-isorhodopsin mixture in Rana pipiens with a λ max in solution of 498 nm. Curve is extrapolated to show the relationship for human rhodopsin P493$_1$. Ordinate, λ max for visual pigments in solution; abscissa, λ max indicated by the right hand limb of the difference spectra of visual pigments in the intact retina, based on the Dartnall nomogram.

between 493 and 497 nm can be explained by suggesting that the absorbance spectrum for human rhodopsin in the intact retina has a right hand limb which fits more closely to a nomogram for a 497 nm pigment and not to a 493 nm nomogram as measured for the pigment in digitonin solution. In fact, from Fig. 6, in which the absorbance curves for visual pigments in solution and in the retina are compared, it could be predicted that there would be a 4 nm difference between the absorbance in solution and in the intact retina of an extractable P493$_1$.

278

Unfortunately, due to the difficulty in obtaining sufficient material, an analysis of the human retina has so far not proved practical. Fig. 6 also predicts that for pigments absorbing further into the red, the difference between the absorbance of the pigment in solution and in the intact retina will be greater than for pigments absorbing in the blue.

The cause of the red shift in the right hand limb of the absorbance curve of the visual pigment in the intact retina compared with the absorbance of the pigment in solution is not apparent. If it is an example of Kundt's rule, it is surprising that in suspensions of the outer segments the difference spectrum of the visual pigment is identical with the difference spectrum obtained from solutions, although perhaps this is not the case with human outer segments (WALD & BROWN, 1958). It would seem more likely that the difference in spectral absorbance is due to the orientation of the visual pigment within the hydrophobic environment of the outer segment disc membranes. In outer segment suspensions the outer segments tend to break up into small stacks of discs and it would not be surprising if the membrane structure was affected by the sucrose medium. In the isolated retina the outer segments remain intact and the environment of the disc membranes will presumably resemble more closely the physiological conditions of the living eye. The enigma of the suspensions of human outer segments (WALD & BROWN, 1958) must still remain, but it is possible that this is a characteristic of mammalian outer segments, although this would place the human visual pigment in a singularly isolated position.

REFERENCES

ARDEN, G. B. Light-sensitive pigment in the visual cells of the frog. *J. Physiol. Lond.* 123:377–385 (1954).

BARER, R. & SIDMAN, R. L. The absorbance spectrum of rhodopsin in solution and in intact rods. *J. Physiol. Lond.* 129:60P (1955).

BAUMANN, C. Sephurpurbleichung und Stabchenfunktion in der isolierten Froschnetzhaut. I. Die Sehpurpurbleichung. *Pflugers Arch. ges. Physiol.* 298:44–60 (1967).

BOWMAKER, J. K. Kundt's rule: the spectral absorbance of visual pigments in situ and in solution. *Vision Res.* 12:529–548 (1972).

BRIDGES, C. D. B. Studies on the flash-photolysis of visual pigments. IV. Dark reactions following the flash-irradiation of frog rhodopsin in suspensions of isolated photoreceptors. *Vision Res.* 2:215–232 (1962).

CRAWFORD, B. H. The scotopic visibility function. *Proc. phys. Soc. Lond.* B. 62:321–334 (1949).

CRESCITELLI, F. The photosensitive retinal pigment system of Gekko gekko. *J. gen. Physiol.* 47:33–52 (1963).

CRESCITELLI, F. The spectral sensitivity and visual pigment content of the retina of Gekko gekko. In: Ciba Foundation Symp. Color Vision. Physiology and Exper. Psychol. London: Churchill. (1965).

CRESCITELLI, F. & DARTNALL, H. J. A. Human visual purple. *Nature, Lond.* 172:195–200 (1953).

DARTNALL, H. J. A. The interpretation of spectral sensitivity curves. *Br. med. Bull.* 9:24–30 (1953).

DARTNALL, H. J. A. The visual pigments. Methuen, London; John Wiley, New York. (1957).

DARTNALL, H. J. A. On the question of the narrow-band pigment of the frog retina. *J. Physiol. Lond.* 45:630–640 (1959).

DARTNALL, H. J. A. Visual pigments before and after extraction from visual cells. *Proc. R. Soc.* B, 154:250–266 (1961).

DOBROWOLSKI, J. A., JOHNSON, B. K. & TANSLEY, KATHERINE. The spectral absorption of the photopigment of Xenopus laevis measured in single rods. *J. Physiol. Lond.* 130:533–542 (1955).

DONNER, K. O & REUTER, T. The photoproducts of rhodopsin in the isolated retina of the frog. *Vision Res.* 9:*815–847* (1969).

GRANIT, R. Sensory mechanisms of the retina. Oxford University Press, London (1947).

LIEBMAN, P. A. & ENTINE, G. Visual pigments of the frog and tadpole (Rana pipiens). *Vision Res.* 8:*761–765* (1968).

RUSHTON, W. A. H. The difference spectrum and the photosensitivity of rhodopsin in the living human eye. *J. Physiol. Lond.* 134:*11–29* (1956).

WALD, G. & BROWN, P. K. Human rhodopsin. *Science N.Y.* 127:*222–226* (1958).

WALD, G., BROWN, P. K. & GIBBONS. I. R. The problem of visual excitation. *J. opt. Soc. Am.* 53: *20–35* (1963).

ANALYSIS OF THE VISUAL RESPONSE OF THE FLY SARCOPHAGA BULLATA DURING PUPAL DEVELOPMENT*

ELLIS R. LOEW**

(Los Angeles)

INTRODUCTION

One of the goals of visual electrophysiology is the resolution of the complex visual response into its various components and the assignment of these components to specific sites in the visual system. By observing the visual response present at different stages in the development of an organism, it is possible to identify those components which, when combined, yield the waveform of the adult response. It is also possible to assign these components to specific neuronal regions based on correlations between structural differentiation and response waveform changes.

The dissection of the insect visual response into its basic components using developmental studies has been limited to only a few species. AUTRUM & GALLWITZ (1951) and AUTRUM (1958) followed the development of the visual response throughout the larval and nymphal instars of the dragonfly Aeschna cyanea. It was found that the initial response was cornea-negative and could be identified with the receptor cell layer. The positivity appearing later in development was associated with the developing ganglionic layers. The assignment of these components to the neuronal layers mentioned had been previously made by many workers studying other species (see FOUCHARD & CARRICABURU, 1972), but these studies all relied upon the adult form of the insect. AUTRUM also found a correlation between the changes in the larval response and the developmental migration of the ganglionic layers toward the receptor cell layer. EGUCHI, NAKA, & KUWABARA (1962) found that the first recordable response during pupal development of the silkworm, Bombyx mori, was a cornea-negative one. This response appeared during the period of retinular microtubule differentiation. These form the rhabdome in the later pupal and adult stages. The authors also mention another negative wave in the adult response which is not identifiable with the receptor cells, however no data were presented indicating when this potential appeared during pupal development. Using the butterfly Heliconus sarae, SWIHART (1967) followed the development of the visual response during pupation and the immediate post-emergent period. The first response found was cornea-negative as in the other studies mentioned. It was also found that a sustained negative wave appeared two hours to 20 minutes before emergence, which was interpreted as an indication of neuronal organization. Changes in the

* This investigation was aided by grant B-1509 from the Division of Research Grants and Fellowships, National Institutes of Health, U.S. Public Health Service.
** From the Department of Biology, University of California, Los Angeles, California, U.S.A.

281

response waveform and spectral sensitivity were also seen during the first 24 hours after emergence indicating continued neuronal changes in the young adult. Similar results were obtained for the beetle, *Tenebrio molitor*, by YINON & AUERBACH (1969).

Specific developmental mutants of *Drosophila* have also been used to dissect the normal adult response. HOTTA & BENZER (1970) and HEISENBERG (1971) found that mutants showing morphological changes in the lamina ganglionaris lacked the fast, positive components of the visual response leaving only a mono-phasic negative wave which they assigned to the normal receptor cell layer.

The present study will rely heavily upon data obtained using CO_2 anesthesia for removal of all but the receptor component from the visual response. LEUT-SCHER-HAZELHOFF & KUIPER (1964) used CO_2 to isolate a component of the *Calliphora* visual response which they interpreted as receptor in origin based upon waveform and electrode advancement data. The waveform seen when their electrodes were recording across the optic ganglion disappeared within 30 seconds after CO_2 administration, while the waveform seen across the receptor cell layer was unaffected. The waveform recorded across the lamina ganglionaris was also altered by CO_2, leaving a mirror image of the receptor response. The origin of their receptor response was at the base of the receptor cells in the region of the basement membrane. WOLBARSHT, WAGNER, & BODENSTEIN (1966) found that treatment of transplanted compound eyes of *Periplaneta*, which lacked all but the receptor cell layer, with CO_2 caused no change in the waveform of the response. They suggested a synaptic mechanism for CO_2 action. In both of these studies, the response remaining after CO_2 treatment was a monophasic, negative one.

While all of the above studies assign a single negative component of the mass visual response to the receptor cell layer, there appears to be little consistent information concerning the number, polarity, and time of appearance of the other components. The purpose of the present study was to follow the development of the visual response during pupation of a dipteran and to determine the number and polarity of the various components as they appeared.

MATERIALS AND METHODS

Flesh-flies, *Sarcophaga bullata*, were raised in the laboratory following the technique of DORMAN, HALE & HOSKINS (1938). The pupa were kept on a 12/12 light-dark diurnal cycle at 22°C. At various times after the start of pupation, pupae were removed from the stock containers and partially inserted into the end of a glass tube and held with wax. A circumferential cut was made in the exposed anterior end of the puparium and the cap removed, exposing the cephalic region. Care was taken to avoid rupture of the pupal membrane during this operation. Two incisions were then made in the pupal membrane exposing the developing compound eyes. One of the eyes, which served for the indifferent lead, was blackened with several coats of enamel paint as were the three developing ocelli. The glass tube was fixed to a moveable platform and placed in the shielded, light-proof recording chamber so that the unpainted eye was at the focus of a

282

condensing lens system present within the chamber. The same basic procedures were used for the adult insect.

The recording chamber consisted of a double-walled copper enclosure mounted on an optical bench. Water circulating between the walls of the enclosure kept the temperature within the chamber at 22°C. A glass window allowed the entry of the stimulating flash while two other openings allowed the atmosphere within the chamber to be controlled experimentally.

Photic stimulation was provided by a Grass PS-2 xenon flashlamp set at its highest intensity. This is referred to as unit intensity and is equivalent to 9×10^5 horizontal candle power as deduced from the figures given by GRASS. Using a photodiode, it was found that 90% of the flash energy was radiated within 10 μsec. The intensity was attenuated with Corning neutral density filters. The flash was directed onto the surface of the compound eye by a system of condensing lenses. To provide a uniform intensity across the surface of the eye, a diffusing screen was placed between the last condensing element and the eye.

The mass visual response was recorded using stainless-steel electrodes having a tip diameter of 10–20 μm. Using a micromanipulator, the recording electrode was advanced into the experimental eye to a depth of approximately 150 μm, which would place the electrode tip near the middle of the receptor cell layer (TRUJILLO-CENOZ & MELAMED, 1966). The indifferent electrode was inserted into the blackened eye which was further shielded from the light by a piece of metal foil. Differential preamplification was provided by a Kiethley 103 AC preamplifier with a band-pass of 0.1 Hz to 30,000 Hz. The amplified signal was displayed on the upper beam of a Tektronix 502 dual-beam oscilloscope and recorded on film for later study. The stimulus marker, provided by a photodiode, and the time marks were displayed on the lower beam.

RESULTS

For ease of presentation, the results will be divided into sections corresponding to stages of pupal development. The four stages are: I, days 1–5; II, days 5–6; III, days 6–9; and IV, days 9–12. An adult section will also be included.

ADULT

A. *Morphology*

The morphology of the adult compound eye and related structures has been previously described (TRUJILLO-CENOZ & MELAMED, 1966; MAZOKHIN-PORSHNYAKOV, 1969).

B. *Electrical Response*

The response of the dark adapted eye to a brief flash of light can be seen in Fig. 1. It consists of a series of waves starting with a fast positive transient which can, by decreasing the intensity, be associated with a positive component. Attenuation of the light flash with a density 1 filter removes a late positive wave and reveals small wavelets on the rising phase of the first negative wave. Further attenuation of the light leads to a loss of the first negative wave followed by the second

283

negative wave. At very low intensities, only a positive wave is present. It can also be seen in Fig. 1 that decreasing the intensity results in an increased latency of the response.

The response of the eye to a flash of unit intensity at various times after administration of CO_2 is shown in Fig. 2. It can be seen that by 30 seconds after exposure, the response has simplified to a fast positive transient followed by a single negative wave. By 120 seconds the positive spike is gone, leaving only the negative wave. No further change occurred until 5 minutes after exposure, at

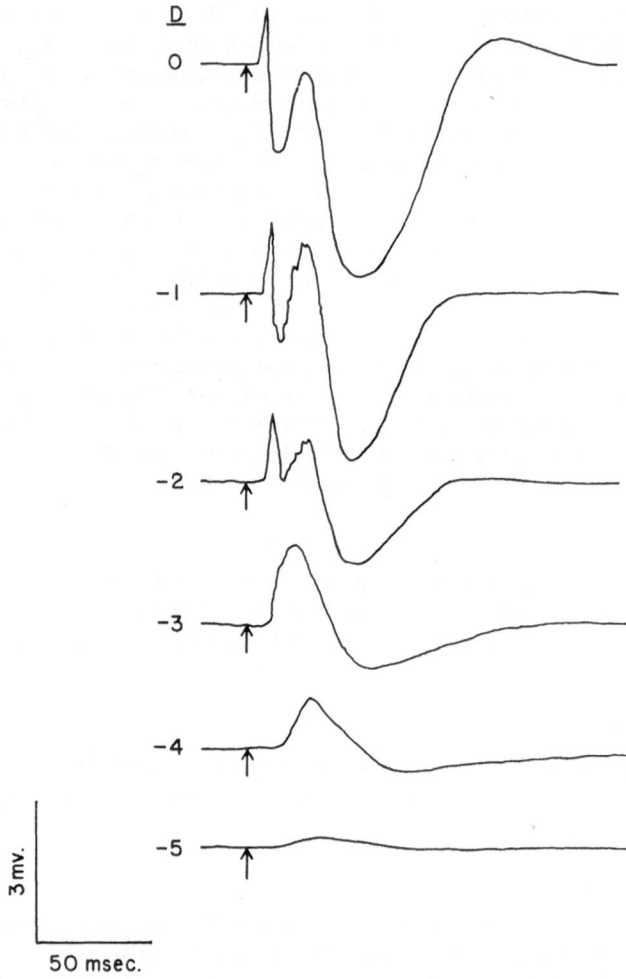

Fig. 1. The visual response of the dark-adapted, adult eye to decreasing flash intensities. The numbers to the left of the tracings indicate the neutral density filter used for attenuation. As with the other figures, a downward deflection indicates corneal negativity.

284

which time the negative wave started to decrease in amplitude. It should be noted that the latency of the response did not change during the experiment.

STAGE I

A. *Morphology*

During this stage the animal was in a semi-fluid state and was incased in a tough, fibrous, opaque pupal membrane containing a relatively large volume of moulting fluid. By day 3 one could discern cephalization by the appearance of bulges on the lateral surfaces of the anterior end of the pupal mass. On day 4 the differentiation of the compound eyes had reached the point where careful examination revealed the faceted nature of the surface. On the 5th day the eye was somewhat firmer than before, but without pigmentation.

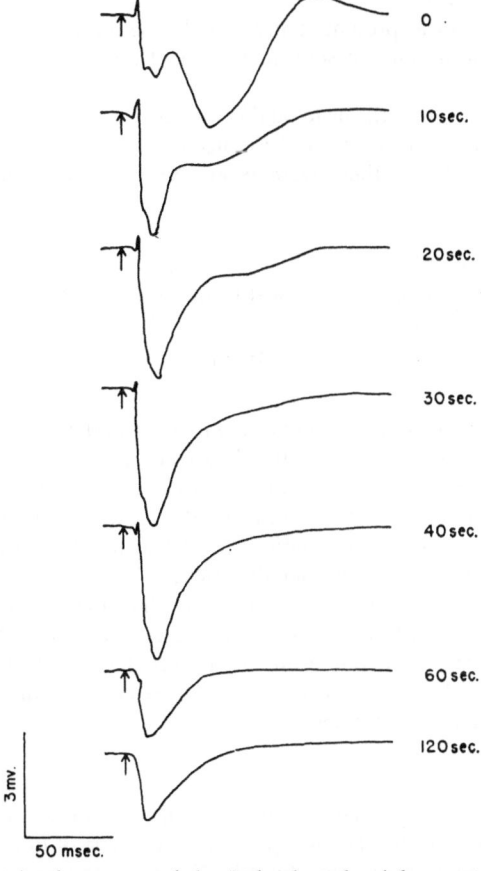

Fig. 2. The visual response of the dark-adapted, adult eye at various times after the introduction of CO_2 gas into the recording chamber.

An incision made in the lateral margin of the eye caused milky-white fluid to escape from the head. Using Giemsa stain, it could be seen to contain many cells both free and in groups. No solid masses could be found in the cephalic contents.

B. *Electrical Response*

Stimulation of 21 pupae in this stage of development failed to elicit any response, even at the highest intensities available.

STAGE II

A. *Morphology*

There was evidence, late on the 5th day, of pigment deposition in the compound eyes. At first this was noticeable as a light orange hue present under oblique illumination with white light. This color intensified over the next two days, until it was a deep orange.

No pseudopupil was present at any time during this period, even though there was a significant amount of screening pigment and the dioptric apparatus was present.

An incision made into the head on the 6th day produced only clear hemolymph with very few free cells. Section of the head revealed that some neural organization had occurred as there were several clear white masses present in the cephalic cavity.

B. *Electrical Response*

As in the previous stage, no electrical response was recorded from 18 pupae in this stage of development.

STAGE III

A. *Morphology*

Early in this stage the development of the pseudopupil was observed. It was first seen as a darkening of the ommatidial surface under illumination striking the eye from the same direction as that used for observation. The depth of the dark area appeared to increase until, on the 9th day, it was easily seen with only low level illumination. The pseudopupil appeared to involve no more than 8 ommatidia when viewed from any one direction.

Other changes in the pupa were also noted. The pupal membrane had become less fibrous and almost transparent. The volume of moulting fluid had also decreased. Opening of the puparium late in this stage resulted in movements of the pupa typical of the flexions of the thorax seen at the time of eclosion. No filling of the ptilinum was noted.

B. *Electrical Response*.

It was during this stage that the first electrical response was recorded. This appeared early on the 7th day as a pure negative wave of low amplitude, which increased in strength during the day. Fig. 3A shows this response, which had a minimum latency of 8 msec. Decreasing the intensity brought the response to

286

the baseline with no positivity noted (Fig. 3B). CO_2 treatment of 6 pupae having this response caused no change in the waveform of the response.

On the 8th day, oscillations appeared in the visual response. They were riding on the negative wave and were always preceded by a fast positive transient (Fig. 3C). These oscillations had a frequency of 150 Hz with a pulse train duration of 50–100 msec. Decreasing the intensity removed the oscillations leaving a positive wave. (Fig. 3D). Treatment of 10 pupae with CO_2 removed the oscillations and the positive transient leaving only a negative wave identical with that recorded on the previous day.

Early on the 9th day the amplitude of the negative wave decreased almost to the baseline, while the oscillations appeared to be almost unaffected (Fig. 3E). It was also found that the positivity produced by an intensity decrease was also lower in amplitude than that seen on the 8th day at the same intensity (Fig. 3F).

Late on the 9th day an increase in the negative wave and oscillation amplitudes was seen (Fig. 3G). The amplitude of the low intensity response also increased (Fig. 3H).

STAGE IV

A. *Morphology*

There were no great changes in the gross morphology of the compound eyes during this stage.

The rest of the pupa was now pigmented, with definite stripes present on the thorax. The pupal membrane was very thin and fragile. The moulting fluid was absent during the last day of this stage.

B. *Electrical Response*

Very early on the 10th day a second negative wave became evident in the visual response, appearing after both the initial negative wave and the oscillations (Fig. 3I). It increased in amplitude during the day, until it was the same amplitude as the initial negative wave. Decreasing the intensity caused a decrease in the second negative component, but at a lower rate than the initial negative wave (Fig. 3J). CO_2 treatment at this stage resulted in a loss of the late negativity, followed by the oscillations and positive transient leaving only a pure negative wave.

On the 11th day the amplitude of the response showed a marked increase, but no new components were noted (Figs. 3K and 3L). The amplitude of the response continued to increase until, by the middle of the 12th day, it was the same as the adult. Accompanying this increase was the appearance of a late positive wave and the loss of the oscillations which were so prominent in the day 11 response (Figs. 3M and 3N). The effect of CO_2 on the day 12 response was the same as that in the adult (see Fig. 2).

DISCUSSION

The results may be interpreted as showing the development of four separate components during pupation (Fig. 4). These correspond to the three proposed by FOUCHARD & CARRICABURU (1972), a rapid negative (NR), a slow negative (NS), and a positive (P); with the additional finding of a late positive potential (PL).

287

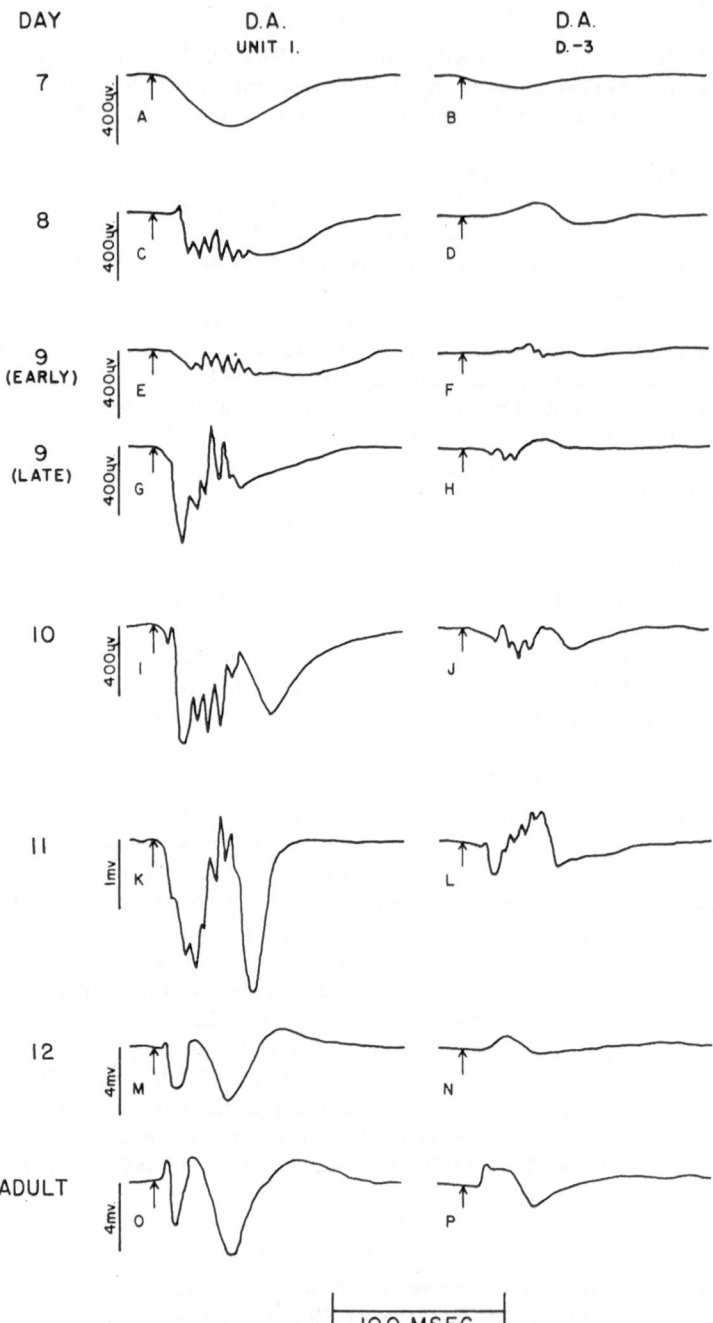

Fig. 3. The visual responses of pupae at different stages of development to a flash of unit intensity and low intensity light.

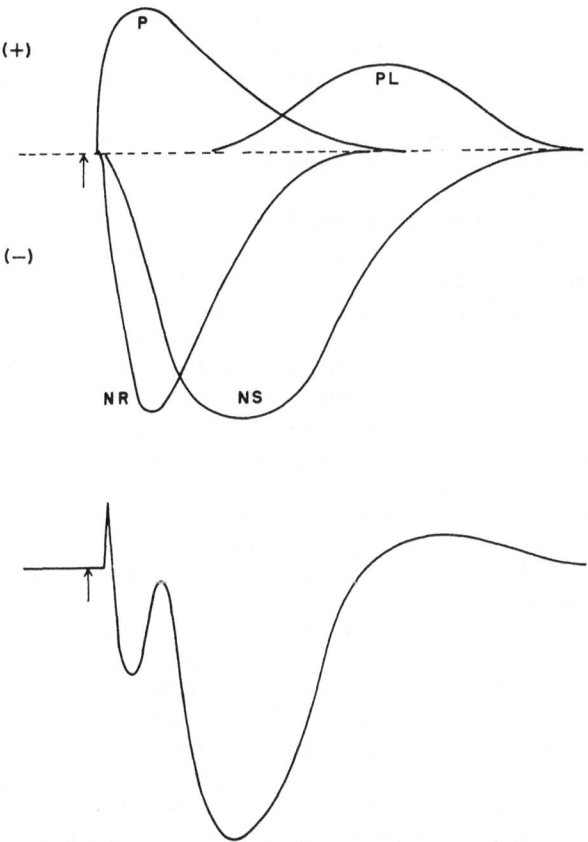

Fig. 4. The upper curves represent the four proposed components developing during pupation and present in the adult, while the lower curve represents the sum of the various components.

It should be mentioned that FOUCHARD & CARRICABURU suggested three components as a minimum number, leaving the possibility open for additional ones in specific cases.

The first response recorded, as in the other developmental studies mentioned, was cornea-negative and probably the receptor component, corresponding to the NR of FOUCHARD & CARRICABURU. Several lines of evidence support the contention that the NR is a receptor potential. Its waveform is not affected by CO_2 treatment which has been shown to be the case for the receptor potential (LEUTSCHER-HAZELHOFF & KUIPER, 1964; WOLBARSHT, WAGNER & BODENSTEIN, 1966). It is also found to be identical in waveform with the receptor potential isolated from adult *Sarcophaga* by selective recording techniques (MOTE, 1968), and from other insect species using drugs and selective recordings (BERNHARD, 1942; AUTRUM, 1958; FOUCHARD & CARRICABURU, 1970; CARRICABURU,

289

1971; HEISENBERG, 1971). Its appearance at a stage in development marked by the formation of the pseudopupil is suggestive of a receptor origin. EGUCHI, NAKA & KUWABARA (1962) failed to record any response before the differentiation of the rhabdome. The presence of a rhabdome is a prerequisite for the formation of the pseudopupil since receptor degeneration mutants of *Drosophila*, which lose the rhabdome soon after formation, also lose the pseudopupil (HOTTA & BENZER, 1970).

A positive component appears next during pupal development as evidenced by the fast positive transient seen preceding the already present negative wave (Fig. 3C). This same transient can be seen in the adult response (Fig. 1) and has been associated with a positive process by HASSENSTEIN (1957).

Isolation of this positive component was accomplished, as in the adult, by decreasing the intensity of the stimulating flash. The resulting positive wave has the form of the proposed P of FOUCHARD & CARRICABURU (1972). It also has the same waveform as the potential recorded across the lamina ganglionaris in adult *Sarcophaga* (MOTE, 1968) and *Drosophila* (HEISENBERG, 1971). This would suggest a laminar origin for the pupal response as well. Indeed, the response first appears at a time when definite neural masses are present in the optic hemispheres, one of which is adjacent to the pupal basement membrane as is the lamina ganglionaris in the adult (TRUJILLO-CENOZ & MELAMED, 1966). That it is not of receptor origin can be shown by its sensitivity to CO_2.

The second negative component, appearing on the 10th day and increasing in amplitude over the next two, has properties similar to the NS of FOUCHARD & CARRICABURU (1972). It is more sensitive to CO_2 than the NR or the P and decreases at a lower rate than the NR with decreasing intensity.

The origin of this potential is probably ganglionic as evidenced by its CO_2 sensitivity. It must originate in layers proximal to the lamina ganglionaris as no evidence of slow negativity has been found in this layer (MOTE, 1968; HEISENBERG, 1971). It is possible that this NS component is the same slow negative potential mentioned by EGUCHI, NAKA & KUWABARA (1962) in the adult silkmoth.

The positive potential (PL), seen developing late in pupation, was not described by HASSENSTEIN (1957) or MOTE (1968) even though it was present in the adult response (Fig. 3M and 3O). It is possible that its occurrence in the present study was due to the high stimulus intensity used, as it was noted that this component disappeared with very small decreases in stimulus intensity (Fig. 1).

The classification of the PL as a separate component from the P is based on the evidence that, while a small intensity decrease removes the late positivity, it does not alter the waveform of the other components (Fig. 1). If the P had been responsible for the late positivity, its width and/or amplitude would have had to substantially change with a small decrease in intensity. This would surely have affected the slopes and latencies of the negative waves which is not seen. There is also some evidence that the PL has a greater CO_2 sensitivity than the P (Fig. 2). While changes in the proposed shapes of the NR, P, and NS components could conceivably account for the late positivity, a separate component best fits the data obtained in the present study.

290

As yet undiscussed are the rapid oscillations present in the pupal response from the 8th day until early in the 12th (Fig. 3). While rhythmic activity as been extensively studied in the insect compound eye starting with the early work of ADRIAN (1937) and CRESCITELLI & JAHN (1939, 1940, 1942), no oscillations with the frequency of those in the pupa have been described. While there is some evidence of rapid oscillations in the response of adult *Lucilia sericata* (FOUCHARD & CARRICABURU, 1970), these are not discussed.

It is possible that these oscillations arise from a negative feedback loop operating over short distances as has been proposed for the mammalian ERG wavelets by Kozak (1971). In fact, the pupal oscillations show a striking similarity to the mammalian wavelets in both frequency and time of appearance in the response. This suggests a similar generating mechanism for both phenomena. It was proposed by KOZAK (1971) that the mammalian wavelets were associated with lateral inhibitory processes affecting the bipolar cell membrane by way of horizontal cell synapses. The delays and distances involved satisfy the boundary conditions required for feedback loop oscillation at the observed frequency (RATLIFF, KNIGHT & GRAHAM. 1969). The same types of interactions hypothesized for the outer plexiform layer in vertebrates have been associated with the lamina ganglionaris of dipterans, especially lateral inhibitory interactions (MAZOHKIN-PORSHNYAKOV, 1969). The pupal oscillations are seen to be associated with the lamina since they appear at a time in development when only this and the receptor layer are active, and they disappear at the same time as the P component after CO_2 treatment. The possibility of some receptor cell-laminar feedback loop being responsible for the oscillations cannot, however, be eliminated. The reason for the disappearance of the oscillations before emergence is unclear, but it may involve some damping applied to the resonating system by other neural mechanisms. This is suggested by the finding that small wavelets can be seen in some of the adult records at low intensities (density 1 and 2) indicating that the feedback loops have not degenerated before emergence (Fig. 1).

This study differs greatly from the other developmental studies in that four separate components were deduced as were oscillations in the visual response. While it is possible that the differences observed are due to technique, it is more probable that they represent basic differences between the animals studied. No evidence was found in this study for any post-emergent alterations of the visual response as seen by SWIHART (1967) and YINON & AUERBACH (1969). This may well be due to the different post-emergent behavior of the fly which would make immediate, total visual function upon emergence a great advantage.

ACKNOWLEDGEMENT

I am indebted to PROFESSOR F. CRESCITELLI for his support and invaluable aid during the course of this investigation, and for reading the preliminary draft of this manuscript.

REFERENCES

ADRIAN, E. D. Synchronized reactions in the optic ganglion of *Dytiscus*. *J. Physiol.* (Lond.) 91:66 (1937).
AUTRUM, H. Electrophysiological analysis of the visual systems in insects. *Exp. Cell Res.* Suppl. 5:426–439 (1958).

291

AUTRUM, H & GALLWITZ, V. Zur analyse der Belichtungspotentiale des Insektenauges. *Z. Vergleich. Physiol.* 33:*407–435* (1951).

BERNHARD, C. G. Isolation of retinal and optic ganglion response in the eye of *Dytiscus*. *J. Neurophysiol.* 5:*32–48* (1942).

CARRICABURU, P. Action du parathion sur l'electroretinogramme de la mouche *Musca domestica*. *C.R. Acad. Sci.* 273:*2576–2578* (1971).

CRESCITELLI, F. & JAHN, T. The effect of temperature on the electrical response of the grasshopper eye. *J. Cell. and Comp. Physiol.* 14:*13–27* (1939).

CRESCITELLI, F. & JAHN, T. Electrical rhythms from the compound eye of insects. *Anat. Rec.* (suppl.) 78:*155* (1940).

CRESCITELLI, F. & JAHN, T. Oscillatory electrical activity from the insect compound eye. *J. Cell. and Comp Physiol.* 19:*47–66* (1942).

EGUCHI, E., NAKA, K-I. & KUWABARA, M. The development of the rhabdome and the appearance of the electrical response in the insect eye. *J. Gen. Physiol.* 46:*143–157* (1962).

FOUCHARD, R. & CARRICABURU, P. La response electroretinographique oscillante chez cinq especes de mouche. *Vision Res.* 10:*655–667* (1970).

FOUCHARD, R. & CARRICABURU, P. Analyse de l'electroretinogramme de l'insecte. *Vision Res.* 12:*1–15* (1972).

HASSENSTEIN, B. Uber Belichtungspotentiale in den Augen der Fliegen *Sarcophaga* und *Eristalis*. *J. Insect Physiol.* 1:*124–130* (1957).

HEISENBERG, M. Separation of receptor and lamina potentials in the electroretinogram of normal and mutant *Drosophila*. *J. Exp. Biol.* 55:*85–100* (1971).

HOTTA, Y. & BENZER, S. Genetic dissection of the *Drosophila* nervous system by means of mosaics. *Proc. Nat. Acad. Sci. Wash.* 67:*1156–1163* (1970).

KOZAK, W. M. Electroretinogram and spike activity in mammalian retina. *Vision Res.* Suppl. 3:*129–149* (1971).

LEUTSCHER-HAZELHOFF, J. T. & KUIPER, J. Response of the blowfly (*Calliphora erythrocephala*) to light flashes and to sinusoidally modulated light. *Docum. Ophthal.* 18:*275–283* (1964).

MAZOKHIN-PORSHNYAKOV, G. Insect Vision, Plenum Press, New York (1969).

MOTE, M. Integrative aspects of the lamina ganglionaris in the compound eye of the fly Sarcophaga bullata. Thesis-UCLA Department of Zoology, Los Angeles (1968).

RATLIFF, F., KNIGHT, B. W. & GRAHAM, N. On tuning and amplification by lateral inhibition. *Proc. Nat. Acad. Sci. Wash.* 62:*733–740* (1969).

SWIHART, S. Maturation of the visual mechanisms in the neotropical butterfly *Heliconus sarae*. *J. Insect Physiol.* 13:*1679–1688* (1967).

TRUJILLO-CENOZ, O. & MELAMED, J. Electron microscopic observations on the peripheral and intermediate retinas of dipterans. In The Functional Organization of the Compound Eye. C. G. Bernhard (Ed.). Pergamon Press, Oxford. pp. 339–361 (1966).

WOLBARSHT, M. L., WAGNER, H. G. & BODENSTEIN, D. Origin of the electrical response in the eye of *Periplaneta americana*, In The Functional Organization of the Compound Eye. C. G. Bernhard (Ed.), Pergamon Press, Oxford. (1966).

YINON, U. & AUERBACH, E. The visual mechanisms of *Tenebrio molitor*: Variations taking place in the ERG of pupa and adults during development. *J. Exp. Biol.* 51:*635–641* (1969).

292